Infection Control in Home Care and Hospice

Second Edition

Emily Rhinehart, RN, MPH, CIC, CPHQ
Vice President
AIG Consultants, Inc., Healthcare Management Division
Atlanta, Georgia

Mary McGoldrick [Friedman], MS, RN, CRNI
Home Care and Hospice Consultant
Home Health Systems, Inc.
Saint Simons Island, GA

JONES AND BARTLETT PUBLISHERS
Sudbury, Massachusetts
BOSTON   TORONTO   LONDON   SINGAPORE

World Headquarters
Jones and Bartlett Publishers
40 Tall Pine Drive
Sudbury, MA 01776
978-443-5000
info@jbpub.com
www.jbpub.com

Jones and Bartlett Publishers Canada
2406 Nikanna Road
Mississauga, ON L5C 2W6
CANADA

Jones and Bartlett Publishers International
Barb House, Barb Mews
London W6 7PA
UK

Jones and Bartlett's books and products are available through most bookstores and online booksellers. To contact Jones and Bartlett Publishers directly, call 800-832-0034, fax 978-443-8000, or visit our Web site www.jbpub.com.

Substantial discounts on bulk quantities of Jones and Bartlett's publications are available to corporations, professional associations, and other qualified organizations. For details and specific discount information, contact the special sales department at Jones and Bartlett via the above contact information or send an email to specialsales@jbpub.com.

Library of Congress Cataloging-in-Publication Data
Rhinehart, Emily.
 Infection control in home care and hospice / Emily Rhinehart, Mary McGoldrick.— 2nd ed.
  p. ; cm.
 Includes bibliographical references and index.
 ISBN 0-7637-4016-0
 1. Home care services. 2. Nosocomial infections—Prevention. 3. Communicable diseases—Prevention.
 [DNLM: 1. Home Care Services. 2. Hospice Care. 3. Infection Control.] I. McGoldrick, Mary II. Title.
 RA645.3.R46 2006 362.14—dc22   2005004500

Production Credits
Acquisitions Editor: Kevin Sullivan
Associate Editor: Amy Sibley
Production Director: Amy Rose
Production Editor: Renée Sekerak
Production Assistant: Rachel Rossi
Marketing Manager: Emily Ekle
Manufacturing and Inventory Coordinator: Amy Bacus
Composition: Graphic World
Cover Design: Kristin E. Ohlin
Printing and Binding: Courier
Cover Printing: Courier

Printed in the United States of America
09 08 07 06 05   10 9 8 7 6 5 4 3 2

Contents

To my fellow Isolation Guideline authors:
Larry, Marguerite, Linda, and Jane,
from whom I have learned so much;
and to my loving husband Randy.

Emily Rhinehart

To my husband Dan,
and our sons,
Evan and Mark,
for their love and support.

Mary McGoldrick [Friedman]

About the Authors

EMILY RHINEHART, RN, MPH, CIC, CPHQ

Emily Rhinehart is the Vice President of AIG Consultants, Inc., Healthcare Management Division (AIGC HMD), providing consultative services to all segments of health care. Services focus on program assessment and development for infection control, patient safety, risk and quality management. Ms. Rhinehart has been a national and international leader in infection control and healthcare epidemiology for over 25 years, providing infection control consultation to healthcare organizations in the United States, Asia, Europe, and Central and South America. Most recently, she has served as a principle author for the revision of the CDC Isolation Guideline, as it is expanded beyond the hospital to all healthcare settings, including home care and hospice. She has published many journal articles and book chapters on a variety of infection control topics. Prior to joining AIGC HMD 12 years ago, she worked in and managed infection surveillance, prevention, and control programs in several hospitals including adult and pediatric tertiary care centers. She is also a past Board Member for the Association for Professionals in Infection Control and Epidemiology.

MARY McGOLDRICK, MS, RN, CRNI

Mary McGoldrick, with over 25 years of home care experience, is a Home Care and Hospice Consultant for Home Health Systems, Inc. *(www.homecareandhospice. com)* where she has provided consultation and education on Joint Commission standards, infection prevention and control activities, patient safety and performance improvement for the past 13 years. Mary served as a home care and hospice nurse surveyor for the Joint Commission on Accreditation of Healthcare Organizations (JCAHO) for over 11 years. She lectures extensively on home care topics and served for 10 years as educational faculty for the JCAHO and five years as an adjunct professor at Mercer University's Graduate School of Business and Economics in Atlanta, GA. Ms. McGoldrick has served as a National Director of Clinical Services where she was responsible for the licensure, certification, accreditation, quality management, training, and clinical operations for over 100 home health care and private duty agencies in 30 states. Her other home care experience includes regional management for Medicare-certified home health agencies, clinical management for a home infusion therapy provider, and other home care clinical and management positions.

Mary has also published over 50 journal articles, and authored several book chapters and manuals on home care topics *(www.infectioncontrolinhomecare.com)*. Ms. McGoldrick [Friedman] is a member of the Editorial Review Boards for the *Journal of Infusion Nursing* and the *Home Healthcare Nurse*. For the past 10 years, Mary has been a department editor and contributing author to the "Accreditation Strategies" column for the *Home Healthcare Nurse* journal and in her "spare time" serves as a hospice volunteer.

Foreword

As health care professionals, we are all concerned with the quality of the care and services we provide. We strive to deliver the most appropriate care in the most effective and efficient manner, optimizing intended outcomes of care and minimizing adverse outcomes. We also strive to provide a safe environment for the patient, his or her family, and for the home care providers. Infection control is critical to these goals for home care and hospice. Prevention and control of home care-acquired infections in patients, as well as exposures and occupational illnesses in staff, is critical to this effort and key to performance measurement and improvement. The Joint Commission's accreditation process for home care and hospice organizations has, since its inception in 1988, included very specific standards related to infection control. In fact, an entire chapter is dedicated to the function.

But, there has been a particular struggle within home care and hospice to develop and implement infection control programs. This challenge is due to the lack of surveillance data on home care-acquired infections as well as the lack of guidelines specifically addressing the prevention and control of infection in home care patients. Nonetheless, home care professionals have made an outstanding effort to address these issues. Now they will have *Infection Control in Home Care and Hospice* to assist them in this important endeavor.

This book will assist home care and hospice organizations in their infection control programs with information for applying and adapting strategies for infection, prevention, control, and surveillance. I applaud the authors for their practical and effective approach as a guide for practice in the home setting. It has been sorely needed and will positively contribute to our mutual goal of improving the quality of health care provided to individuals in the home!

Maryanne L. Popovich, RN, BSN, MPH
Executive Director
Home Care Accreditation Services
Joint Commission on
*   Accreditation of Healthcare Organizations*

Preface

The application of infection control principles in home care and hospice continues to be challenging. As home care has expanded its scope of services to include more high technology services and care for acutely ill patients, the risk of healthcare-associated infection continues to increase. Hospice providers have also expanded, both in the number of hospice organizations—which is now over 3,200—as well as the number of patients and families they serve. The Joint Commission on Accreditation of Healthcare Organizations (JCAHO) acknowledged the need for a systematic infection control program with the advent of the home care accreditation program and standards in 1988. The infection control standards, which have evolved over the past 15 years with significant revision in 2005, require an organized approach to infection surveillance, prevention, and control. Whether a home care or hospice organization is accredited or not, the professionals within these organizations recognize the need for a comprehensive approach to preventing infections in patients and staff members. This book is intended to provide information and guidance in the effort to develop, implement, and manage infection control in home care and hospice organizations.

Infection control programs were initiated in United States hospitals in the early 1970s. Thus, the majority of infection control experience, information, and published literature focuses on acute care settings. The Association for Practitioners in Infection Control and Epidemiology (APIC) was founded in 1972 to support hospital-based infection control practitioners (ICP). In the early 1990s, APIC recognized the need to support infection control professionals in other healthcare set-

tings and initiated various membership sections to provide an opportunity for those outside of hospitals to discuss and advance their infection control efforts. Home care was one of the original APIC membership sections and it remains active.

While infection control and nursing professionals recognize that although the principles of infection control should be applied in home care and hospice, their actual application in organizational policies and procedures will be different. Thus, the challenge is to read and interpret the infection control literature for adaptation in non-acute care settings. Home care and hospice have special challenges in this endeavor. The home is not a clinical setting and does not ordinarily have either the benefits or risks of an institutional setting. The home environment may not include sufficient bathing or handwashing facilities or adequate air handling. There is no central supply or reprocessing nor a utility room stocked with patient care supplies and personal protective equipment. Space in the home may be limited; maintenance of aseptic techniques may be difficult, and there is no support staff available for on-site consultation or assistance. Home care and hospice providers do their best to provide comprehensive, safe patient care in a challenging environment that was not intended for the high-tech procedures and equipment that are now common.

We hope that this book will support and assist in advancing the application and adaptation of strategies for infection surveillance, prevention, and control in home care and hospice. We have attempted to incorporate scientific knowledge, data, and information from the infection control literature into the 14 chapters of this book to formulate an appropriate approach for home care and hospice providers.

Since the first edition was published in 1999, there has been increasing interest and effort in the expansion of infection control beyond hospital settings. As mentioned above, APIC initiated a home care section in the early 1990s. In 2000, this group published a set of draft definitions for home care-acquired infections (Embry, 2000). Although to date the definitions have not been finalized, they provide a good resource for home care organizations. Surveillance in home care has also benefited from the efforts of the Missouri Home Care Alliance and its Infection Surveillance Project that supports the sharing of data for comparison of infection rates for central line-associated urinary tract infections, blood stream infections, and surgical site infections. There are a number of publications in medical literature that are focused on home infusion therapy. There are now three reports of outbreaks of central line-associated bloodstream infections (Danzig, 1995; Do, 1999; Kellerman, 1996) and a number of papers that report the epidemiology of IV-related infections in various home care populations (Gorksi, 2004; Moureau, 2002; Skeist, 1998). Researchers from the Centers for Disease Control and Prevention (CDC) have evaluated and published risk-factors for infection in home infusion therapy (Tokars, 1999). Others have published surveillance methods and results for other device-related infections in home care (Rosenheimer, 1998; Leuhm, 1999; Long, 2002). Although there is still considerable work to be done in standardizing surveillance of healthcare-associated infections in home care and hospice, progress is being made. The revised chapter on surveillance (Chapter 11) provides a review of the published data as well as guidance in its application and the development of a surveillance system for a home care or hospice organization.

In addition to surveillance, there have been other efforts to expand and improve infection prevention and control in home care. As discussed in Chapter 4, the CDC revised its Guideline for the Prevention of Intravascular Catheter-Related Infections (CDC, 2002a). The revised recommendations are applicable in home care and hospice. The CDC also released a revised guideline on hand hygiene, which also has a significant impact on home care and hospice as discussed in Chapter 3 (CDC, 2002b).

The Draft Guideline on Isolation: Prevention of Transmission of Infectious Agents in Healthcare Settings (CDC, 2004a) will provide significant information and support to infection control in home care and hospice. One of us (ER) was invited to be a principal author for the revised Guideline. This Guideline has been researched and developed to incorporate strategies to prevent transmission of infectious agents, including multidrug-resistant organisms, in all healthcare settings including home care and hospice. The Guideline was published in draft form in June 2004 to elicit public comments. At the time of publication of this book, the Guideline was undergoing final review and clearance. It will be available in its final form at the CDC website (http://www.cdc.gov/ncidod/hip).

Home care infection control has not escaped the potential involvement in the management of new infection threats including those posed by agents of bioterrorism, as well as SARS (Sudden Acute Respiratory Syndrome or Avian Influenza). The CDC has developed and published plans for management of a smallpox outbreak that includes a role for home care (CDC, 2003). This is discussed in Chapter 13 in relationship to occupational health issues. The JCAHO has also incorporated requirements for preparedness for outbreaks related to terrorism in its revised standards for home care in 2005.

The CDC has also published guidance for care of the SARS patients in the home, as discussed in Chapter 8 on isolation precautions (CDC, 2004b). Additional government decisions and publications impacting occupational health in home care and hospice are also discussed in Chapter 13, including the revised approach to tuberculin skin testing. Thus, there have been many new publications, guidelines, and requirements for home care since the first edition of this book. We have tried to identify and incorporate them into this second edition. There certainly will be ongoing discussion of infection control in home care and hospice with additional publication of the epidemiology of healthcare- associated infections in these settings as well as other experiences.

We are hopeful that this book will accomplish several goals. First, we hope that it will serve as a reference and guide for home care and hospice nurses as they develop policies and procedures, implement surveillance programs, and continue to provide safe care for their patients. In addition, we hope the book's content will help those who read it to understand the principles of infection control in order to better adapt and apply strategies in home care and hospice. Although we have attempted to provide guidance in the areas of patient care practices, every potential situation that might be encountered cannot be anticipated nor discussed. If nurses have a comprehensive understand-

ing of the principles of infection prevention and control, they should be able to make sound decisions when faced with a situation requiring an infection control intervention. Finally, we have tried to update the text to incorporate the most recent events and publications that have an impact on infection control in home care and hospice.

REFERENCES

Centers for Disease Control and Prevention. Guidelines for the prevention of intravascular catheter-related infections. (2002a). Recommendations of the Hospital Infection Control Practices Advisory Committee (HICPAC).

Morbidity and Mortality Weekly Report. August 9, 2002. Vol. 51. (No. RR-10), 1–36.

Centers for Disease Control and Prevention. (2002b). Guideline for Hand Hygiene in Health-Care Settings: Recommendations of the Healthcare Infection Control Practices Advisory Committee and the HICPAC/SHEA/APIC/IDSA Hand hygiene Task Force. MMWR. 51 (No. RR-16), 1–56.

Centers for Disease Control and Prevention. (2003). Smallpox Response Plan and Guidelines (Version 3.0), Guide C—Infection Control Measures for Healthcare and Community Settings and Quarantine Guidelines. *http://www.bt.cdc.gov/agent/smallpox/response-plan/index.asp#guidec*

Centers for Disease Control and Prevention. (2004a). Draft Guideline for Isolation: Preventing Transmission of Infectious Agents in Healthcare Settings. Retrieved June 15, 2004 from *http://www.cdc.gov/ncidod/hip/hicpac*.

Centers for Disease Control and Prevention (2004b) Severe Acute Respiratory Syndrome; Supplement I: Infection Control in Healthcare, Home and Community Settings. *http://www.cdc.gov/ncidod/sars/guidance/I/pdf/patients_home.pdf*

Danzig, L. Short, L., Collins, K. Mahoney, M., Sepe, S., Bland, L., & Jarvis, W. (1995). Bloodstream infections associated with a needleless intravenous infusion system in patients receiving home infusion therapy. *Journal of the American Medical Association, 23,* 1862–1864.

Do, A.N., Banerjee, R, Barnett B, Jarvis W. (1999). Bloodstream infection associated with needleless device use and the importance of infection control practices in home health care setting. *Journal of Infectious Diseases, 179,* 442–4428.

Embry, F., Chinnes, L. (2000). Draft definitions for surveillance of infections in home health care. *American Journal of Infection Control, 28,* 449–453.

Gorski, L. (2004). Central venous access device outcomes in a homecare agency: a 7-year study. *Journal of Infusion Nursing, 27*(2), 104–11.

Kellerman, S., Shay, D., Howard, J., Goes, C., Feusner, J., Rosenberg, J., Vugia, D., & Jarvis, W. (1996). Bloodstream infections in home infusion patients: The influence of race and needleless intravascular access devices. *Journal of Pediatrics, 129,* 711–717.

Leuhm, D., Fauerbach, L., (1999). Task force studies infection rates, surgical management, and foley catheter infections. *Caring, 18*(11), 30–34.

Long, C., Anderson, C., Greenberg, E., Woomer, N. (2002). Defining and monitoring indwelling central line-associated urinary tract infections. *Home Healthcare Nurse, 20*(4), 255–262.

Moureau, N., Poole, S., Murdock, M., Gray, S., Semba, C. (2002). Central venous catheters in home infusion care: outcomes analysis in 50,470 patients. *Journal of Vascular and Interventional Radiology, 13*(10), 1009–16.

Rosenheimer, L., Embry, F., Sanford, J., Silver, S. (1998). Infection surveillance in home care: device-related incidence rates. *American Journal of Infection Control, 26*(3), 359–363.

Skiest, D., Grant, P., Keiser, P. (1998). Nontunneled central venous catheters in patients with AIDS are associated with lower infection rate. *Journal of Acquired Immune Deficiency Syndrome, 17*(3), 220–226.

Tokars, J., Cookson, S., McArthur, M., Boyer, C., McGeer, A., Jarvis, W. (1999). Prospective evaluation of risk factors for bloodstream infection in patients receiving home infusion therapy. *Annals of Internal Medicine, 131*(5), 340–351.

CHAPTER 1

Infection Control as a Health Care Discipline

HISTORICAL PERSPECTIVE

Although the modern era of infection control began in the early 1950s, the recognition and awareness that the provision of medical and nursing care in an institutional setting (e.g., a hospital) could result in an increased risk for the acquisition of infection occurred more than 100 years ago. In the 1840s, Dr. Ignaz Philip Semmelweiss was caring for postpartum women in a lying-in hospital in Vienna. He was concerned about the incidence of puerperal fever and its related mortality. Eighteen percent of the women who acquired the infection died. As the first hospital epidemiologist, Semmelweiss observed and studied postpartum infection and proved that it was related to care provided by the medical students. His theory was that the medical students carried an infectious agent from the autopsy suite to the maternity wards, where they infected patients through direct transmission via their unwashed hands. Because the science of microbiology was in its infancy, Semmelweiss could not perform cultures to identify the source of the infection (cadavers), the mode of transmission (hands of the medical students), or the causative agent of infection (*Streptococcus* organisms) in the postpartum women. Through a simple case-control study, however, he did demonstrate the relationship (time, place, and person) between the medical students' work in the necropsy suite and their directly subsequent work in the postpartum ward, where they transmitted infection. Semmelweiss showed that the uninfected private patients (controls) had significantly less risk for puerperal fever than did the ward patients (cases), who were cared for by the medical students. When medical students began washing their hands before going from their anatomic studies to the patient ward, the incidence of puerperal fever declined measurably (Rotter, 1996). This classic epidemiological study is the earliest evidence we have of the identification and analysis of nosocomial infection. *Nosocomial* specifically refers to hospital-acquired infections. More recently, the term health care-associated has been used to reflect iatrogenic infections that occur in settings such as long-term care, home care, and other ambulatory care settings.

Some time after Semmelweiss reported his observations and findings, other physicians and scientists furthered his work; among these were Louis Pasteur, who developed the germ theory, and Robert Koch, who contributed to the science of microbiology. In England, Joseph Lister added to the work of Semmelweiss with his study and development of surgical asepsis. These scientific pioneers provided the initial scientific theories and foundations for modern infectious disease epidemiology.

INFECTION CONTROL PROGRAMS IN THE UNITED STATES

Infection control as an organized discipline in American health care dates back to the 1950s. In the post–World War II years, hospital-based outbreaks of infection caused by *Staphylococcus aureus* were being frequently recognized and reported. Many of these outbreaks were occurring in newborn nurseries. The increased incidence of nosocomial infection in outbreak situations demanded an organized response for investigation and control. Thus the discipline of hospital infection control was born. Teams of nurses, physicians, and microbiologists worked together to investigate the occurrence of the outbreaks and to develop and implement measures to control them. Strategies to prevent further outbreaks were developed and implemented, as were methods to reduce the risk of endemic infection.

In 1958, the American Hospital Association (AHA) recommended that surveillance of nosocomial infections be undertaken in all hospitals. Many large hospitals undertook this task. It was not until 1970, however, when the Center for Disease Control (CDC), as it was then called, recommended that hospitals establish and support specific job descriptions and roles for an infection control nurse (ICN) and a hospital epidemiologist that formal programs and training for infection control began to emerge. The CDC held its first course for ICNs (course 1200G) in 1972. Support for the role of the ICN and the discipline of infection control was enhanced in 1976, when the Joint Commission on Accreditation of Hospitals (now the Joint Commission on Accreditation of Healthcare Organizations, or JCAHO) included in its accreditation standards a requirement for a formal, organized infection control program.

Because there was little in the scientific literature to guide prevention and control strategies, early hospital infection control programs concentrated time and effort on surveillance of nosocomial infections. The CDC, through the National Nosocomial Infection Surveillance (NNIS) study, supported this effort. Using standardized definitions and methods for nosocomial infection surveillance, ICNs performed continuous, hospitalwide surveillance (Garner, Jarvis, Emori, Horan, & Hughes, 1988; Horan, Gaynes, Martone, Jarvis, & Emori, 1992). Some hospitals reported their results to the CDC NNIS program for aggregation and analysis, establishing a national database. This provided the opportunity to develop benchmarks for the incidence of nosocomial infection, which allowed individual hospitals to compare their data with those of other institutions [National Nosocomial Infections Surveillance (NNIS) System, 2003].

In addition to surveillance, infection control programs developed policies and procedures for the prevention and control of nosocomial infections. Initially these policies and procedures focused on patient care practices such as handwashing, care of surgical wounds, insertion and care of urinary catheters, care of tracheotomies and endotracheal tubes, and other inva-

sive procedures. Surveillance data provided early recognition of risk related to the use of indwelling medical devices.

Isolation precautions were also developed and implemented by the infection control program. Again, the CDC provided guidance and standardization through its publication *Isolation Techniques for Use in Hospitals* (CDC, 1970). Isolation precautions were used to prevent the transmission of infection from a patient known to have a potentially communicable disease to other patients and health care providers. As infection control programs grew and developed, increased attention to the prevention of occupationally acquired infections among hospital staff was expanded and is currently a major part of any infection control program (see Chapter 13).

In 1972, the Association for Practitioners in Infection Control (APIC), a national professional organization, was chartered to support communication among infection control professionals through conferences, meetings, and newsletters. In 1983, the APIC published its first major document to support infection control and assist individuals in their preparation for certification in infection control. Through the development of the *APIC Curriculum for Infection Control Practice* (Soule, 1983), APIC established eight essential domains for infection control practice:

1. Patient care practices
2. Microbiology
3. Infectious diseases
4. Occupational health
5. Sterilization, disinfection, and cleaning
6. Epidemiology and statistics
7. Communication and management
8. Education

These eight distinct areas continue to provide the foundation for the professional practice of infection control in all segments of health care delivery.

EPIDEMIOLOGY OF NOSOCOMIAL INFECTION

The current epidemiology of nosocomial infection is based on more than 25 years of NNIS data and many studies in the published literature, and is therefore well known. Descriptive information about the endemic (usual) rate of nosocomial infection as well as epidemics (instances of a greater-than-expected number of infections or unusual occurrences) is easily obtained.

Nosocomial infection is defined by the site of infection. Although both intrinsic (host) factors and extrinsic (environmental) factors must be considered, endemic rates of nosocomial infection are well established. The reliability of these data depends on the application of standard definitions and methods as developed and published by the CDC NNIS study (Garner *et al.,* 1988; Horan *et al.,* 1992). Therefore, if a hospital infection control program applies these definitions and methods (Emori, Culver, & Horan, 1991), it can compare its endemic rate at specific body sites with national data to determine whether its rate is significantly higher or lower than that of other hospitals. Epidemiological methods to control for additional factors that are known to affect the rate of infection can be applied to ensure a more reliable comparison. Such extrinsic factors include the type and size of the hospital, the level of care, the length of surgery, and the duration of exposure to medical devices. Intrinsic factors may include such considerations as underlying severity of illness, age, immunologic status, other infections, and current antibiotic therapy. Some of these risk factors are well studied (e.g., duration of indwelling urinary catheter), whereas many others require further investigation and analysis.

STATUS OF INFECTION CONTROL IN HOME CARE AND HOSPICE

It is evident that the discipline of hospital infection control is well developed and has a significant body of knowledge and epidemiologic data. The practice has been an acute care–based discipline and has evolved with the support of the CDC, NNIS, APIC, and other professional organizations, such as the Society for Healthcare Epidemiologists of America (SHEA) and the American Society for Microbiology. Physicians, nurses, microbiologists, and others have worked diligently to perform original research on risks related to the acquisition of nosocomial infection and to report outbreak investigations. These approaches have resulted in a body of knowledge on which the discipline is based and that has provided support to the CDC in its guidelines development. Since the publication of the first guideline, *Guideline for the Prevention of Catheter-Associated Urinary Tract Infections* (Wong, 1981), the CDC (through the Healthcare Infection Control Policy Advisory Committee, or HICPAC) and APIC have supported the development of additional guidelines and updates (Table 1-1).

The collective efforts of the CDC and HICPAC as well as professional organizations, i.e., APIC and SHEA

Table 1-1 CDC Guidelines for the Prevention of Health Care-acquired Infections

Guideline Title	Year of publication
Guideline for Isolation Precautions: Preventing Transmission of Infectious Agents in Healthcare Settings	Pending publication 2005
Guideline for Sterilization and Disinfection	Pending publication 2005
Guidelines for Preventing Health Care–Associated Pneumonia	2003
Guideline for Environmental Infection Control in Health-Care Facilities	2003
Recommendations for Using Smallpox Vaccine in a Pre-event Vaccination Program	2003
Guidelines for the Prevention of Intravascular Catheter-Related Infections	2002
Guideline for Hand Hygiene in Healthcare Settings	2002
Management of Occupational Exposures to Hepatitis B, Hepatitis C, and HIV and Recommendations for Postexposure Prophylaxis	2001
Guidelines for the Prevention of Surgical Site Infections	1999
Guidelines for Infection Control in Healthcare Personnel	1998
Immunization of Healthcare Workers	1997
Guideline for the Prevention of Catheter-Associated Urinary Tract Infections	1981

(All guidelines can be found on the CDC website at *www.cdc.gov.*)

have contributed significantly to the improvement of care and the reduction of risk of infection in hospitalized patients. There are no comparable comprehensive efforts or epidemiologic data pertaining to other health care-associated infections, including home care–acquired infection, however. Because the health care delivery system continues to shift more severely ill patients with greater high-tech care needs into home care and hospice, home care providers and infection control professionals need to develop a body of knowledge and data more specific to the risks of infection in the home care setting. Risk analysis for infections and outbreak investigations will be reported. Surveillance systems and databases will eventually be developed and improved. Organizations such as APIC and SHEA will focus more attention on home care and hospice; agencies such as the CDC and the Department of Health and Human Services (HHS) will support efforts to write guidelines and develop surveillance systems. The National Association for Home Care (NAHC) will provide information, education, and services as its members demand them. The Joint Commission continued its requirements for an organized infection control and surveillance program in home care and hospice, updating its standards in January 2005. These standards are very comprehensive, addressing organizational issues, surveillance, prevention of infections in patients and staff, and education. A consideration has been added to require home care organizations to plan for a sudden influx of patients resulting from an infectious disease outbreak (JCAHO, 2004). This is a new requirement for home and hospice care and is related to the focus on emergency preparedness for bioterrorism by hospitals, which was introduced after 9/11 and the anthrax exposures of 2001.

Until this evolution occurs, home care providers and infection control professionals must rely on previously established principles found within the eight core areas of infection control practice. Principles and knowledge of infectious diseases and their transmission can be directly applied. Practices related to the prevention and control of infection in patient care, however, require modification and adaptation. Although the principles of microbiology remain the same, application and use of microbiologic methods for identification and diagnosis of home care–acquired infection must be modified or developed. New sterilization and disinfection methods are needed for easy and safe application in home care as well as other ambulatory settings. Occu-

pational health practices for the prevention and control of exposure and infection in staff members can generally be applied to home care. The basic principles of adult education as well as management and communication for infection control can also be directly applied to home care and hospice.

Perhaps the greatest challenges are in the areas of epidemiology and statistics. First, increased effort to describe and analyze the epidemiology of home care–acquired infections is critically needed. Before this body of data-based evidence can be produced, however, definitions and methods for the surveillance of home care–acquired infections must be developed and standardized (Embry, 2000). Although definitions of nosocomial infection are standardized (Garner *et al.,* 1988; Horan *et al.,* 1992), these definitions are not feasible for unmodified application in home care. Surveillance methods that were developed for hospitals also require significant modification for use in home care and hospice. Fortunately, investment in information systems and databases for home care is increasing. These efforts will help support the implementation of home care surveillance systems.

Surveillance data, once they are standardized and have become widespread, can be used to begin to measure the incidence of home care–acquired infection. Additional risk analysis efforts can be instituted to determine what practices in what patients increase the risk for home care–acquired infections and what practices in what patients decrease risk (Danzig, 1995; Do, 1999; Kellerman, 1996). These data and the information they provide will be used to reduce risk. Specific patient care practices, especially those involving an indwelling device, will be modified and improved.

It has been demonstrated that health care-associated infection increases the overall cost of health care. As more skilled care and a higher intensity of services shift to the home setting, home care–acquired infection will correspondingly increase the cost of home care and may increase the utilization of acute care and other resources. Without sufficient data on the incidence of home care–acquired infections, the actual cost of this adverse outcome will remain unknown. As more information about the incidence and cost of home care–acquired infection becomes available, more informed decisions will lead to the lowest-risk care in the most appropriate setting.

REFERENCES

Centers for Disease Control and Prevention. (1970). *Isolation techniques for use in hospitals.* Atlanta, GA: Department of Health, Education, and Welfare.

Danzig, L., Short, L., Collins, K., Mahoney, M., Sepe, S., Bland, L., & Jarvis, W. (1995). Bloodstream infections associated with the needleless intravenous infusion system in patients receiving home infusion therapy. *Journal of the American Medical Association, 12,* 1862–1864.

Do, A., Ray, B., Banerjee, R., Barnett, B., Jarvis, W. (1999). Bloodstream infection associated with needleless device use and the importance of infection control practices in home health care setting. *Journal of Infectious Diseases, 179,* 442–448.

Embry, E. & Chinnes, L. (2000). Draft definitions for surveillance of infections in home health care. *American Journal of Infection Control, 28,* 449–453.

Emori, G., Culver, D., & Horan, T. (1991). National Nosocomial Infections Surveillance (NNIS) system: Description of surveillance methods. *American Journal of Infection Control, 19,* 259–267.

Garner, J., Jarvis, W., Emori, T., Horan, T., & Hughes, J. (1988). CDC definitions for nosocomial infection, 1988. *American Journal of Infection Control, 23,* 128–140.

Horan, T., Gaynes, R., Martone, W., Jarvis, W., & Emori, T. (1992). CDC definitions of nosocomial surgical site infections, 1992: A modification of CDC definitions of surgical wound infections. *Infection Control and Hospital Epidemiology, 13,* 606–608.

Joint Commission on the Accreditation of Healthcare Organizations (2004). *2005 Home Care Surveillance, Prevention and Control of Infection.* Retrieved 7/21/04, from *www.jcaho.org.*

Kellerman, S., Shay, D., Howard, J., Goes, C., Feusner, J., Rosenberg, J., et al. (1996). Bloodstream infections in home infusion patients: The influence of race and needleless intravascular access devices. *Journal of Pediatrics, 129,* 711–717.

National Nosocomial Infections Surveillance (NNIS) system (2003). National Nosocomial Infections Surveillance (NNIS) system report, data summary from January 1992 through June 2003. *American Journal of Infection Control, 31* (8), 481–498.

Rotter, M. (1996). Hand washing and hand disinfection. In G. Mahall (Ed.), *Hospital epidemiology and infection control* (pp. 1052–1068). Baltimore: Williams & Wilkins.

Soule, B. (Ed.). (1983). *The APIC curriculum for infection control practice.* Dubuque, IA: Kendall/Hunt.

Wong, E. (1983). Guideline for the prevention of Central Line-Associated urinary tract infections. *American Journal of Infection Control, 11,* 28–31.

CHAPTER 2

The Infectious Disease Process

AGENT, HOST, AND ENVIRONMENT

Humans live in their environment with many other species. Many members of the animal and plant kingdoms are microscopic and can cause human illness, called an infection. The presence of microscopic organisms does not always cause infection, however. The physical environment is abundant with microscopic organisms, such as bacteria, fungi, molds, and viruses. Under certain circumstances, some microorganisms cause disease; under the same circumstances, others do not. There are many microorganisms regularly found on and within human beings; these are referred to as normal or resident flora.

The infectious disease process provides a scientific explanation for the factors that determine the relationships among humans, the many microorganisms that are in the environment, and normal flora. There are many variables that determine the relationship between microorganisms and the human host. This interaction has been illustrated in various ways, including the epidemiologic triangle (Figure 2-1). The triangle portrays the three key elements in infection—agent, host, and environment—and their dynamic interaction. This model demonstrates this interaction for other types of disease as well. In this chapter, we discuss specific characteristics or changes in any one of the three elements that can lead to the development of an infectious disease.

TYPES OF INFECTION

The term *infection* refers to the presence and multiplication of microorganisms in the tissue of a host. The host's response to this invasion and replication varies. When there are signs and symptoms caused by this in- vasion, such as fever, swelling, pain, and inflammation, we recognize these as characteristics of infection. Some infectious diseases are evident and produce acute signs and symptoms. For example, an acute urinary tract infection in a normal host results in pain; frequency, urgency, and burning on urination. An acute skin infection produces pain, swelling, warmth, and redness of the tissue. Other infections, referred to as subclinical infections, may occur without observable signs. For example, a mild case of chicken pox may go unrecognized in a child if no rash occurs or if there are so few concealed lesions that they go unnoticed.

Some viruses can cause asymptomatic, chronic infections. For example, approximately 10% of individuals infected with hepatitis B virus become chronically infected, and the majority remain asymptomatic. Hepatitis C virus is thought to result invariably in a chronic infection. Either of these viral infections may remain asymptomatic for a long period of time. This condition is referred to as a carrier state. The infection can be diagnosed or documented by serologic blood testing, which detects the viral antigen or antibody to show evidence of the infection. Although no signs and symptoms of an illness are evident, the host potentially can transmit hepatitis to another susceptible individual. Carriers of hepatitis B and hepatitis C viruses can transmit infection to others through sexual contact or contact with their blood.

NORMAL FLORA

The term *normal flora* describes the bacteria frequently found in everyone in specific parts of the body. For example, millions of *Escherichia coli* are normally found in the bowel. *Streptococcus viridans* is

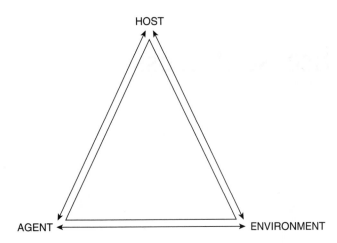

Figure 2-1 The Epidemiologic Triangle

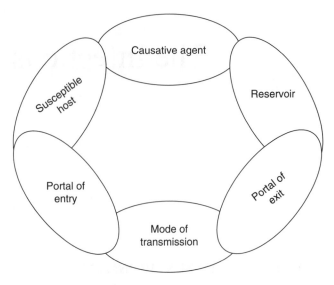

Figure 2-2 The Chain of Infection

also a normal flora present in the upper respiratory tract and mouth. *Colonization* is the term that describes the presence of bacteria without multiplication and damage to the host tissue. Sometimes bacteria that are not normal flora can be isolated from patients who are colonized. An example is found in patients who become colonized with multidrug-resistant microorganisms, such as methicillin-resistant *Staphylococcus aureus* (MRSA) or vancomycin-resistant enterococci (VRE). Patients with these organisms may have infections or may be colonized; as asymptomatic carriers, like asymptomatic hepatitis carriers, they can serve as the source of infection or colonization of others.

CHAIN OF INFECTION

The interaction among the agent, the host, and the environment leading to infection has been described in a model called the chain of infection (Figure 2-2). Specific conditions and characteristics affecting each element in the chain and each element's interaction with the other elements determine whether an infection will result.

CAUSATIVE AGENT

The causative agent of infection may be one of several classes of microorganisms causing human infectious disease. These include bacteria, viruses, fungi, protozoa, rickettsia, chlamydia, mycoplasma, prions, and helminths. Each has characteristics that influence its ability to cause an infection (Table 2-1). First, a suffi-

cient number of organisms (an infective dose) must be present to cause an infection. It takes only a few *Shigella* bacteria to cause an infection in the gastrointestinal (GI) tract, leading to severe diarrhea. In contrast, it takes many *Salmonella* organisms to cause a GI tract infection. Pathogenicity is the ability of the agent to cause disease (*Staphylococcus epidermidis* has low pathogenicity); the term *virulence* refers to the severity of the disease. *Shigella* species are considered more virulent than *Salmonella* species because they cause a more severe form of diarrhea. Invasiveness is the abil-

Table 2-1 Characteristics of Causative Agents

Characteristic	Definition
Infective dose	Number of organisms required to cause infection
Pathogenicity	Likelihood that exposure to an organism will lead to infection
Virulence	Capacity to produce disease
Invasiveness	Ability of organism to breech natural barriers
Viability	Ability of organism to survive in the environment
Host specificity	Ability of organism to infect specific animal hosts
Antigenic variation	Changes in organism makeup
Resistance	Ability of organism to develop resistance to antimicrobials through molecular changes

ity of the organism to enter the host tissues. Viability is the organism's ability to survive in the environment. Viruses, for example, are like parasites because they cannot survive independently; thus they require a living host (such as blood cells) to replicate. Other organisms, such as spore-forming bacteria, can survive in hostile environments and endure a wide range of conditions, such as high and low temperatures or exposure to low-level disinfectants. *Mycobacteria tuberculosis* (MTB) is a spore-forming bacterium that can survive for many years in dust particles.

Infectious agents cause disease in specific animal hosts. This is referred to as host specificity. There are various viruses, such as canine parvovirus, that cause disease in certain animals but do not affect humans. Others, such as varicella virus, cause human infectious disease (chicken pox) but are harmless to animals. In addition, viruses such as influenza A virus and bacteria such as streptococci can change their virulence through natural alterations in their antigen makeup. Thus in some years the severity of the flu is worse than in others, as a result of antigenic variation in the influenza virus in those years.

Finally, the organism's ability to develop resistance to specific antimicrobial agents may also affect its ability to cause an infection. There are many biological mechanisms by which organisms such as bacteria can acquire resistance. Once resistance develops, the frequency of colonization and infection by the organism may increase, as has been observed with MRSA over the past two decades (see Chapter 8).

A list of common microorganisms that cause human infections is provided in Table 2-2. Bacteria are divided into categories of Gram negative and Gram positive based on their appearance when a particular stain—Gram's stain—is applied to them and they are examined under a microscope. Their shape can also be determined with a Gram's stain test. Round organisms are called *cocci*. Bacteria that are longer and in the shape of a rod are called *bacilli*. There are Gram positive cocci, such as streptococci, and Gram negative bacilli, such as *Pseudomonas* species. Many other variations and shapes also exist. The results of a Gram's stain are used as a preliminary test to determine the type of bacteria that are present. For some sites of infection, the stain is used to determine whether white blood cells are also present, providing further evidence of infection. Other microorganisms can be initially identified by different microscopic examinations and

staining techniques. For example, MTB in the sputum is identified by an acid-fast stain. These various stains may be used for a preliminary identification of an infectious organism. In most cases, however, the identification of the specific organism causing an infection is made by performing a culture.

RESERVOIR OF INFECTION

The source of a causative agent (e.g., bacterium, fungus, or virus) is referred to as the reservoir. In a reservoir, the organism can survive but may or may not multiply. Organisms causing infectious disease may be found in other humans, animals, or the physical environment. Human reservoirs may have a symptomatic or asymptomatic infection, or they may be colonized with a potentially infective agent. In health care settings, the human reservoir includes other patients as well as health care providers. In home care, because there are usually no other patients in the setting, that particular reservoir is less important. Home care staff, however, can transmit from their hands organisms from one patient who is infected or colonized to other patients. Animals can also carry or be infected with agents of human infection. This reservoir is more important in home care settings than in other settings (see Chapter 5). Animals infected with rabies can transmit the disease to humans; turtles and other reptiles are frequently colonized with *Salmonella* organisms, which can be transmitted to humans and cause disease.

The environment, including patient care equipment and devices, can also serve as a reservoir for infectious agents. Although this has not been studied or confirmed as an important source of infectious organisms in home care, there are many examples from other settings. In intensive care units, outbreaks have been traced to antibiotic-resistant, Gram-negative bacteria that contaminate sinks (Dandalides, Rutala, & Sarubbi, 1984). When health care workers used these sinks, their hands became contaminated, and they transmitted the organisms to patients. Ventilator tubing frequently becomes contaminated with bacteria from the patient's respiratory tract that can be transmitted to other patients via the hands of health care workers. Reusable devices can also serve as reservoirs of potentially infectious agents. If a bronchoscope used to examine a patient with tuberculosis is not sufficiently cleaned and disinfected, it can serve as the reservoir of infection for a patient who is subsequently examined with the same instrument.

Table 2-2 Common Pathogenic Agents

Agent	Type	Disease or Infection
Bacteria		
Acinetobacter spp.	Gram-negative rod	Upper respiratory tract infection, urinary tract infection (UTI), wound infection
Campylobacter jejuni	Gram-negative rod	Diarrhea, abdominal pain, fever
Clostridium difficile	Gram-positive rod (forms spores)	Diarrhea, pseudomembranous colitis
Clostridium tetani	Gram-positive rod (forms spores)	Tetanus
Cornybacterium diptheriae	Gram-positive rod	Cause of diptheria; skin, eye, ear infections
Enterobacter aerogenes	Gram-negative rod	UTI; respiratory tract, wound, blood, central nervous system (CNS) infections
Enterococcus faecalis (formerly Streptococcus faecalis)	Gram-positive coccus	UTI, subacute endocarditis
Escherichia coli	Gram-negative rod	Diarrhea, UTI, septicemia
Klebsiella pneumoniae	Gram-negative rod	Bacterial pneumonia, UTI, respiratory tract infections
Listeria monocytogenes	Gram-positive rod	Meningitis, encephalitis, septicemia
Mycobacterium tuberculosis	Acid-fast mycobacterium	Tuberculosis
Proteus vulgaris	Gram-negative rod	UTI, burn wound infection, respiratory tract infection
Proteus mirabilis	Gram-negative rod	UTI, bacteremia
Pseudomonas aeruginosa	Gram-negative rod	Eye, wound, burn wound infections; diarrhea
Salmonella choleraesuis, S. paratyphi, S. schottmuelleri	Gram negative rod	Gastroenteritis, enteric fever, bacteremia, pneumonia
Serratia marcescens	Gram-negative rod	Wound, blood, CNS, respiratory tract infections; UTI
Shigella dysenteriae	Gram-negative rod	Bacterial dysentery
Staphylococcus aureus	Gram-positive coccus	Wound infection, boils, carbuncles, impetigo, pneumonia, bacteremia, food poisoning, toxic shock syndrome
Staphylococcus epidermidis	Gram-positive coccus	Skin abscesses, ventriculitis, meningitis, bacteremia
Streptococcus pneumoniae	Gram-positive coccus	Pneumonia, scarlet fever, meningitis
Streptococcus pyogenes	Gram-positive coccus	Tonsillitis, impetigo, rheumatic fever, skin infection
Streptococcus salivarius	Gram-positive coccus	Endocarditis
Viruses		
Adenovirus	Intermediate	Upper and lower respiratory tract infection, conjunctivitis
Coxsackievirus	Hydrophilic	Herpangina, aseptic meningitis, pleurodynia, myalgia
Cytomegalovirus	Lipophilic	Usually asymptomatic in immunocompetent adults (may infect unborn fetus)
Echovirus	Hydrophilic	Aseptic meningitis, encephalitis, exanthema, respiratory disease
Hepatitis A (formerly infectious hepatitis)	Hydrophilic	Low-grade fever, fatigability, myalgia, anorexia, vomiting
Hepatitis B (formerly serum hepatitis)	lipophilic	Acute and chronic hepatitis
Hepatitis C (formerly non-A, non-B hepatitis)	lipophilic	Acute and chronic hepatitis
Herpes simplex type 1	lipophilic	Skin lesions; eye, ear, face infections
Herpes simplex type 2	lipophilic	Skin lesions on and around genitalia
Human immunodeficiency virus	Lipophilic	Acquired Immunodeficiency Syndrome

Table 2-2 continued

Agent	Type	Disease or Infection
Influenza A2 and B	Lipophilic	Headache, chills, fever, muscular pain, lower respiratory tract infection, pneumonia
Parainfluenza	Lipophilic	Upper respiratory tract infection
Poliovirus	Hydrophilic	Poliomyelitis, aseptic meningitis
Respiratory syncytial virus	Lipophilic	Lower respiratory tract infection
Rhinovirus 39	Hydrophilic	Common cold, upper respiratory tract infection
Rotavirus	Hydrophilic	Diarrhea, vomiting, fever
Rubella	Lipophilic	German measles
Vaccinia	Lipophilic	Used as model for smallpox virus
Fungi		
Aspergillus niger	Mold	Lower respiratory tract infection in immunosuppressed patients
Candida albicans	Yeast	Mouth, skin, hand, lung infections; thrush
Tricophyton mentagrophytes	Fungus	Athlete's foot

Courtesy of Reckitt & Colman, Inc., Wayne, New Jersey.

PORTAL OF EXIT

If a human is serving as the reservoir of an infectious agent, the means by which the agent leaves the original host is the portal of exit. Orifices that are part of each body system can serve as portals of exit. For example, the portal of exit for influenza is the mouth and nose (upper respiratory tract), from which secretions carrying the virus are excreted through coughing and sneezing. The upper respiratory tract (coughing through the mouth) is the portal of exit for pulmonary tuberculosis. Viruses and bacteria that cause diarrhea leave the host via the GI tract through feces and, occasionally, vomitus. Sexually transmitted diseases exit via the genitourinary tract. Blood and other body secretions that are contaminated with blood are also reservoirs of infectious disease. In this case, the portal of exit may vary. Blood can exit a wound or a break in the skin, or it can exit via bloody respiratory secretions.

PORTAL OF ENTRY

The portal of entry is the means by which the infectious agent enters the susceptible host. The portal of entry can be the respiratory tract, GI tract, genitourinary tract, or skin or mucous membranes. Breaks in the skin or mucous membranes can create a portal of entry, such as can occur with injuries from needlesticks or sharps.

MODE OF TRANSMISSION

The mechanism by which an organism moves from the portal of exit (from an infected or colonized person) or an environmental reservoir through a susceptible host's portal of entry is referred to as the mode of transmission. Recognizing the mode of transmission is a critical component of infection control. There are four modes of transmission: contact, airborne, vehicle, and vector. Contact spread and airborne transmission are the most common modes of transmission in the home care setting.

Contact Transmission

Infections can be transmitted through direct or indirect contact with the infected or colonized source. Direct contact occurs when there is actual person-to-person physical contact. Sexually transmitted diseases are spread through direct contact. Infectious droplets from the upper respiratory tract that go from one person to another is another form of direct contact transmission. This is called droplet spread or droplet transmission, and it is the mode of transmission for common upper respiratory infections such as colds and flu. These respiratory droplets can travel about 3 feet before gravity causes them to fall. This makes droplet transmission different from airborne transmission (discussed in the next section).

Indirect contact transmission occurs when the infectious agent is carried from one person to another on an object. As mentioned above, a contaminated bronchoscope may be the inanimate object involved in indirect contact transmission. The hands of a home care staff member may also be involved in the indirect contact transmission of multidrug-resistant organisms such as MRSA or VRE.

Airborne Transmission

Airborne transmission can occur with a few infectious agents that can travel through the air on tiny respiratory particles called droplet nuclei. Other organisms, such as MTB, may be carried on dust particles and through ventilation systems. Some fungi and molds, such as *Aspergillus* species, may also be airborne. Tuberculosis can be droplet spread or airborne spread, as can measles and varicella.

Vehicle Transmission

Vehicle transmission refers to infections that are spread through a common reservoir, such as food. Foodborne illnesses are frequently caused by vehicle transmission and occur when a number of people ingest the same contaminated food (e.g., staphylococcal food poisoning related to potato salad) or contaminated water. Infection from contaminated blood is also considered to occur from vehicle transmission. In home care settings, vehicle transmission can occur in contaminated intravenous fluid.

Vector Transmission

Vectorborne spread refers to infectious diseases that are transmitted through insects or rodents. For example, deer ticks transmit Lyme disease, and West Nile virus is transmitted by mosquitoes. Vectorborne spread is not a common occurence in home care or hospice in the United States.

REDUCING THE RISK OF INFECTION

Many home care and hospice policies and procedures for infection control are adopted to prevent infection by breaking the chain of transmission. That is why it is so important for home care and hospice staff to understand the chain of transmission model. Once it is understood, there can be better comprehension of many of the infection control strategies, such as transmission-based precautions. Not all circumstances can be addressed in written policies and procedures, but if the basic principles of infection control and the chain of infection are understood, home care and hospice staff will be better prepared to make decisions and to apply interventions to protect themselves and patients. In addition, this understanding may reduce practices that are unnecessary and costly. In applying these principles, however, home care and hospice staff must also understand that each patient is different and that his or her particular risk for infection also may be different.

SUSCEPTIBLE HOST

The host is the final and most important link in the chain of transmission. There are many variables that determine whether a host will be susceptible to an infectious agent. Home care and hospice staff routinely assess patients for host factors to determine their specific risk for acquiring an infection. Some factors, referred to as intrinsic risk factors, are specific to the patient (host). The risk for infection is also dependent on extrinsic factors, the external factors in the delivery of care—including the devices and procedures, the care provider, and the environment—that may increase or decrease risk.

The home care or hospice nurse can also recognize increased risk based on the physical assessment. Any break in the natural barriers to infection, including the skin and mucus membranes, can increase risk. Any indwelling catheters, tubes, or drains increase risk by breaching normal barriers and providing a portal of entry for infecting organisms. Such breaches can be caused by catheters anywhere in the urinary system, wound drains and catheters, tracheotomies, or gastrostomy tubes for enteral feeding.

Intrinsic Risk Factors

There are many recognized factors that can increase a patient's risk for developing or acquiring an infection. One basic consideration is age. It is well recognized that there is greater risk for infection at the extremes of age; that is, in the very young and the very old. In newborns and infants, increased risk is related to the immaturity of the immune system as well as the lack of experience with and exposure to infectious agents.

Newborns and infants have not yet developed antibodies to common agents. Even a full-term infant does not have a fully functioning immune system, which is usually around the age of 6 months. Infants, toddlers, and children frequently get community-acquired infections, especially as they enter day care and preschool, because they have not been exposed to these agents before and do not have immunity to them. The most common of these are called childhood diseases because most individuals used to get them sometime during their childhood, before vaccines were widely available.

In older people, increased susceptibility is related to the aging of the immune system. White blood cell function is not as efficient or effective in older individuals. Changes in anatomic structures, including the integumentary system, also increase risk among older people because the natural physical barriers to infection are not as effective. Older patients are also more likely to have poor cough reflexes and therefore are more prone to aspiration; this increases risk for pneumonia. Poor circulation delays healing, which also increases risk for infection.

Gender may also increase a patient's risk for infection. Females have a greater risk for urinary tract infections than males do as a result of an anatomically shorter urethra. In addition to gender, a person's ethnic background may increase risk for certain diseases, including sickle-cell anemia and Tay-Sachs disease, which may increase risk for infection.

Many studies have demonstrated the effect of socioeconomic status on risk for infection. Cytomegalovirus infection occurs more frequently at a younger age in people of lower socioeconomic status than in those of higher status; this is attributed to crowded living conditions. There are many other infections that are acquired as a result of crowded living conditions. In addition, poor nutrition in groups of lower socio-economic status increases risk for infection. Similarly, lifestyle and marital status may affect risk for infection. Increased stress (e.g., as a result of homelessness) appears to affect the immune system. Other lifestyle issues, such as sexual behaviors, may also increase risk through increased exposure to infectious agents.

Occupation may also increase risk. Individuals involved in occupations that expose them to hazardous or carcinogenic agents that may affect the function of their immune system can have increased risk. Chronic pulmonary diseases (e.g., brown lung) increase risk for pulmonary infection. Health care workers experience occupational exposures to infectious diseases.

The overall immune status of an individual is extremely important in determining risk for infection. Immune status can be affected by nutrition as well as by inherited and acquired-immune diseases. Other chronic diseases, such as diabetes mellitus, affect immune system function. Some treatments, such as chemotherapy and radiation therapy, cause immunosuppression, as can drugs. Pregnancy also affects the immune system and increases risk for infection; anatomic changes may also be related to increased risk.

In assessing home care and hospice patients for risk of infection, the home care or hospice nurse considers the patient's history (congenital, underlying, acute, or chronic illness) and immune status as well as any current treatments or medications that may reduce immune response or increase susceptibility. It is well recognized that a patient who has an infection at one site is at significantly greater risk for infection at another. There may be some interventions that home care staff can undertake to reduce this intrinsic risk (e.g., provide education to improve nutritional status, provide influenza vaccine, etc.), but for the most part there is little that home care or hospice staff can do to improve host immunity.

Extrinsic Risk Factors

There are various extrinsic risk factors that may affect a home care or hospice patient, including devices, invasive procedures, exposure to home care or hospice staff, and the environment. Home care minimizes the extrinsic risk of exposure to other patients that exists in inpatient care. It is assumed that this is one reason the incidence of home care–acquired infection is lower than that of nosocomial infection. Home care or hospice staff, however, may transfer organisms from an infected or colonized patient to another patient with their hands, clothing, or inanimate objects used from one patient to another. Again, this occurs less frequently in home care than in hospitals or long-term care facilities because most of the inanimate objects used from one patient to another are noncritical items (see Chapter 9).

Devices are the most important extrinsic risk for home care–acquired infections. Devices that are left in place present the greatest risk because they breach a natural barrier and serve as a portal of entry for microorganisms. Indwelling urinary drainage catheters (i.e., urethral and suprapubic), intravenous devices, drainage tubes in surgical sites (e.g., Jackson-Pratt closed-wound drainage systems), feeding tubes (e.g., gastrostomy tubes), and breathing tubes (e.g., tracheotomy tubes) relate to an increased risk for infection. Various interventions are necessary to reduce this extrinsic risk. First, the placement of a device into a sterile space (e.g., urinary bladder or venous system) must include preparation of the site using aseptic technique and antiseptic solutions to reduce the number of bacteria that could be introduced with the device. For this purpose, for example, antiseptics are used to prepare the skin or to cleanse the area around the urinary meatus before the device is introduced. If a device is left in place and involves a sterile space, the drainage or infusion system must be maintained in a sterile fashion. Other tubes and drains that are not introduced into a sterile space (e.g., gastrostomy tubes) must be maintained in a clean fashion to decrease extrinsic risk (see Chapter 3). Appropriate care of the insertion site, such as an intravenous catheter exit site, or a surgical wound drain site, is also important.

A single invasive event or procedure may also increase extrinsic risk. This can occur when a blood sample is obtained or when a urine sample is obtained from a urinary catheter. These procedures also include skin preparation or cleansing of the local area with an antiseptic to reduce the number of bacteria. When some devices, such as electronic thermometers, are used, protective covers (e.g., probe covers) are applied as a barrier to contamination and to reduce the risk of transmitting infectious organisms to the patient.

The experience and skill of the home care or hospice staff member can also increase or decrease extrinsic risk for infection. A more experienced, skillful nurse will likely provide sterile, invasive procedures in an efficient manner thus reducing the risk of introduction of bacteria. Skill may also reduce the risk of trauma to the surrounding area or tissue.

Many times, home care staff must provide care in a home environment that is not well maintained or clean; the home may be infested with rodents and insects, for instance. Although this is frequently perceived as creating an increased extrinsic risk for infection, there is no evidence that it does. If the lack of sanitary facilities, such as sinks with running water and toilets, negatively affects the patient's and family's ability to maintain an appropriate level of personal hygiene, this may affect risk for infection. For example, if there is no running water, handwashing may not be accomplished by caregivers in the home in an effective manner.

IMPACT OF HOME CARE AND HOSPICE STAFF

Home care and hospice staff can identify both intrinsic and extrinsic risks, but their ability to control and reduce risk is limited. As discussed earlier, there are limited interventions that can be undertaken to improve the patient's ability to resist infection. Many of these strategies are related to patient and family education; provision of vaccines for prevention of infection may also contribute to reducing risk. Home care staff also have limited ability to control or reduce risks related to the patient's environment. Therefore, the focus of risk reduction is directed at the delivery of care. Hand hygiene (see Chapter 3) is the most important factor for minimizing the risk of transmission of organisms from one patient to another and from home care and hospice staff members to patients. Use of gowns and gloves as a Standard Precaution and transmission-based precaution is also important. When home care involves skilled nursing procedures, risk is reduced by using the level of technique (e.g., clean or aseptic) that is appropriate to the specific procedure and level of risk. When inanimate objects are used, cleaning is the minimal risk reduction strategy. If the item is semicritical or critical, then disinfection or sterilization may be necessary (see Chapter 9).

REFERENCE

Dandalides, P., Rutala, W., & Sarubbi, F. Jr., (1984). Postoperative infection following cardiac surgery: Association with an environmental reservoir in a cardiothoracic intensive care unit. *Infection Control, 5,* 378–384.

CHAPTER 3

Patient Care Practices

Any home or hospice care that involves direct, hands-on patient care faces infection control issues. Responses to these issues may be as simple as performing hand hygiene or may involve strict adherence to sterile technique. As a home care or hospice organization develops policies and procedures for care, it must determine its standard of practice. This is guided by the experience of the nursing staff as well as by written resources and references. Much of the written material on infection control is based on care provided in hospitals; thus, home care and hospice professional staff must adapt these practices to make them appropriate for the home care setting. Although many of the structural advantages of an institutional setting are not present in the home, neither are many of the potential risks for infection. In most home care situations, there are no other patients being cared for in the same room or area. Although this decreases the transmission risk of microorganisms from one patient to another, it does not totally eliminate the sources of infection risk. Transmission can still occur from one patient to another on the hands of the home or hospice care staff member. Potential environmental reservoirs that have been implicated in infections within hospitals and other care settings—such as contaminated sinks, shared urine measurement devices, contaminated ventilator tubing, and other inanimate objects—are eliminated in the home care situation. Although practices should be performed in such a manner as to decrease infection risk, patient care practices in the home must also be feasible, sensible, practical, and cost effective. Infection control principles should be employed in a manner appropriate to the level of risk. The following discussion and recommen-

dations for patient care practices have been developed with these guiding principles in mind.

HAND HYGIENE

Hand hygiene is the single most important patient care practice that a home care or hospice staff member can perform to prevent cross-contamination and health care–associated infection resulting from their home care or hospice services. In home care, the staff member's hands are the greatest potential source for transmission of potentially infectious organisms to other patients.

Resident and Transient Microorganisms

The skin on the hands carries both resident and transient microorganisms. The resident (colonizing) microorganisms are normally located on the skin, whereas transient (noncolonizing) microorganisms are recent contaminants that survive only for a limited amount of time on the skin and are readily removed by handwashing. Resident microorganisms (e.g., *Staphylococcus epidermidis*) rarely cause infections unless they enter sterile body spaces through an invasive procedure, such as during the placement of a peripherally inserted central catheter. Most resident microorganisms are located in the superficial skin layers, but 10% to 20% can invade the deep epidermal layers. Handwashing with plain soaps or detergents and water will not remove resident microorganisms in the deep epidermal layers, but will remove many transient microorganisms. Only antimicrobial soaps can kill or inhibit resident microorganisms in the deep epidermal layers. For patients at high risk for infection, resident microorganisms can cause infections. *Staphylococcus aureus (S. aureus)* is an example of a resident organism. Home care staff members may carry *S. aureus* on their hands and can spread the infection to the home care or hospice patient if the microorganism comes in contact with a portal of entry (e.g., IV port, urinary drainage system, etc.).

Transient microorganisms survive less than 24 hours on the skin and can be removed easily by handwashing. Examples of transient microorganisms are *Escherichia coli* and *Pseudomonas, Salmonella,* and *Shigella.* These transient organisms can be found on home and hospice care staff members' hands and may cause a health care–associated infection. The reservoir of transient microorganisms is usually col-onized in infected patients or contaminated patient care equipment.

Hand Hygiene Terminology

In October 2002, the CDC published *The Guideline for Hand Hygiene in Health-Care Settings* (CDC, 2002a). This guideline contains a review of data regarding handwashing and hand antisepsis in health care settings, as well as specific recommendations to promote improved hand hygiene practices and reduce the transmission of pathogenic microorganisms to patients and personnel. The CDC guideline's framework comprises a number of important terms and definitions related to effectively implementing hand hygiene procedures in the home care or hospice setting. A listing of hand hygiene definitions is found in Table 3-1.

Table 3-1 Hand Hygiene Terminology Definitions

Alcohol-based hand rub. An alcohol-containing preparation designed for application to the hands for reducing the number of viable microorganisms on the hands. Such preparations in the United States usually contain 60% to 95% ethanol or isopropanol.

Antimicrobial soap. Soap (i.e., detergent) containing an antiseptic agent.

Antiseptic agent. Antimicrobial substances applied to the skin to reduce the number of microbial flora. Examples include alcohols, chlorhexidine, chlorine, hexachlorophene, iodine, chloroxylenol (PCMX), quaternary ammonium compounds, and triclosan.

Antiseptic handwash. Washing hands with water and soap or other detergents containing an antiseptic agent.

Antiseptic hand rub. An antiseptic hand-rub product applied to all surfaces of the hands to reduce the number of microorganisms present.

Cumulative effect. A progressive decrease in the number of microorganisms recovered after repeated applications of a test material.

Decontaminate hands. To reduce bacterial counts on hands by performing an antiseptic hand rub or antiseptic handwash.

Detergent (or surfactant). A compound that possesses a cleaning action. Although products used for hand hygiene or antiseptic handwash in health care settings represent various types of detergents, the term *soap* is used to refer to such detergents.

Hand antisepsis. Either antiseptic handwash or antiseptic hand rub.

Hand hygiene. A general term that applies to hand washing, antiseptic handwash, antiseptic hand rub, or surgical hand antisepsis.

Handwashing. Washing hands with plain (i.e., nonantimicrobial) soap and water.

Persistent activity. Prolonged or extended antimicrobial activity that prevents or inhibits the proliferation or survival of microorganisms after application of the product. Also referred to as *residual activity.*

Plain soap. Detergents that do not contain antimicrobial agents or with low concentrations of antimicrobial agents that are effective solely as preservatives.

Visibly soiled hands. Hands showing visible dirt or visibly contaminated with proteinaceous material, blood, or other body fluids.

Waterless antiseptic agent. An antiseptic agent that does not require use of exogenous water. After applying such an agent, the hands are rubbed together until the agent dries.

Source: Adapted from Centers for Disease Control and Prevention. *Guideline for Hand Hygiene in Health-Care Settings: Recommendations of the Healthcare Infection Control Practices Advisory Committee and the HICPAC/SHEA/APIC/IDSA Hand Hygiene Task Force.* MMWR 2002; 51 (No. RR–16): [pages 1–45].

Indications for Handwashing and Hand Antisepsis

The home and hospice care staff member can serve as a role model for the patient and his or her family to promote hand hygiene while performing the patient's care. The indications for hand hygiene depend on the type, intensity, duration, and sequence of home care activities. The indications for handwashing and hand antisepsis are listed in Exhibit 3-1.

Hand hygiene is not required for the following activities:

- superficial contact with a source not suspected of being contaminated (e.g., touching an object that is not visibly soiled, such as the doorknob of a patient's front door to enter the home)
- routine home visit activities that do not involve direct patient contact or contact with frequently touched items in the patient's immediate care environment (e.g., completing paperwork or talking with the patient and family)

When to Use Plain Soaps Versus Antiseptic Agents for Hand Hygiene

Home care and hospice staff members face the dilemma of deciding when to use an antimicrobial soap and which agent to use. The choice of using plain soap, an antimicrobial soap, or a waterless antiseptic agent should be based on the degree of hand contamination (soiling with organic material), whether it is important to maintain a minimal number of resident microorganisms or to decrease the number, and whether it is important to remove the transient microorganisms mechanically. For routine hand hygiene, washing the hands with plain soap and water for 15 seconds is sufficient to remove most transient contaminants from the skin. Plain soap removes microorganisms from the skin by suspending them and allowing them to be rinsed off the skin.

The Food and Drug Administration considers antimicrobial soaps to be drugs because they kill or inhibit both transient and resident microorganisms. Even when an antimicrobial soap is used, there is a maximum level of reduction in bacterial counts that can be reached regardless of handwashing frequency or intensity (Larson, 2001). Antimicrobial soap not only kills microorganisms, but it also can bind to the skin and continue to suppress microbial growth. The antimicro-

Exhibit 3-1 Indications for Hand Antisepsis or Handwashing

Wash hands with soap and water using either an antimicrobial soap or plain soap in the following circumstances:

- Hands are visibly dirty or contaminated with proteinaceous material
- Hands are visibly soiled with blood or other body fluids
- Before eating and after using a restroom
- When there has been exposure to *Bacillus anthracis* (suspected or proven)
- When removing gloves after caring for a patient with *C. difficile*–associated diarrhea

Decontaminate the hands using an alcohol-based hand rub, or wash hands with an antimicrobial soap and water when the hands are not visibly soiled and:

- Before having direct contact with patients
- Before donning sterile gloves when inserting a central intravascular catheter
- Before inserting indwelling urinary catheters, peripheral venous catheters, or other invasive devices that do not require a surgical procedure
- After contact with a patient's intact skin (e.g., when taking a pulse or blood pressure or when lifting a patient)
- After contact with body fluids or excretions, mucous membranes, nonintact skin, and wound dressings
- After removing gloves
- Before and after contact with a patient who has a tracheostomy tube in place, and before and after contact with any respiratory device used on the patient, whether or not gloves are worn

When possible, decontaminate the hands using an alcohol-based hand rub, or wash hands with an antimicrobial soap and water when the hands are not visibly soiled and:

- When performing patient care and moving from a contaminated-body site to a clean-body site
- After having contact with inanimate objects (including medical equipment) in the immediate vicinity of the patient

Source: Adapted from Centers for Disease Control and Prevention. *Guideline for Hand Hygiene in Health-Care Settings: Recommendations of the Healthcare Infection Control Practices Advisory Committee and the HICPAC/SHEA/APIC/IDSA Hand Hygiene Task Force.* MMWR 2002; 51 (No. RR-16): [pages 1-45] and Tablan, O. C., Anderson, L. J., Besser, R., Bridges, C. Hajjeh, R. (2004). *Guidelines for Preventing Health-Care–Associated Pneumonia, 2003.* MMWR, March 26, 2004 53(RR03), 1–36.a.

bial spectrum and characteristics of hand-hygiene antiseptic agents are listed in Table 3-2.

Antimicrobial products that are used as waterless antiseptic agents kill transient microorganisms but do not

Table 3-2 The Antimicrobial Spectrum and Characteristics of Hand-Hygiene Antiseptic Agents*

Group	Gram-positive bacteria	Gram-negative bacteria	Mycobacteria	Fungi	Viruses	Speed of action	Comments
Alcohols	+++	+++	+++	+++	+++	Fast	Optimum concentration 80%–95%; no persistent activity
Chlorhexidine (2% and 4% aqueous)	+++	++	+	+	+++	Intermediate	Persistent activity; rare allergic reactions
Iodine compounds	+++	+++	+++	++	+++	Intermediate	Causes skin burns; usually too irritating for hand hygiene
Iodophors	+++	+++	+	++	++	Intermediate	Less irritating than iodine; acceptance varies
Phenol derivatives	+++	+	+	+	+	Intermediate	Activity neutralized by nonionic surfactants
Tricolsan	+++	++	+	—	+++	Intermediate	Acceptability on hands varies
Quaternary ammonium compounds	+	++	—	—	+	Slow	Used only in combination with alcohols; ecologic concerns

Note: +++ = excellent; ++ = good, but does not include the entire bacterial spectrum; + = fair; — = no activity or not sufficient.
*Hexachlorophene is not included because it is no longer an accepted ingredient of hand disinfectants.

Source: Centers for Disease Control and Prevention. *Guideline for Hand Hygiene in Health-Care Settings: Recommendations of the Healthcare Infection Control Practices Advisory Committee and the HICPAC/SHEA/APIC/IDSA Hand Hygiene Task Force.* MMWR 2002; 51 (No. RR-16): [pages 1–45].

remove soil or organic material. If the home care staff member's hands are visibly soiled and there is no running water available, single-use towelettes can be used to remove the physical dirt, and then the hands can be cleaned with a waterless antiseptic agent. If an alcohol-based hand rub is used, an alcohol concentration of between 60% and 95% by weight is the most effective. An alcohol concentration of greater than 70% by weight should not be used, however, because (1) it can cause the skin to dry out and result in a chemical dermatitis (Larson, 2001) and (2) higher concentrations are less potent because the proteins are not denatured as easily in the absence of water (and it is the alcohol's ability to denature proteins that makes it antimicrobial).

Bar Soap Versus Liquid Soap

Bar soap should not be carried by staff members making home visits because it may not have sufficient time to dry. Pooled moisture in a staff member's home care supply bag may support the growth of Gram-negative bacteria. Plain soap is acceptable, but it should be used in liquid form.

Liquid soap pump dispensers may become contaminated as well. For that reason, a small soap container is recommended because liquid soap containers can serve as a reservoir of microorganisms. A small container can be cleaned when empty and brought back to the office to be refilled. A container that is almost empty should be completely emptied, cleaned, and dried before it is refilled. Liquid soap should not be added to a partially full soap dispenser. Refilling a pump dispenser is a more cost-effective approach and can serve as an indicator of the frequency with which the home and hospice care staff members are washing their hands in the home (i.e., if they do not use the patient's soap).

Hand Hygiene Facilities

Home care staff members do not have the luxury of working in a health care facility where there is access to needed equipment and supplies. Staff members may find themselves caring for a patient who has no access to clean or running water or having to bring water to the patient's home to give the patient a bath. When running water is not available, staff members should use a waterless antiseptic agent for routine hand hygiene. The waterless antiseptic agent should be used when it would be appropriate to decontaminate the hands, such as after performing patient care. As long as the staff member has used a waterless antiseptic agent for hand hygiene, there is no need for the staff member to wash his or her hands with soap and running water as soon after as feasible, unless the staff member's hands are visibly dirty or contaminated with proteinaceous material, the hands are soiled with blood or other body fluids, or the staff member has just cared for a patient with *C. difficile*–associated diarrhea.

Side Effects of Hand Hygiene

Frequent hand hygiene with plain soap or antimicrobial soap can cause skin dryness, cracking, irritation, or dermatitis, especially in geographical locations where the weather is cold and dry. This is caused by the soap stripping away the skin's natural oils. Home and hospice care staff members with cracked skin or dermatitis are at increased risk for infection from contact with blood or other potentially infectious body fluids because there has been a break in the skin's integrity. Patients may also be placed at an increased risk for infection because handwashing does not effectively decrease the bacterial counts on irritated, dry, or cracked skin or dermatic skin because of the high numbers of microorganisms present in dermatic skin (Larson, 2001).

To prevent the skin from becoming cracked or developing dermatitis, soap must be thoroughly rinsed off and the skin dried thoroughly. Staff members should try not to use excessive amounts of soap or antimicrobial soaps when washing the hands. Home and hospice care staff members providing patient care must be provided with a product that has a low potential of irritancy. For example, a hand hygiene product that contains iodophor (an antibacterial additive) should be avoided because iodophor dries the skin.

Home care staff members should be provided with hand creams or lotions to minimize the occurrence of irritant contact dermatitis associated with hand antisepsis or handwashing. When selecting a hand cream or lotion, information should be obtained from the manufacturer regarding any interactions that these products may have on the persistent effects of antimicrobial soaps being used by the home or hospice care staff. Hand creams and lotions can be helpful, but they also can become contaminated. If lotion is provided, the purchase of small, individual-use containers or pump dispensers that can be discarded when empty should be considered.

Considerations When Purchasing Hand Hygiene Products

When selecting non-antimicrobial soaps, antimicrobial soaps, or alcohol-based hand rubs, the following guidelines apply:

1. Obtain information from the manufacturers regarding
   - any possible effects on the persistent activities of antimicrobial soaps being used by home care staff members.
   - any known interactions between products used to clean hands, skin care products, and the types of gloves used in home health agencies or hospices.
2. Obtain input from staff members regarding their opinions of the products' fragrance, feel, and skin tolerance.
3. Cost should not be the primary factor.
4. Evaluate the products' dispenser systems to ensure that they function adequately and deliver an appropriate volume of product. Obtain information about recommended storage methods (CDCa, 2002).

Other Hand Hygiene Considerations

Staff having direct contact with high-risk patients (i.e., immunosuppressed patients or infants less than six months of age) should not wear artificial fingernails or extenders. For staff with natural nails, the tips should be kept to less than 1/4-inch long (CDCa, 2002).

Behavioral Aspects of Hand Hygiene

Compliance with hand hygiene guidelines has been a problem for a long time. Home care staff members with cracked skin or dermatitis might avoid hand hygiene. The following factors may promote the frequency of hand hygiene:

- informing staff members of infection rate(s) and presence of multidrug-resistant organisms
- involving staff in the selection of hand hygiene products

- observing hand hygiene technique during competence assessment activities
- having hand hygiene supplies readily available
- promoting hand hygiene practices
- involving staff in planning for hand hygiene education

National Infection Control Week is observed during October of each year. This may be a good time to focus on hand hygiene by providing buttons, posters, in-service education, or written information about hand hygiene to home care and hospice staff, patients, and families.

Hand Hygiene Supplies Needed by Home Care Staff

Hand hygiene supplies may be brought to the patient's home by home and hospice care staff members, or if appropriate, the patient's supplies may be used. Staff members providing direct, hands-on patient care activities should have the following supplies:

- plain soap and antimicrobial soap or antimicrobial soap only
- a waterless antiseptic agent
- paper towels
- skin lotion

Staff members who do not provide hands-on patient care (e.g., social workers, dietitians) and do not anticipate patient contact should have a waterless antiseptic agent in their possession during home visits in case the need for hand hygiene arises.

Using the Patient's Hand Hygiene Supplies

It is preferred that, when performing hand hygiene in a patient's home, home care staff members use their own hand hygiene supplies. When this is not possible, the patient's liquid soap may be used if the dispenser appears to be clean and the home environment is clean. If hands-on patient care is to be provided, the staff member should verify that the patient's soap is an antimicrobial agent so that the hands can be properly decontaminated as needed for direct patient care activities. The patient's bar soap should not be used if it has been resting in a pool of accumulated water, because it may be contaminated with bacteria.

When drying the hands, staff members may use either their own paper towels or the patient's paper tow-

Table 3-3 How to Wash the Hands with Soap and Water

1. Wet the hands under running water. To reduce the risk of dermatitis, avoid using hot water.
2. Apply to the hands the amount of soap recommended by the manufacturer.
3. Vigorously rub the hands together for a minimum of 15 seconds, covering all surfaces of the hands and fingers.
4. Rinse the hands under running water to remove residual soap.
5. Dry the hands with a clean, disposable (or single-use) towel.
6. Use the towel to turn off the faucet.
7. Discard the used towel in a trash container.
8. Apply hand lotion to prevent chapping of the hands.

Source: Friedman, M. M., Home Health Systems, Inc. (2005). *Infection Control Policies and Procedures.* Marietta, GA: self-published.

els. The patient's cloth towels may be used if they are clean and have not been used previously by anyone in the home. Hand drying is an integral part of cleaning the hands. The friction created by hand drying can remove many bacteria by rubbing away transient microorganisms and dead skin cells, and it can remove bacteria from deeper skin layers.

After performing hand hygiene, hand lotion may be used to prevent chapping of the hands. If lotions are used, liquids or tubes that can be squirted are recommended, so that the hands do not come into direct contact with the container spout. Direct contact with the spout could contaminate the lotion inside the container. Staff members should never use lotion from jars or containers into which the hands must be dipped. Refer to Table 3-3 for instructions on how to wash the hands and Table 3-4 for information on how to decontaminate the hands.

Antiseptic Hand Rub

Failure to use a sufficient volume of alcohol for hand hygiene may result in an ineffective effort to cleanse the skin. One study documented that 1 mL of alcohol was substantially less effective than 3 mL (Larson et al., 1987). Another study verified that the volume of hand hygiene agent used was a factor affecting the efficacy of hand hygiene (Sickbert-Bennett, E., Weber, D., Gergen-Teague, M., & Rutala, W., 2004). The ideal volume of product to apply to the hands is not known

Table 3-4 How to Decontaminate the Hands with an Alcohol-Based Hand Rub

1. If the hands are visibly soiled with dirt or blood or body fluids and there is no running water available in the home, clean the hands with an individual-use antimicrobial-impregnated towelette.

2. Apply product to the palm of one hand and rub the hands together. Follow the manufacturer's recommendations regarding the volume of product to use.

3. Cover all surfaces of the hands and fingers with product until the hands are dry.

The efficacy of an alcohol-based hand hygiene product is affected by:

- the type of alcohol used
- the concentration of alcohol
- the contact time with the skin
- the volume of alcohol used
- whether the hands were wet when the alcohol was applied
- whether all parts of the hand surface were covered

Source: Friedman, M. M., Home Health Systems, Inc. (2005). *Infection Control Policies and Procedures.* Marietta, GA: self-published.

and may vary for different formulations. However, if the hands feel dry after rubbing them together for 10 to 15 seconds, there was not a sufficient volume of alcohol applied to the hands.

Alcohol-impregnated towelettes may be used when hand hygiene with a non-antimicrobial agent is indicated. Although the product label states that the towelettes are "antimicrobial," they are not as effective as alcohol-based hand rubs or washing with an antimicrobial soap and water for reducing bacterial counts on the hands because they contain a limited volume of alcohol (CDCa, 2002). Therefore, the towelettes should be used only as an alternative to washing the hands with non-antimicrobial soap and water.

Some home care staff members have expressed concern regarding a "buildup" of emollients on their hands after using alcohol-based hand rubs repeatedly. For that reason, some manufacturers have recommended that users of their products wash their hands with soap and water after a certain number (i.e., between 5 and 10) of product applications. This recommendation is aimed more at maximizing staff members' acceptance and use of the product than it is at further reducing the bacterial count on the hands. Therefore, home care policies should identify this as an optional step in the product's use.

Fire Hazards and Storage of Alcohol-Based Hand Rubs

Most home care and hospice organizations routinely use antiseptic hand rubs, primarily an alcohol-based hand rub, for hand hygiene. For antiseptic hand rubs to be effective, the CDC requires that they contain over 60% alcohol by volume (CDCa, 2002). According to the National Fire Protection Association (NFPA), this concentration of alcohol classifies the product as

- a Flammable Liquid Class 1B (flash point less than 73°F; boiling point equal to or greater than 100°F)
- a Flammable Level 1 Aerosol (for foam products) (NFPA, 2003)

Some manufacturers advertise that their products are not flammable. These products may contain as little as 10% alcohol by volume, however, which does not meet the CDC's recommendations for effectiveness.

There has been a report in the United States of a flash fire that resulted from the use of alcohol-based products. A health care worker applied an alcohol gel to her hands, immediately removed a polyester isolation gown, and then touched a metal door before the alcohol had evaporated. The removal of the polyester gown created a substantial amount of static electricity, which generated an audible static spark when the worker touched the metal door. The spark ignited the unevaporated alcohol on her hands (Bryant, 2002). Although this was an isolated event, it emphasizes the need to stress to home care and hospice staff the importance of rubbing their hands together after applying alcohol-based products until their hands are dry and *all* the alcohol has evaporated.

Most home care and hospice offices would be classified as business occupancies (i.e., as being used for accounting and record keeping, with no sale of merchandise). According to the NFPA, business occupancies may store up to 10 gallons of a flammable liquid, Class 1B (such as an alcohol-based hand rub solution) out in the open without special storage requirements such as safety cans.

Aerosolized hand rub containers should be stored at ambient indoor conditions—not at high temperatures. The containers should be kept sealed and away from heat sources or open flames. Although there is no specific NFPA prohibition against storing aerosolized containers or foam dispensers in the trunk of a vehicle, common sense would indicate this to be unwise, as extreme heat can accumulate and become a safety factor.

The limited quantities of alcohol-based hand rub products typically stored in a home care or hospice office, in staff's supply bags taken into the home, and in staff's vehicles would be considered of minimal danger in causing a fire or contributing to its spread (Friedman, 2003).

ASSESSMENT OF THE PATIENT AND HOME ENVIRONMENT

During the initial assessment and on an ongoing basis thereafter, the patient should be evaluated for factors that may predispose him or her to infection (see Chapter 2). These factors include immunization status, past and present infectious diseases, age, nutritional status, immune status, substance abuse, financial resources available to purchase needed medication, equipment and supplies, motivation to learn, learning needs, mental status, and overall physical condition. Patients at high risk for infection should be encouraged to receive pneumococcal and influenza vaccines unless contraindicated by their physician. The findings of the initial and ongoing assessments should be incorporated into the plan of care.

The home environment should be assessed on admission not only for safety issues, but also from an infection control perspective. Conditions and facilities to be assessed in this regard include general cleanliness, availability of refrigeration, health status of other individuals residing in the home (e.g., the presence of acute or chronic infectious diseases), availability of running water, utility systems (e.g., electricity for refrigeration), heat and air conditioning (so that equipment and supplies can be stored under proper temperature and humidity conditions), availability of toilet facilities, and the presence of pets and pests. Even in the new millennium, some home environments have dirt floors and no running water or indoor toilet facilities. Frequently, home care organizations must take extra steps to work within particular home situations. For example, some home care organizations must bring water to the patient's home to bathe the patient because running water in the home is not available. During staff members' initial home visits, handwashing facilities should be assessed so that appropriate hand hygiene supplies can be available and appropriate hand hygiene can be performed.

Pets (e.g., dogs and cats) and pests (e.g., cockroaches) present another infection control concern over which home care and hospice organizations do not have direct control. Although there are situations in which the home environment is infested with roaches, these insects are not usually disease vectors. The infection risk related to this unpleasant and distasteful situation may be more perceived than actual, although no data on this subject exist. In an insect-infested home, the home care staff should educate the patient and family in general principles of hygiene and cleanliness and provide reinforcement and guidance whenever possible.

Rodents, too, can be an environmental risk factor in home care. Hantavirus pulmonary syndrome (HPS) is a deadly disease transmitted by infected rodents through urine, droppings, or saliva. Humans can contract the disease by breathing in the aerosolized virus. HPS was first recognized in 1993 and has since been identified throughout the United States. Although rare, HPS is potentially deadly. Rodent control in and around the home remains the primary strategy for preventing Hantavirus infection (CDC, 2002b).

In setting up for patient care activities, to the best of the home care staff member's abilities the patient's direct care environment (not the entire home) should be cleaned or, if necessary, barriers should be used to maintain the area as clean as possible (refer to Chapter 6 for additional information about the use of barriers in the home). When invasive procedures are performed in an unsanitary environment, efforts must be made to provide the care in as safe a manner as possible.

WOUND CARE

The types of wounds typically cared for in the home include infected surgical or acute wounds and chronic wounds, such as pressure ulcers and stasis ulcers the healing of which is slow or difficult. An acute wound heals either by regeneration or in a timely and orderly process (Lazarus et al., 1994). A surgical wound primarily heals when the wound edges have been drawn together to achieve closure (Stotts et al., 1997). A surgical wound may also be considered an acute wound. Surgical wounds seal quickly, and unless they are left open, do not heal, or have adjacent drains, there is minimal risk for contamination. A chronic wound is a wound that has "failed to proceed through an orderly and timely process to produce anatomic and functional integrity" (Lazarus et al., 1994). When performing wound care in the home, the staff member may have to adapt patient care practices to determine which technique, clean or sterile, is appropriate.

Clean Technique Versus Sterile Technique

The term *clean technique* refers to the strategies used in patient care to reduce the overall number of microorganisms present or to prevent or reduce the transmission of microorganisms from one person to another or from one place to another. It is also called *nonsterile technique* and the "sterile to sterile" rule does not apply. Clean technique involves meticulous hand hygiene with either an antiseptic hand rub product or an antibacterial soap and water with adequate rinsing; using barriers and sterile materials and supplies; maintaining a clean environment; and preparing a clean field to prevent the direct contamination of materials and supplies. Barriers involve using no-touch techniques to avoid contamination of sterile supplies; wearing clean gloves; or wearing personal protective equipment, such as a gown and gloves, to avoid direct contact with infectious materials (refer to Chapter 6 for additional information about personal protective equipment). Other components of clean technique include using a detergent to remove soil and a disinfectant agent to clean up a spill of blood or other potentially infectious material (APIC & WOCN, 2001). The no-touch technique is a method of changing surface dressings without touching the wound or the surface of any dressing that might be in contact with the wound. Dressings that adhere to the skin are grasped by the corner and slowly removed, whereas gauze dressings can be pinched in the center and lifted off.

The APIC defines *aseptic technique* as sterile technique (DeCastro, 2005). *Sterile technique* refers to strategies used in patient care to render and maintain objects and areas maximally free from microorganisms. Sterile technique involves meticulous hand hygiene, use of sterile barriers, and use of sterile instruments. The "sterile to sterile" concept must be adhered to, and only sterile instruments and materials should be used during wound care procedures. During the use of sterile technique, there should be no contact with any nonsterile surface or product. Equipment used in procedures requiring sterile technique must be maintained as sterile and discarded after one-time use. (Refer to Chapter 4 for additional information about how to prepare a patient's skin for an invasive procedure.)

When sterile technique is used in the home, a sterile field should be established to prevent the transmission of microorganisms from the environment or from the staff member to the patient. This involves using a sterile barrier or drape and, at minimum, wearing sterile gloves. Additional attire, such as a sterile gown or a mask, should be worn if appropriate. For example, if a peripherally inserted central catheter is being placed, maximum barrier protection, which includes a cap, a mask, a sterile gown, sterile gloves, and a large sterile drape, must be used (CDC, 2002c). As is the case with clean technique in the home, maintaining a clean environment is not within the direct control of the home care organization, but the immediate environment in which care is provided should be maintained as clean as possible. When a procedure requiring sterile technique is performed in the home, the staff member should close the door(s) to the room where the procedure is being performed and turn off any ceiling fan(s) to reduce the potential for airborne transmission of microorganisms. In addition to general housecleaning, maintaining a clean environment includes using a detergent to remove soil and a disinfectant agent to clean up a spill of blood or other potentially infectious material.

Selecting the "Right" Technique

The definitions of *clean technique* and *sterile technique* are not as important as making the appropriate choice of intervention for a procedure when managing acute and chronic wounds. There is no evidence-based research to support either clean or sterile management of chronic wounds in the home. Therefore, it is left to the discretion of the home care or hospice organization to determine the appropriate approach for performing wound care. Guidelines for the use of clean technique versus sterile technique in providing care to chronic wounds—not surgical wounds—are presented in Table 3-5. Anecdotally, the clean, no-touch technique is used most often in home care.

The Agency for Health Care Policy and Research (AHRQ) has published the *Clinical Practice Guidelines* for the treatment of pressure ulcers (Bergstrom, 1994). The guidelines recommend the use of clean gloves and clean dressings, as opposed to sterile dressings, when providing wound care in the home setting. If a wound needs to be debrided, however, the instrument used must be sterile. The practice of using clean gloves and dressings may be followed until research demonstrates otherwise and as long as this complies with the home care or hospice organization's policies

Table 3-5 Technique for the Management of Chronic Wounds

Intervention	Handwashing	Gloves	Supplies (solutions and dressing supplies)	Instruments
Wound cleansing	Yes	Clean/nonsterile	Normal saline or commercially prepared wound cleanser—sterile; maintain clean as per care setting policy [a]	Irrigation with sterile device; maintain clean as per care setting policy
Routine dressing change without debridement	Yes	Clean/nonsterile	Sterile; maintain clean as per care setting policy	Sterile; maintain clean as per care setting policy
Dressing change with mechanical, chemical, or enzymatic debridement	Yes	Clean/nonsterile	Sterile; maintain clean as per care setting policy	Sterile; maintain clean as per care setting policy
Dressing change with sharp, conservative bedside debridement	Yes	Sterile	Sterile	Sterile

[a] "Maintain clean as per care setting policy" means that each care setting must address the parameters for maintenance, such as expiration dates for supplies, consideration of cost, and correct interpretation of the manufacturer's recommendations.

Source: Adapted from Association for Professionals in Infection Control and Epidemiology, Inc. (APIC) and the Wound Ostomy Continence Nurses Society (WOCN). 2001. Position Statement Clean vs. Sterile: Management of Chronic Wounds. Retrieved March 30, 2004, from *http://www.apic.org/resc/ppcleansterile.cfm.*

and procedures and physician's orders. The recommendation for using clean dressings also takes into account the expense of sterile dressings and the dexterity often required of the patient's family members when applying them. It is important to note that the AHRQ's guideline is based on expert opinion and not founded on evidenced-based research (Bergstrom *et al.*, 1994). The use of clean technique versus sterile technique is an area needing further research.

Wound Care Procedures

Various dressing techniques and wound care procedures may be performed in the home setting. Frequently, dressing changes are delegated to the patient or a family member. Either clean technique or sterile technique may be used to perform wound care in the home. Sterile technique should be performed when required by the physician's orders. The CDC's Guideline for the Prevention of Surgical Site Infections (Mangram, 1999) states that when a surgical incision dressing must be changed within the first 24 to 48 hours, sterile technique should be used. Beyond 48 hours, the guideline does not contain any recommendations for the type of incision care and method. The guideline further notes that "the lack of optimum

protocols for home incision care dictates that much of what is done at home by the patient, family, or home care agency practitioners must be individualized" and that patients and family must be educated in proper incision care, symptoms of a surgical site infection, and the need to report the symptoms (Mangram *et al.*, 1999). Regardless of the technique used, the wound itself should never be touched with any item that is not sterile. Home care staff members should not touch an open wound directly unless they are wearing sterile gloves or are using no-touch technique.

When wounds are measured in the home with nonsterile measuring devices, special care should be taken to avoid touching the wound directly. When dressings are removed, nonsterile examination gloves may be worn when there is no direct touching of the wound itself; a new dressing may be applied with either new, sterile gloves or nonsterile gloves using no-touch technique. Dressings over closed wounds should be removed or changed if they are wet or if the patient has signs or symptoms suggestive of infection (e.g., fever or unusual wound pain). When the dressing is removed, the wound should be evaluated for signs of infection, and if necessary the physician should be contacted. Any purulent drainage should be reported to the physician, and a culture and sensitivity smear as well as a Gram's stain smear obtained if ordered.

Home and hospice care staff members and the patient and family members should wash their hands before and after taking care of a wound (refer to Chapter 7 for information about isolation precautions and Chapter 9 for information about storing wound care supplies in the home).

Irrigating Solution Maintenance

Currently, there are no home care or hospice industry standards prescribing a specific time frame for which an irrigating solution, such as normal saline or sterile water, may be used after it is opened. Thus, current practice varies. Although it seems logical to have some policy setting a time limit, the contamination of irrigation fluid is not dependent on time. It is an event-related risk that depends on how the solution and its container are handled. If the inside of the container or the fluid is contaminated, the container and fluid should be discarded immediately. If the container is handled carefully and contamination does not occur, the fluid will probably remain sterile. Without specific data, it is impossible to determine what time frame for use is safe or necessary. To address this issue, the home care organization should incorporate some commonsense strategies to avoid arbitrary discarding of irrigation fluid, which increases the cost of care. The guiding principles noted in Table 3-6 should also be considered to improve patient safety by reducing the risk of infection.

Preparing Irrigation Solutions in the Home

Most home care or hospice organizations provide patients with commercially prepared, sterile irrigating solutions for their use. If a patient cannot afford to purchase the commercially prepared products, the patient or family member can prepare sterile water in the home as follows (Luebbert, 2000):

1. Place a small (quart-size or smaller), closeable glass jar and its lid into a pan of boiling water.
2. Submerge the jar and lid, and boil the jar and the lid for 10 minutes.
3. Fill a separate pan with a sufficient amount of distilled water to fill the jar of water.
4. Boil the distilled water for 10 minutes.
5. Remove the jar and the lid from the pan, being careful not to touch the top of the jar or the inside of the lid (tongs or pick-ups may be used), and allow them to cool.
6. Pour the boiled distilled water into the jar, close tightly, and store.

Table 3-6 Guiding Principles for Irrigation Fluid Storage

Use smaller (for example, 50 to 100 ml) containers of irrigation solution designed for single use whenever possible. If irrigating solution is left over in the smaller container after the intended amount has been removed, do not save the leftover content and combine it for later use.

Do not use any container of irrigation solution that has visible turbidity, leaks, cracks, or particulate matter, or if the manufacturer's expiration date has passed.

When using larger (500 ml to 1000 ml) containers of irrigation solution that will be used on multiple, separate occasions, take the following precautions:

- Date the container with the date it was opened.
- Write the "discard by" date, according to the time set by the organization.

Open the container without contaminating the fluid, the inside neck of the bottle, or the inside of the top of the cap.

Place the cap face up when the container is open and being used, and replace the cap as soon as possible.

Pour the intended amount of irrigation solution into a secondary container, if necessary. Do not place a syringe inside the container to remove the contents, unless the syringe is sterile.

Store the irrigation solution in a safe place that minimizes the possibility of tampering.

Consider refrigerating the irrigation solution after the initial use to reduce bacterial growth; warm to room temperature just prior to use.

Discard the container of irrigation solution if the integrity is compromised or the solution is contaminated.

Source: Friedman, M. M. Home Health Systems, Inc. (2005). *Infection Control Policies and Procedures.* Marietta, GA: self-published.

The patient or family member can prepare 0.9% normal saline by following these steps (Luebbert, 2000):

1. Place a small (quart-size or smaller), closeable glass jar and its lid into a pan of boiling water.
2. Submerge the jar and lid, and boil the jar and the lid for 10 minutes.
3. Fill a separate pan with approximately 1 quart of distilled water and add 1.5 teaspoons of salt.
4. Boil the salt water for 10 minutes.
5. Remove the jar and the lid from the pan, being careful not to touch the top of the jar or the inside of the lid (tongs or pick-ups may be used), and allow them to cool.
6. Pour the boiled salt water into the jar, shake well, and store.

If any solution is left over two days, a new mixture should be prepared. If a family member prepares the normal saline or sterile water, a new mixture should be prepared daily. The patient and family should be instructed never to pour any leftover solution back into the container.

Patient Education Related to Wound Care

Patient and family education related to infection control and wound care should include the following topics:

- hand hygiene
- clean technique versus sterile technique
- proper storage and setup of equipment and supplies
- proper use of irrigation solutions
- wound care procedure
- wound assessment
- signs and symptoms of a localized or systemic infection
- disposal of soiled dressings

The CDC's Guideline for the Prevention of Surgical Site Infections further states that patients and families must be educated on proper incision care, symptoms of a surgical site infection, and the need to report the symptoms (Mangram et al., 1999).

REUSING EQUIPMENT IN THE HOME

Items that directly or indirectly contact mucous membranes are considered semicritical items (see Chapter 9). According to Spaulding's classification system for cleaning and disinfecting medical equipment (Spaulding,

1968), semicritical items should be sterilized or subjected to high-level disinfection before reuse (except for thermometers and tubs used for soaking nonintact skin). In the home environment, however, it is not possible to sterilize equipment or perform high-level disinfection. Many patients being cared for at home are chronically ill and do not have the financial resources to afford a new sterile item, such as a tracheal suction catheter or intermittent urethral catheter, for each use. For many years, these catheters have been safely reused without reports of infectious complications. As in most home care situations, scientific data are not available to support this practice, but reuse of tracheal suction catheters and intermittent urethral catheters after meticulous cleaning and disinfection is acceptable for most (not all) patients. Each patient and situation must be evaluated for the potential risk versus the cost of using disposable catheters.

URINARY TRACT CARE

Catheter-associated urinary tract infection (CAUTI) is the most common health care-associated infection, comprising more than 40% of all nosocomial infections. CAUTI also contributes to the incidence of bloodstream infection as the second most common cause of nosocomial secondary bloodstream infection. Each year, urinary catheters are inserted in more than 5 million patients in acute-care hospitals and extended-care facilities in the United States; more than 1 million patients in these hospitals and extended-care facilities acquire a catheter-associated urinary tract infection. Studies suggest that patients with CAUTI have an increased institutional death rate, unrelated to the development of urosepsis (Maki & Tambyah, 2001). Minimal data suggest that CAUTI may be the most common type of infection in home care patients as well. Although not all CAUTI can be prevented, proper placement and management of the indwelling catheter can contribute to the prevention of associated infections. Long-term indwelling catheterization, which usually is more prevalent in home care patients than intermittent or condom catheterization, is generally associated with a higher urinary tract infection rate. The incidence of infection in acute care is directly related to the duration of catheterization. Prolonged catheterization beyond 6 days was the most important, potentially modifiable risk factor identified in every study; by the 30th day of catheterization, infection is near universal. (Maki, Knasinski, & Tambyah, 2000). Other data show that 50% of patients develop a urinary tract infection by day 15 of catheterization and that almost 100% of patients develop a urinary tract infection by the end of 1 month (Kunin, 1987).

The risk of acquiring a urinary tract infection depends on the method and duration of catheterization, the quality of catheter care, and host susceptibility. Host factors that increase the risk for a urinary tract infection include advanced age, female gender, general debilitation, meatal colonization by urinary pathogens, and bowel incontinence. CAUTI is caused by various pathogens, including *Escherichia coli, Candida albicans,* enterococci, and various species of *Klebsiella, Proteus, Pseudomonas, Enterobacter,* and *Serratia.* Many of these microorganisms are part of the patient's normal bowel flora, but they also can be acquired by cross-contamination from staff members or by exposure to contaminated solutions or nonsterile equipment (Wong, 1983). Whether from endogenous or exogenous sources, infecting microorganisms gain access to the urinary tract by several routes. Microorganisms that inhabit the distal urethra can be directly introduced into the bladder when the catheter is inserted. With indwelling catheters, infecting microorganisms can migrate on biofilm to the bladder along the outside of the catheter or along the inside lumen of the catheter if the collection bag or catheter drainage tube junction has been contaminated.

One of the most important strategies for preventing a urinary tract infection is to limit the use of urinary catheters and the number of days they are in place, thereby reducing exposure risk. If possible, alternative techniques of urinary drainage, such as the placement of a suprapubic catheter or intermittent urethral catheterization, should be considered before an indwelling urethral catheter is inserted. The physician will make these determinations, with input from the home or hospice care staff member.

Condom Catheter Drainage

Condom catheter drainage, although not free from risk for urinary tract infections, appears to be associated with a lower risk than indwelling urethral catheters in incontinent males who do not have a bladder outlet obstruction (Maki & Tambyah, 2001). Condom catheters should be used to manage incontinence in men only where the benefits to the patient outweigh the potential risks. When a condom catheter is used for external uri-

nary drainage, it should be applied and managed to minimize skin breakdown and ensure unobstructed drainage. Condom catheter leg bags should also be disinfected and dried prior to reuse (Nicolle et al., 2001). Refer to the "Catheter Maintenance" section, which provides instruction for cleaning and disinfecting urine collection tubing and bags.

Indwelling Catheter Insertion and Replacement Frequency

With many home care patients, it is difficult to avoid long-term urinary catheterization. In these patients, it has become routine to change the catheter and drainage system arbitrarily every 30 days. Prior to the implementation of Periodic Payment System (PPS), this practice had been supported by the Health Care Financing Administration (HCFA), which reimbursed Medicare-certified home health agencies for skilled nursing services on a per-visit basis for catheter insertion, sterile irrigation, and replacement of catheters, as well as for care of suprapubic catheters and, in selected patients, urethral catheters. The frequency of catheter-related services that is considered reasonable and necessary is as follows: "Absent any complications, Foley catheters generally require skilled care once approximately every 30 days, and silicone catheters generally require skilled care once every 60 to 90 days" (HCFA, 1996, pp. 14–15). Therefore, most Medicare-certified home health agencies replaced patients' Foley catheters at 30-day intervals because it was considered a billable skilled nursing visit rather than it being a clinical need. This is still considered a Medicare-covered service, but the home health agency is no longer reimbursed on a per-visit basis.

The CDC's Guideline for the Prevention of Catheter-Associated Urinary Tract Infections states that indwelling catheters should not be changed at arbitrary fixed intervals (Wong, 1983) in the absence of leakage, malfunction, or palpable concretions in the catheter lumen. The Society of Healthcare Epidemiologists of America (SHEA) position paper addressing the prevention of urinary tract infections held that there were insufficient data to make a recommendation for or against routine catheter changes in chronic indwelling urethral catheters (Nicolle et al., 2001). Indications for the replacement of an indwelling catheter include catheter damage or leakage, an obstruction that is not relieved by irrigation (Wong, 1983), and physician's orders. Insertion or replacement of an indwelling catheter should be performed using aseptic/sterile equipment and as small a catheter as possible, consistent with good drainage, to minimize urethral trauma.

Catheter Maintenance

Hand hygiene using an antiseptic agent should be performed immediately before and after any manipulation of a catheter site or apparatus. As much as possible, a closed urinary catheter drainage system (where the collection tube is fused to the drainage bag) should be maintained. Closed drainage systems reduce the incidence of bacteriuria from 95% after 96 hours of open drainage to 50% after 11 days of closed drainage for men and 11 days of closed drainage for women (Kunin & McCormick, 1966). The catheter and drainage tube should not be disconnected unless the catheter must be irrigated, the catheter tubing and bag must be changed for routine maintenance, or the patient uses a temporary leg bag. If the system must be disconnected, the catheter–tubing junction should be disinfected with 70% isopropyl alcohol or povidone-iodine solution. The collection tubing and bag should always remain below the level of the patient's bladder, but the drainage tubing should always be above the level of the collection bag and be kept free of kinks, to prevent a reflux of urine into the bladder. The collection bag should be emptied on a regular basis using a separate collection container. The draining spigot on the collection bag should not come in direct contact with the urine collection container. After use, the urine collection container should be cleaned and disinfected with a bleach solution or sprayed/rinsed with a commercial disinfectant, with the solution remaining on the container for the time recommended by the manufacturer. Indwelling catheters should be properly secured after insertion to prevent movement and urethral traction.

Meatal Care

Data has not supported that performing routine meatal care in patients by cleaning with povidone-iodine twice a day or cleansing daily with soap and water reduces the risk of catheter-associated urinary tract infection (Wong, 1983). Meatal care and cleansing in the perineal area should be performed with soap and water during the bathing and care of the incontinent patient. In females, cleansing should be performed by wiping from the front to the back.

Indwelling Catheter Irrigation

Indwelling catheters may require frequent irrigation because of obstructions caused by clots, mucus, or other causes. Routine irrigation should be avoided, however, because it interrupts a sterile system and increases the risk for contamination and infection. When intermittent catheter irrigation must be performed, the catheter–tubing junction should be disinfected before disconnection, and the catheter should be irrigated using aseptic technique. If the catheter becomes obstructed and can be kept open only by frequent irrigation, the catheter should be changed if it is likely that the catheter itself is contributing to the obstruction (e.g., by the formation of concretions) (Wong, 1983). Catheter irrigation has been found to be an ineffective strategy against the prevention of CAUTI as catheter-associated biofilm will not be dislodged by a saline rinse (Trautner & Darouiche, 2004).

Suprapubic Catheters

Suprapubic catheterization may be associated with a lower incidence of CAUTI and according to patients is more comfortable and acceptable (Maki & Tambyah, 2001); there is also evidence that patients placed with suprapubic catheters more frequently experience certain mechanical complications, however (AHRQ, 2001). Suprapubic catheters are inserted in the lower abdomen, an area with less bacterial colonization than the periurethral region. It is not known what proportion of patients who require indwelling urinary catheters receive suprapubic catheters; however, it is known to be a much less common practice than the use of indwelling urethral catheters. The lower incidence of suprapubic catheter use likely is associated with its cost of placement (because it is necessary that a urologist surgically insert the catheter) versus the cost of a nurse inserting an indwelling urethral catheter. Anecdotally, the use of suprapubic catheters varies by geographic location.

The primary problem associated with suprapubic catheter use involves mechanical complications during insertion, most commonly catheter dislodgement or obstruction. On the other hand, urethral catheters are likely to lead to a higher incidence of urethral strictures. Given these mixed results, conclusions regarding the overall benefit of routine suprapubic catheterization cannot currently be made (AHRQ, 2001).

Intermittent Catheterization

For patients with certain types of bladder-emptying dysfunction, such as those caused by spinal cord injuries or other neurological disorders (e.g., muscular sclerosis), intermittent catheterization is commonly used. Clean technique is acceptable for intermittent catheterization (Nicolle *et al.,* 2001). The intermittent urethral catheter may be reused as long as the cleaning and disinfection process is performed effectively and does not change the structural integrity or function of the urethral catheter. Another option for patients requiring intermittent catheterization is a catheterization system with an introducer tip, such as the MMG/O'Neil™ Catheter System. The MMG/O'Neil™ Catheter System is a closed-system intermittent catheter designed to help protect against recurring urinary tract infections; it is used on a one-time basis. The catheter system consists of a sterile, plastic catheter enclosed in a prelubricated plastic sleeve and a urethral introducer tip that protects the catheter from contamination by the colonized first 1.5 cm of the urethra—the area most commonly associated with urethral bacteria. The use of this sterile system has significantly decreased the urinary tract infection rate in hospitalized men with spinal cord injuries on intermittent catheterization, although the costs were significantly higher than the cost of continuous catheterization (Bennett *et al.,* 1997).

Cleaning and Disinfecting Intermittent Urethral Catheters

Urethral catheters for intermittent catheterization used by a single patient may be reused after cleaning and disinfection. Methods used by home care organizations include either boiling or microwaving the catheter. When the boiling method is used, the catheter is cleaned with soap and tap water, rinsed with tap water, boiled for 15 minutes, dried on a clean towel or paper towels, and allowed to cool before use or stored in a clean, closeable container or a new plastic bag. When the microwaving method is used, the catheter is cleaned with soap and tap water on the inside and outside, rinsed with tap water on the inside and outside, placed in a bowl of water and mi-

crowaved on high for 15 minutes, dried on a clean towel or paper towels, and allowed to cool prior to use or stored in a clean, closeable container or a new plastic bag (Luebbert, 2000).

Cleaning and Disinfecting Urine Collection Tubing and Bags

Several methods, including the following, may be used to clean and disinfect the urine collection system.

1. Drain the urine from the bag and rinse the tubing and bag with tap water until clear.
2. With a catheter tip syringe, clean the tubing and bag with soapy water and rinse with tap water until clear.
3. With a catheter tip syringe, instill either 1:3 white vinegar solution or a bleach solution of 1 teaspoon bleach to 1 pint of water.
4. Soak for 30 minutes.
5. Empty the collection system and allow the tubing and bag to air dry.
6. Cover the ends aseptically, such as with a sterile gauze pad, and store in a clean, dry place.

The tubing must be completely filled with the selected disinfectant for it to be properly disinfected. When the tubing is submerged, caution should be used to avoid getting air bubbles trapped in it.

Specimen Collection

If small volumes of urine are needed for laboratory analysis, the distal end of the catheter, or preferably the sampling port, if present, should be used to obtain the specimen. If the catheter–tubing junction must be disconnected, it should be disinfected before disconnection with a 70% isopropyl alcohol preparation pad. If the sampling port is used, it should be cleansed with a 70% isopropyl alcohol preparation pad, and the urine should be aspirated through a sterile syringe.

Patient Education for Prevention of Urinary Tract Infection

Patient and family education specifically related to infection control and prevention of urinary tract infection should include hand hygiene; indwelling, condom, or suprapubic catheter care and maintenance; drainage-bag-emptying procedures; cleaning and disinfecting procedures for catheter care equipment and supplies; and signs and symptoms of urinary tract infections.

RESPIRATORY THERAPY AND INFECTION CONTROL

Prevention of Health Care-Associated Bacterial Pneumonia

Mechanically Assisted Ventilation

Pneumonia is the second most common type of nosocomial infection in the United States and is associated with substantial morbidity and mortality (Tablan *et al.,* 1994). Although patients receiving mechanically assisted ventilation do not represent a major proportion of home care patients, they are at highest risk for acquiring pneumonia because mechanical ventilation alters first-line patient defenses. In fact, patients receiving continuous, mechanically assisted ventilation have 6 to 21 times the risk for acquiring pneumonia compared with patients not receiving ventilatory support (Tablan *et al.,* 1994). Other risk factors for pneumonia include host factors (e.g., extremes of age and severe underlying conditions, including immunosuppression), factors that enhance colonization of the oropharynx and/or stomach by microorganisms (e.g., administration of antimicrobials, underlying chronic lung disease, or coma), and conditions favoring aspiration or reflux (e.g., insertion of a nasogastric tube or lying in a supine position). Most bacterial pneumonias occur through aspiration of bacteria colonizing the oropharynx or upper gastrointestinal tract. Bacteria can invade the lower respiratory tract through aspiration of oropharyngeal organisms, inhalation of aerosols containing bacteria, or less frequently, hematogenous spread from a distant body site (Tablan *et al.,* 1994).

Breathing Circuits

A breach of a breathing circuit occurs anytime the ventilator is disconnected from the patient's tracheostomy tube to perform suctioning, to change the ventilator circuit, or to empty condensate that accumulates in the ventilator circuit. Each time the circuit is breached, the patient is placed at risk for infection. Therefore, the Centers for Disease Control and Prevention (CDC) recommends that the breathing circuit with a humidifier

(i.e., ventilator tubing and exhalation valve and the attached humidifier) not be changed routinely on the basis of a fixed interval when it is in use on an individual patient. The breathing circuit is to be changed only when it is visibly soiled or malfunctioning mechanically (Tablan *et al.,* 2004).

The American Association of Respiratory Care's clinical practice guideline on long-term mechanical ventilation in the home recommends that ventilator circuits should not be changed more often than once each week (AARC, 1995). When the breathing circuit is in use, home care staff should periodically drain and discard any condensate that collects in the tubing of a mechanical ventilator, being careful not to allow the condensate to drain back towards the patient. Gloves are to be worn when handling the fluid or draining the breathing circuit. The internal machinery of mechanical ventilators is not considered an important source of bacterial contamination of inhaled gas; therefore routine sterilization or high-level disinfection of the ventilator's internal machinery is not necessary (Tablan *et al.,* 2004). If it is necessary to use resuscitation equipment (an ambu resuscitation bag) on a patient, a new sterile bag is to be obtained and replaced in the home for subsequent emergency use.

Suctioning of Respiratory Tract Secretions

Removal of tracheal secretions by gentle suctioning using aseptic technique has traditionally been used to help prevent pneumonia in patients. Tracheal suction catheters can introduce microorganisms into a patient's lower respiratory tract, however, which could lead to pneumonia. Currently, there are two types of suction catheter systems in use: the open, single-use catheter system and the closed, multiuse catheter system. The CDC's guidelines do not recommend one system over the other for preventing pneumonia nor do they contain recommendations for how often the in-line suction catheter of a closed suction system used on one patient should be changed (Tablan *et al.,* 2004).

Practices regarding the reuse of tracheal suction catheters and the use of clean versus sterile technique may differ between home care settings and other settings. A tracheal suction catheter may be reused as long as the cleaning and disinfection process is effective and does not change the structural integrity or function of the catheter. Obviously, the main patient care concern is infection from the introduction of bacteria into the lungs, which could lead to pneumonia. In day-to-day practice, most home care organizations use a new sterile suction catheter each time the patient is suctioned. Other home care organizations rinse the catheter after suctioning, store it a manner to keep it dry and avoid contamination, and then replace it with a new, sterile catheter every 8 to 24 hours. Yet other home care organizations soak or disinfect the catheters at the end of the day, rinse them, and then reuse them. If the patient is an infant, is immunocompromised, or develops a respiratory infection, the use of a new sterile suction catheter for each suctioning procedure while maintaining sterile technique is recommended. In most other cases, clean technique is acceptable, although the care of each patient must be evaluated individually. It should be the mutual decision of the home care organization and the patient's physician whether clean or sterile technique will be used and the frequency with which a new suction catheter will be replaced.

The CDC's guideline does not contain recommendations for the use of sterile versus clean gloves (Tablan *et al.*, 2004); minimally, clean nonsterile gloves should be worn by home and hospice care staff when suctioning a patient's respiratory secretions. If sterile technique is used to suction the patient and a new sterile suction catheter is used for each episode of suctioning, sterile gloves should be worn. Fresh tap water for each episode of suctioning (Luebbert, 2000), or 3% hydrogen peroxide, or a solution of equal parts normal saline and 3% hydrogen peroxide may be suctioned through the suction catheter to remove secretions if the catheter is going to be used again to suction the patient.

Cleaning and Disinfecting Tracheal Suction Catheters

If it is the home care organization's and the physician's mutual decision to reuse tracheal suction catheters, the catheters must be cleaned and disinfected between uses. One of two methods may be used for cleaning and disinfecting tracheal suction catheters between uses. The first method of disinfection involves soaking the tracheal suction catheter in 3% hydrogen peroxide, and the other involves boiling the catheter. Hydrogen peroxide may lose its disinfecting capabilities if it is exposed to air and light. Therefore, if hydrogen peroxide is poured into a secondary container, it should be changed daily.

When the hydrogen-peroxide-soaking method is used, the tracheal suction catheter should be:

1. cleaned with soap and tap water
2. rinsed with tap water
3. flushed with 3% hydrogen peroxide
4. placed in a container of 3% hydrogen peroxide to soak for a minimum of 20 minutes
5. rinsed and flushed with sterile water before use
6. stored in a clean, closeable jar that has been boiled, or in a new plastic bag

The suction tubing must be completely filled with hydrogen peroxide for complete disinfection of all internal and external surfaces. When the suction tubing is submerged in the hydrogen peroxide, caution should be taken to avoid getting air bubbles trapped in the tubing.

When the boiling method is used, the tracheal suction catheter should be:

1. cleaned with soap and tap water
2. boiled in water for 10 minutes
3. dried on a clean towel or paper towels and allowed to cool before use
4. stored in a clean, closeable jar that has been boiled, or in a new plastic bag

Cleaning and Disinfecting the Inner Tracheal Cannula

One of two methods may be used for disinfecting the inner tracheal cannula. The first method involves soaking the inner tracheal cannula in 3% hydrogen peroxide, and the other involves boiling the inner tracheal cannula. When the hydrogen-peroxide-soaking method is used, the inner cannula should be:

1. cleaned with soap and cold water and friction (if there is a buildup of mucous inside the inner cannula, 3% hydrogen peroxide may be used to remove crusted exudate)
2. soaked in 3% hydrogen peroxide or 70% isopropyl alcohol for 20 minutes
3. rinsed with sterile water or tap water, with care taken to ensure that all hydrogen peroxide or alcohol has been removed
4. allowed to air dry on a clean towel or paper towels
5. stored in a clean, closeable jar that has been boiled, or in a new plastic bag

When the boiling method is used, the inner cannula should be:

1. cleaned with soap and cold water and friction (if there is a buildup of mucous inside the inner cannula, 3% hydrogen peroxide may be used to remove crusted exudate)
2. rinsed with tap water
3. boiled for 10 minutes
4. allowed to air dry on a clean towel or paper towels and allowed to cool before use
5. stored in a clean, closeable jar that has been boiled or in a new plastic bag

The frequency with which the inner cannula is cleaned and tracheostomy stoma site care provided should adhere to the organization's policies and procedures or the physician's orders, but minimally it should be frequent enough to keep the skin clean and dry and to prevent excoriation around the stoma. The outer tracheal cannula should be changed regularly to prevent tissue granulation around the stoma and to avoid infection. The frequency of tracheostomy tube changes (inner and outer cannulas) should be consistent with the physician's orders. When changing a tracheostomy tube, the home care staff member should wear a gown, use aseptic technique, and replace the tube with a new, sterile one each time (Tablan *et al.,* 2004).

Cleaning and Disinfecting Respiratory Equipment and Supplies

Devices used on the respiratory tract for respiratory therapy (e.g., nebulizers used to deliver morphine sulphate to hospice patients) represent potential reservoirs and vehicles for infectious microorganisms. Proper cleaning and disinfection of reusable equipment will reduce infections associated with respiratory therapy equipment. All respiratory equipment and devices must be cleaned before disinfection. Once the equipment is cleaned and disinfected, care must be taken not to contaminate the equipment in the process of rinsing, drying, and packaging. Preferably, sterile water should be used for rinsing reusable semicritical respiratory equipment and devices after they have been chemically disinfected. If this is not feasible, staff members should rinse the device with tap water, rinse with isopropyl alcohol (Tablan *et al.,* 2004), and air dry.

Between treatments on the same patient using small-volume medication in-line and a hand-held nebulizer, home care staff should clean and disinfect the equipment and then rinse it (if rinsing is needed) and dry. Only sterile fluid is to be used for nebulization, and the fluid must be dispensed into the nebulizer aseptically. Whenever possible, aerosolized medications should be used in single-dose vials or containers. If multidose medication vials are used, the manufacturers' instructions are to be followed for handling, storing, and dispensing the medications.

A suction collection canister should be emptied and cleaned with soap and water on a daily basis. The suction cannula, tubing, and glass and plastic containers should be disinfected once a week or more often using a 1:3 vinegar solution or a 1:10 bleach solution (Feenan & Voutroubek, 1997). The manufacturers of some of the newer portable suction machines recommend placing the suction machine components into a dishwasher for cleaning and disinfecting.

Low-flow oxygen systems without humidifiers do not present a clinically important risk for infection and do not need to be routinely replaced. High-flow systems that employ heated humidifiers or aerosol generators, however, especially when applied to patients with artificial airways, should be cleaned and disinfected on a regular basis. Any respiratory equipment tubing (including that for any nasal cannula or masks), regardless of whether humidification is used, should be cleaned or replaced, and the cannula should be changed or replaced when it is visibly contaminated (Tablan *et al.,* 2004). To clean the tubing (not the nasal cannula), a solution of 1 part white vinegar to 3 parts water can be used. This vinegar solution should not be used to clean any tubing or reusable objects that touch mucous membranes. The tubing must be completely filled with the vinegar solution to be properly disinfected. When the tubing is submerged, caution should be taken to avoid trapping air bubbles in it.

The preferred humidification fluid used with the oxygen system should be sterile water rather than distilled nonsterile water (Tablan *et al.,* 2004), which is commonly used in home care and hospice settings.

Other Measures to Prevent Respiratory Infection

Traditional preventive measures for pneumonia include decreasing the risk of aspiration; preventing cross-contamination or colonization via the hands of home care staff members; appropriately disinfecting respiratory therapy devices; and educating staff members, patients, and family members. Regardless of whether gloves are worn, the hands should be decontaminated with an antiseptic agent after contact with mucous membranes, respiratory secretions, or objects contaminated with respiratory secretions; both before and after contact with a patient who has a tracheostomy tube in place; and before and after contact with any other respiratory device used on the patient. Gloves should be worn when respiratory secretions or objects contaminated with respiratory secretions are handled. Gloves should be changed and hands should be washed after contact with a patient; after respiratory secretions or objects contaminated with secretions from one patient are handled and before contact is made with another object or environmental surface; and between contacts with a contaminated body site and the respiratory tract of, or respiratory device on, the same patient. A gown should be worn if soiling with respiratory secretions from the patient is anticipated, and the gown should be changed after contact (Tablan *et al.,* 1994; refer to Chapter 6 for additional information about when personal protective equipment should be worn in the home).

Preventing Aspiration

When a home care patient is receiving enteral feedings or mechanical ventilation, measures should be taken to prevent a respiratory infection caused by aspiration. These measures may include the following:

- elevating the head of the bed to 30° to 45° for patients at high risk for aspiration pneumonia (unless medically contraindicated)
- verifying the appropriate placement of the enteral feeding tube
- assessing the patient's intestinal motility by auscultating for bowel sounds
- measuring residual gastric volume or abdominal girth, with a physician's order, adjusting the rate and volume of the enteral feeding to avoid reflux aspiration
- providing meticulous mouth care
- cleaning and decontaminating the patient's mouth with an antiseptic agent (e.g., Listerine)

Patient Education for the Prevention of a Respiratory Tract Infection

Patient and family education related to infection control and the prevention of a respiratory tract infection should include hand hygiene, use of personal protective equipment, tracheostomy care, suctioning procedures, cleaning and disinfecting procedures for respiratory care equipment and supplies, and signs and symptoms of a respiratory infection.

Patients who have had surgery may be discharged to continue their health care at home. Patients at high risk for postoperative pneumonia include those who:

- had abdominal aortic aneurysm repair, thoracic surgery, or emergency surgery
- received general anesthesia
- are 60 or more years old
- have totally dependent functional status
- have had a weight loss of more than 10%
- are using steroids for chronic conditions
- have a recent history of alcohol use or COPD, or have smoked during the preceding year
- have impaired sensorium, a history of cerebrovascular accident with residual neurologic deficit, or low (less than 8 mg/dL) or high (more than 22 mg/dL) blood urea nitrogen level; also those who received more than 4 units of blood before surgery (Tablan *et al.,* 2004)

Patients at high risk for pneumonia should continue the use of an incentive spirometer postoperatively if ordered by their physician.

All patients receiving home care services postoperatively should receive teaching aimed at preventing postoperative pneumonia. Areas of education for such patients include taking deep breaths, moving about in bed, and ambulating (unless otherwise ordered by their physician).

PREVENTION AND CONTROL OF INFLUENZA

Modifying the Host Risk for Infection Through Vaccination

An influenza vaccine should be offered annually, beginning in September and throughout the influenza season, to home care patients at high risk for influenza-related complications. Refer to Chapter 13 for information related to the use of influenza vaccine for home and hospice care staff members. High-risk patients include the following:

- all children aged 6–23 months;
- adults aged ≥65 years;
- persons aged 2–64 years with underlying chronic medical conditions;
- all women who will be pregnant during the influenza season;

- residents of nursing homes and long-term care facilities;
- children aged 2–18 years on chronic aspirin therapy;
- health care workers involved in direct patient care; and
- out-of-home caregivers and household contacts of children aged <6 months (CDC, 2004c).

In addition, an influenza vaccine should to be offered to the following non-high-risk persons:

- out-of-home caregivers and household contacts of persons in high-risk groups (e.g., persons aged ≥65 years; persons with chronic conditions such as diabetes, heart or lung disease, or weakened immune systems because of illness or medication; and children aged <2 years); and
- all adults aged 50–64 years (CDC, 2005).

ENTERAL THERAPY

Enteral feedings may be a source of infection through contaminated enteral formula. Enteral nutrition may be administered either intermittently or continuously. Intermittent feeding may be administered as a bolus, rapidly infused via a syringe, or given slowly via gravity or an infusion pump. Unopened enteral therapy formula may be stored at room temperature in the home. When formulas are reconstituted or diluted, the label instructions for preparation, storage, and stability should be closely followed. Most reconstituted or diluted formulas should be covered, refrigerated, and used within 24 hours from the time the container was opened. Expiration dates should always be checked before the container is opened and the formula is administered to the patient. Refrigerated formula should sit at room temperature for 30 minutes before administration because room-temperature feedings avoid abdominal cramping and discomfort. The enteral feeding bag and its tubing should be rinsed with tap water until clean in between intermittent feedings. Newly prepared enteral feeding formula should not be added to the bag of existing enteral formula that has been hanging. "Topping off" the bag with new feeding formula is discouraged because the new formula may become contaminated with bacteria from old formula that has been left hanging for too long. During the feeding, the bag and tubing should be checked intermittently for foreign matter, mold, and leakage.

Cleaning Enteral Feeding Equipment and Supplies

Proper handling and cleaning of enteral formula, equipment, and supplies using clean technique are important for reducing the risk of formula contamination. Equipment used to prepare enteral feeding should be washed in a dishwasher or cleaned with hot water and soap. If a blender is used to prepare the enteral feeding solution, all washable components should be washed in a dishwasher or cleaned with hot water and soap. Blender parts that contain electrical components and cannot be placed in the dishwasher or submerged in water should be hand washed with hot water and soap. Enteral feeding bags and tubing should not be used for more than 24 hours. After that they should be either discarded or washed thoroughly with soap and water, drained, and allowed to air dry.

Patient Education Related to Enteral Therapy

Patient and family education related to infection control and enteral therapy should include hand hygiene, clean technique, setup and administration, formula hang time, infusion method, proper storage, cleaning and disinfecting enteral therapy equipment and supplies, signs and symptoms of a local infection at the gastrostomy tube site indications of contaminated formula (e.g., diarrhea or vomiting), mouth care, assessment of residual feedings, assessment of feeding tube placement, gastrostomy tube site care (if applicable), and prevention of aspiration pneumonia.

POST-MORTEM CARE

Precautions for Handling the Deceased Body

In home care and hospice, it is not uncommon for the patient to request that the place of death be in the home setting. In providing routine post-mortem care and handling the body post mortem, the home care and hospice staff should maintain Standard Precautions and protect themselves from blood or body fluids as they would if the patient were still alive. If the patient was on airborne or droplet precautions prior to death, wearing a mask post mortem is not necessary unless the staff anticipate that aerosols may be generated during the handling of the body.

If there is concern that the patient's death was caused by an agent of bioterrorism, the following precautions should be taken in addition to standard ones:

- Droplet precautions for pneumonic plague
- Airborne precautions for smallpox
- Contact Precautions for smallpox and viral hemorraghic fever

The room in the home where the patient resided should be cleaned and disinfected, especially high-touch items, and the linens used by the patient washed in hot soap and water. If a patient had a viral hemorrhagic fever, the surfaces in the patient's vicinity should be cleaned and disinfected with a 1:10 bleach solution (Johnson, 2003).

The funeral home personnel or other individuals accepting possession of the body (e.g., medical examiner's office) should be informed if additional precautions, other than Standard Precautions, need to be taken during the handling and release of the body from the home and during transport.

REFERENCES

Agency for Healthcare Research and Quality (AHRQ). Evidence Report/Technology Assessment No. 43, Making health care safer: A critical analysis of patient safety practices, AHRQ Publication No. 01-E058. July 2001. Subchapter 15.2., Prevention of nosocomial urinary tract infections. Use of suprapubic catheters. Accessed March 30, 2004, *http://www.ahrq.gov/clinic/ptsafety/chap15b.htm.*

American Association of Respiratory Care. (1995). AARC clinical practice guideline: Long-term invasive mechanical ventilation in the home. *Respiratory Care, 40,* 1313–1320.

Association for Professionals in Infection Control and Epidemiology, Inc. (APIC) and the Wound Ostomy Continence Nurses Society (WOCN). (2001). *Clean vs sterile: Management of chronic wounds. Position Statement.* Retrieved March 30, 2004, from *http://www.apic.org/resc/pp-cleansterile.cfm.*

Bennett, C., Young, M., Razi, S., Adkins, R., Diaz, F. & McCrary, A. (August 1997). The effect of urethral introducer tip catheters on the incidence of urinary tract infections: Outcomes in spinal cord injured patients. *The Journal of Urology, 158,* 519–527.

Bergstrom, N., Bennett, M. A., Carlson, C. et al., (1994). *Treatment of pressure ulcers: Clinical practice guideline number 15:59–60.* AHCPR Publication 95-0652. Rockville, MD: Agency for Health Care Policy and Research, Public Health Service, U.S. Department of Health and Human Services.

Bryant, K. A., Pearce, J., & Stover, B. (2002). Flash fire associated with the use of alcohol-based antiseptic agent [Letter to the editor]. *American Journal of Infection Control, 30,* 256–57.

Centers for Disease Control and Prevention. (2002a). Guideline for hand hygiene in health-care settings: Recommendations of the Healthcare Infection Control Practices Advisory Committee and the HICPAC/SHEA/APIC/IDSA hand hygiene task force. *Morbidity and Mortality Weekly Report, 51* (RR16), 1–45.

Centers for Disease Control and Prevention. (2002b). Hantavirus Pulmonary Syndrome—United States: Updated recommendations for risk reduction. *Morbidity and Mortality Weekly Report, 51* (RR09), 1–12.

Centers for Disease Control and Prevention. Guidelines for the prevention of intravascular central line-associated infection. (2002c). Recommendations of the Hospital Infection Control Practices Advisory Committee (HICPAC). Morbidity and Mortality Weekly Report. August 9, 2002. Vol. 51. No. RR-10.

Centers for Disease Control and Prevention (2004). Prevention and Control of Influenza. Recommendations of the Advisory Committee on Immunization Practices (ACIP). Morbidity and Mortality Weekly Report. May 28, 2004/53 (RR06); 1–40.

Centers for Disease Control and Prevention (2005). Updated Interim Influenza Vaccination Recommendations—2004–2005 Influenza Season. Retrieved from *http://www.cdc.gov/flu/protect/whoshouldget.htm* on March 25, 2005.

DeCastro, M. G. & Iwamoto, P., (2005). *Aseptic technique. APIC text of infection control and epidemiology: Principles and practice* (20–1 to 20–3). Washington, DC: Association for Professionals in Infection Control and Epidemiology, Inc.

Feenan, L., & Voutroubek, W. L. (1997). Alterations in respiratory functions. In W. Voutroubek & J. Townsend (Eds.), *Pediatric home care* (pp. 59–94). Gaithersburg, MD: Aspen Publishers, Inc.

Friedman, M. M. (2005). *Infection Control Policies and Procedures.* Marietta, GA: Home Health Systems, Inc.

Friedman, M. (November 2003). Infection control update for home care and hospice organizations. *Home Healthcare Nurse,* 753–760.

Health Care Financing Administration. (April 1996). *Medicare home health agency manual,* rev. ed. Washington, DC: Government Printing Office. Transmittal no. 277.

Jarvis, W., Gaynes, R., Horan, T., Alonso-Echanove, J., Emori, T., Fridkin, S., Lawton, R., Richards, M., Wright, G., Culver, D., Abshire, J., Henderson, T., Peavy, G., Toslon, J., & Wages, J. (1998). National Nosocomial Infections Surveillance (NNIS) system report: Data summary from October 1986–April 1988, issued June 1988. *American Journal of Infection Control, 26,* 522–533.

Johnson, S., (2003). Bioterrorism Infection Control: Guidelines for Patient Management. Walter Reed Army Medical Center. Retrieved from *http://www.semp.us/biots/biot49.html* on February 5, 2005.

Kunin, C. M. (1987). *Detection, prevention and management of urinary tract infections,* 4th ed. Philadelphia: Lea & Febiger.

Kunin, C., & McCormick, R. (1966). Prevention of catheter-associated urinary tract infections by sterile closed drainage. *New England Journal of Medicine, 274,* 1154–1161.

Larson, E. (March–April 2001). Hygiene of the Skin: When is Clean Too Clean? *Emerging Infectious Diseases, 7*(2), 225–229.

Larson, E. (1996). Hand washing and skin preparation for invasive procedures. In R. Olmsted (Ed.), *APIC infection control and applied epidemiology: Principles and practice* (pp. 19-1–19-7). Washington, DC: Association for Professionals in Infection Control and Epidemiology, Inc.

Larson, E. L., Eke, P. I., Wilder M. P., & Laughon, B. E. (1987). Quantity of soap as a variable in handwashing. *Infection Control, 8,* 371–375.

Lazarus, G., Cooper, D., Knighton, D., Margolis, D., Pecoraro, R., Rodeheaver, G., & Robson, M. (1994). Definitions and guidelines for assessment of wounds and evaluation of healing. *Archives of Dermatology, 130*(4), 489–493.

Luebbert, P. (2000). Home Care. In R. Olmsted (Ed.), *APIC text of infection control and epidemiology: Principles and practice* (pp. 44–47). Washington, DC: Association for Professionals in Infection Control and Epidemiology, Inc.

Maki, D., & Tambyah, P. (March–April 2001). Engineering out the risk of infection with urinary catheters. *Emerging Infectious Diseases, 7*(2), 1–6.

Maki, D. G., Knasinski, V., & Tambyah, P. A. (2000). Risk factors for catheter-associated urinary tract infection: a prospective study showing the minimal effects of catheter care violations on the risk of CAUTI. *Infection Control and Hospital Epidemiology.* 4th Decennial International Conference on Nosocomial and Health-Care–Associated Infections, Atlanta, Georgia, March 2000.

Mangram, A., Horan, T., Pearson, et al. (1999). Guideline for the prevention of surgical site infection, 1999. *American Journal of Infection Control, 27*(2), 97–134.

National Fire Protection Association [NFPA]. (2003). FAQs on NFPA 30 flammable and combustible liquids code. Retrieved May 30, 2003, from *http://www.nfpa.org/Codes/interpretations/faq30/faq30.asp.*

Nicolle, L., SHEA Long-Term Care Committee. (2001). Urinary tract infections in long-term care facilities. *Infection Control and Hospital Epidemiology, 22*(3), 167–175.

Sickbert-Bennett, E., Weber, D., Gergen-Teague, M., & Rutala, W. (2004). The effects of test variables on the efficacy of hand hygiene products. *American Journal of Infection Control, 32*(2) 69–83.

Spaulding, E. H. (1968). Chemical disinfection of medical and surgical materials. In C.A. Lawrence & S.S. Block (Eds.), *Disinfection, sterilization, and preservation* (pp. 517–531). Philadelphia: Lea & Febiger.

Stotts, N., Barbour, S., Griggs, K., Bouvier, B., Buhlman, L., Wipke-Tevis, D., & Williams, D. (1997). Sterile versus clean technique in postoperative wound care of patients with open surgical wounds: A pilot study. *Journal of Wound, Ostomy, and Continence Nursing, 24*(1), 10–18.

Tablan, O. C., Anderson, L. J., Besser, R., Bridges, C., & Hajjeh, R. (2004). Guidelines for Preventing Health Care–Associated Pneumonia, 2003. *Morbidity and Mortality Weekly Report, 53*(RR03), 1–36.

Tablan, O. C., Anderson, L. J., Arden, N. H., Breiman, R. F., Butler, J. C., & McNeil, M. M. (1994). Guideline for prevention of nosocomial pneumonia. *American Journal of Infection Control, 22,* 247–292.

Trautner, B., Darouiche, R. (2004). Role of biofilm in central line-associated urinary tract infections. *American Journal of Infection Control, 32,* 177–183.

Wong, E. S. (1983). Guideline for prevention of central line-associated urinary tract infections. *American Journal of Infection Control, 11,* 28–31.

CHAPTER 4

Infection Control in Home Infusion Therapy

OVERVIEW

The economic pressures to reduce health care costs have contributed to the growth of the home infusion therapy industry. This treatment modality probably puts home care patients at greatest risk for home care–acquired infection, however. If a home care or hospice organization provides infusion therapy, risk reduction efforts must be undertaken to ensure that the therapy is provided in a safe manner that is also cost effective. It is also imperative that surveillance for local and systemic IV-related infections be conducted. Systemic infections include bloodstream infection (BSI), septic thrombophlebitis, and endocarditis. If an intravenous catheter becomes colonized by pathogenic organisms, these organisms can be spread through the bloodstream and cause infections at distant sites (e.g., endocarditis). Local infections related to venous access devices include exit-site infections (related to percutaneously placed catheters), pocket infections (related to implanted access devices), and tunnel infections (related to surgically placed central venous catheters). Local site infections may also lead to BSIs.

Catheter-related infections in hospitalized patients, especially catheter-related bloodstream infections, are of great concern. They have been associated with increased morbidity, mortality rates of 10% to 20%, prolonged hospital stays, and increased medical costs (Pittet, Tarara, & Wenzel, 1994). If entire hospitals, rather than only ICUs, were assessed for central venous catheter (CVC)-associated BSIs, an estimated total of 250,000 cases would be recorded annually, with an attributable mortality of an estimated 12% to 25% per infection, and the marginal cost to the health care system of $25,000 per infection (Kluger & Maki, 1999).

The incidence of catheter-related bloodstream infections for patients cared for in the home is not well studied or reported. One study representing 50,470 home infusion patients and 2.83 million catheter days was conducted. This study reviewed and assessed the rate and type of complications in home infusion therapy patients that used venous access devices. The rates of catheter complications (per 1000 catheter days) for the most common events were as follows: catheter dysfunction (0.83), total; thrombotics (0.23) and nonthrombotics (0.6); catheter-site infections (0.26); and BSIs (0.19). The total rates of complications were by types of catheter and are as follows: midline catheter (4.5), peripherally inserted central catheter (PICC) (2.0), nontunneled central catheter (1.1), tunneled catheter (1.0), and chest ports (0.52). Catheter dysfunction from thrombotic occlusion resulting in loss of patency was the most common complication, most commonly occurring within the first seven days of catheter insertion. It is noteworthy that catheter dysfunction occurred almost twice as much as catheter infection. Catheter dysfunction primarily resulted in a disruption of the infusion therapy (43%), catheter replacement (29%), premature CVC removal (14%), unscheduled emergency room visits (9%), and unplanned hospitalizations (6%) (Moreau et al., 2002).

Another study of home infusion therapy analyzed 110,869 catheter days of central venous catheter complications for 447 patients on home parenteral nutrition. Infectious complications occurred in approximately one fourth of the 447 patients, necessitating catheter removal in about one half of those patients (Bozzetti et al., 2002).

In another study, the incidence of infection in HIV/AIDS patients that had nontunneled, nonimplanted central venous catheters was analyzed. The authors found a low infection rate with the use of these catheters in this population. The total infection rate was 2.8 per 1000 catheter days, with a BSI rate of 1.4 per 1000 catheter days. Neither the patient's HIV status nor the number of catheter ports, indication for the catheter, anatomic site of catheter insertion, medication administered via the catheter, or presence of neutropenia was found to be a contributing factor in catheter complications. The rate of infection in patients with nontunneled, nonimplanted catheters was similar to that for patients with tunneled and totally implanted central venous catheters. The results of this study indicate that nontunneled, nonimplanted central venous catheters may be a safe, cost-effective alternative to other central venous access devices in these patients (Skiest, Grant, & Keiser, 1998).

The organisms that cause health care–associated BSI have changed over time. In the 1980s there was a predominance of Gram negative bacilli, such as *Enterobacter* and *Pseudomonas* species. Fungal BSIs were seen in severely ill patients with many risk factors, including immunosuppression. In the 1990s, however, there was a shift in the etiology of health care–associated BSIs from Gram-negative to Gram-positive organisms. From 1986 through 1989, coagulase-negative staphylococci, followed by *Staphylococcus aureus*, were the most frequently reported causes of BSIs, accounting for 27% and 16% of BSIs, respectively. Pooled data from 1992 through 1999, however, identified that coagulase-negative staphylococci, followed by enterococci, are now the most frequently isolated causes of health care–associated BSIs in hospitals. Coagulase-negative staphylococci account for 37% and *S. aureus* for 12.6% of reported health care–associated BSIs. Also notable was the susceptibility pattern of *S. aureus* isolates. In 1999, for the first time since National Nosocomial Infections Surveillance (NNIS) has been reporting susceptibilities, more than 50% of all *S. aureus* isolates from ICUs were resistant to oxacillin. In 1999, enterococci accounted for 13.5% of BSIs, an increase from 8% reported to NNIS during the period from 1986 to 1989. The percentage of enterococcal ICU isolates resistant to Vancomycin has also increased, escalating from 0.5% in 1989 to 25.9% in 1999 (CDC, 2002). A study conducted on BSIs associated with needless devices in the home care setting found that 49% of the organisms were hydrophilic Gram-negative bacteria (i.e., *Pseudomonas*, *Stenotrophomonas*, *Acinetobacter*,

and *Serratia* species), 17% were of the *Staphylococcus* species, 12% gram-negative bacteria, 8% fungi, 3% other Gram-positive bacteria, and 11% other mixed organisms (Do *et al.*, 1999). Although there are limited data on the epidemiology of IV-related infections in home care, the risk related to these skin organisms must be noted. Policies and procedures must be designed and implemented to control this known risk.

CAUSES OF IV CATHETER–RELATED INFECTIONS

The causes and sources of IV catheter-related infections are both intrinsic and extrinsic. An IV catheter may be seeded and colonized if bacteria or fungi travel through the bloodstream from another site of infection or colonization within the patient. This can lead to a catheter-related bloodstream infections. Host factors such as immunosuppressive diseases (e.g., cancer) or treatments (e.g., chemotherapy) can also increase the intrinsic risk for infection.

Based on scientific evidence, however, experts agree that most catheter-related infections result from the migration of microorganisms on the skin (e.g., *S. epidermidis*) around the catheter insertion site into the catheter's insertion tract. This migration can eventually lead to colonization of the catheter tip as well (Snydman *et al.*, 1982). The catheter hub may also be an important source of contamination leading to the colonization of catheters, particularly long-term central venous catheters (Linares *et al.*, 1993). Another source of extrinsic infection is catheter contamination at the time of insertion. This risk seems to be greatest in catheters placed during an emergency. Based on this data, the CDC recommends that catheters be replaced as soon as possible and no longer than 48 hours after emergency insertion (CDC, 2002). Contaminated IV fluid is also a risk for catheter-associated bloodstream infection, but this rarely actually occurs (Maki, 1982). Figure 4-1 shows potential sources of contamination for IV access devices.

TYPES OF IV CATHETERS AND DEVICES
Peripheral Venous Catheters

Peripheral venous catheters are the devices most commonly used for vascular access. A peripheral venous (short-line) catheter is 3 inches or less in length and in adults is inserted into a vein of the forearm or hand. Al-

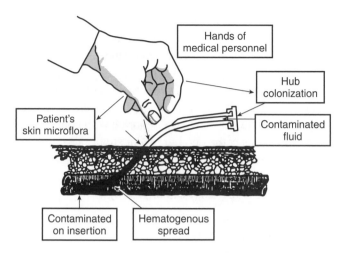

Figure 4-1 Potential Sources of Contamination of IV Access Devices. *Source:* Reprinted with permission from M. L. Pearson, Guideline for the prevention of intravascular device-related infections, *American Journal of Infection Control,* pp. 262–293, © 1996, Mosby-Year Book, Inc.

Exhibit 4-1 Factors Associated with Infusion-Related Phlebitis Among Patients with Peripheral Venous Catheters

Catheter material
Catheter size
Size of catheter insertion
Experience of person inserting catheter
Duration of catheterization
Composition of infusate
Frequency of dressing change
Catheter-related infections
Skin preparation
Host factors
Emergency department insertion

Source: Reprinted with permission from M. L. Pearson, Guideline for the prevention of intravascular device-related infections, *American Journal of Infection Control,* pp. 262–293, © 1996, Mosby-Year Book, Inc.

though the incidence of local infections or BSIs associated with peripheral venous catheters is usually low, serious infectious complications produce considerable annual morbidity because of the frequency with which peripheral venous catheters are used. The majority of serious catheter-related infections are associated with central venous catheters (CDC, 2002). The low incidence of local infections or BSIs may be due to the short period of time that a peripheral venous catheter is in place. Phlebitis is the most important complication associated with the use of peripheral venous catheters. Phlebitis is an inflammation of the vein caused by a chemical or mechanical process rather than an infectious process. Exhibit 4-1 lists the risk factors associated with infusion-related phlebitis for patients with a peripheral venous catheter.

Midline Catheter

A midline catheter is also a peripheral catheter, but it is 3 to 8 inches in length and is inserted via the antecubital fossa into the proximal basilic or cephalic vein or the distal subclavian vein. The catheter tip does not enter a central vein, however. The tip of the midline catheter resides below the axilla, and the actual insertion site should not be more than 1 to 2 inches above or below the antecubital fossa. A midline catheter should be considered when the duration of therapy will likely exceed

6 days (Ryder, 1995). Midline catheters have been associated with lower rates of phlebitis than short-line peripheral venous catheters and with lower rates of infection than central venous catheters (CDC, 2002). In one prospective study of 140 midline catheters, the catheters were in place a median of 7 days and up to 49 days. The BSI rate in this study was 0.8 per 1000 catheter days, with no specific risk factors identified, including the catheter dwell time (Mermel, Parenteau, & Tow, 1995). The study's findings suggest that midline catheters can be changed only when there is a specific indication. However, no prospective, randomized studies have assessed the benefit of routine replacement of midline catheters as a strategy to prevent a catheter-related bloodstream infection (CDC, 2002).

Central Venous Catheters

Nontunneled Central Venous Catheters

Percutaneously inserted, nontunneled, central venous catheters are used in the home setting, but they are not found as often in home care as tunneled central venous catheters or implanted ports are. Central venous catheters account for an estimated 90% of all health care-associated catheter-related bloodstream infections (Maki, 1992). Among the factors that influence the risk of infection associated with the use of central venous catheters are the number of catheter lumens, whether there is repeated catheterization, the presence of an infectious focus elsewhere in the body, exposure of the catheter to bacteremia, absence of systemic antimicrobial therapy, duration of catheterization, type of dressing, and the experience of the health care personnel inserting the device (Pearson, 1996).

Peripherally Inserted Central Catheters

A peripherally inserted central catheter (PICC) may be placed in the home setting by a competent registered nurse. A PICC is inserted in the antecubital space via the cephalic or basilic vein with the catheter tip ending in the superior vena cava. This area is usually less colonized, less oily, and less moist than is the skin on the chest and neck. A PICC should be considered for insertion when the duration of IV therapy will likely exceed 6 days (Ryder, 1995; CDC, 2002). The advantages of inserting a PICC over other catheters are that PICCs:

- cost less than other central venous catheters
- are easier to maintain than short-line peripheral venous catheters (e.g., less frequent site rotation, infiltration, and phlebitis)
- have been associated with fewer mechanical complications (e.g., thrombosis, hemothorax)
- have a lower rate of infection than that associated with other nontunneled central venous catheters

The lower rates of infection observed with PICCs may be partially accounted for by the use of the antecubital fossa as the insertion site area. The optimal length of time for a PICC line to remain in place is not known, but data have shown that PICCs have been used successfully for extended periods, in some cases longer than 300 days (Merrill et al., 1994; Raad et al., 1993).

Tunneled Central Venous Catheters

The most commonly used tunneled central venous catheters include the Hickman, Broviac, closed-tip catheter (e.g., Groshong), and Quinton catheters. These catheters are surgically implanted and are used to provide venous access to patients who require prolonged infusion therapy (e.g., chemotherapy, TPN, and hemodialysis). In contrast to nontunneled central venous catheters, tunneled catheters have a Dacron cuff just inside the exit site, which prevents the spread of microorganisms into the tunneled catheter tract by stimulating growth of the surrounding tissue, sealing the catheter tract, and providing a natural anchor for the catheter. Tunneling of central venous catheters also serves to prevent dislodgment of the catheter, reduce the incidence of catheter-related bloodstream infection (by increasing the distance between the sites where the catheter exits the skin and where it enters the subclavian vein), and protect the catheter from potentially contaminated sites, such as tracheostomies (Pearson, 1996). According to the CDC, the rates of infection with tunneled catheters have been significantly lower than those reported with nontunneled central venous catheters, but recent studies (Andrivet et al., 1994; Raad et al., 1993) have found no significant difference in the rates of infection among tunneled and nontunneled catheters (Pearson, 1996).

Hemodialysis Catheters

Approximately 150,000 patients a year undergo maintenance hemodialysis for chronic renal failure. Central venous catheters have gained popularity as a convenient, rapid way of establishing temporary vascular hemodialysis access (until placement or maturation of a permanent arteriovenous fistula) or permanent access in the case of patients without alternative vascular access. Catheter-related bloodstream infections in hemodialysis patients, as in other patient populations, are caused most frequently by S. epidermidis. Because of their high rates of colonization with S. aureus, however, hemodialysis patients have a greater proportion of catheter-related bloodstream infection due to S. aureus than other patient populations do. In some studies, as many as 50% to 62% of hemodialysis patients have been found to be carriers of S. aureus (Yu et al., 1986). Therefore, skin antisepsis is a crucial component of home care for the prevention of hemodialysis-catheter-associated infections.

The use of catheters for hemodialysis is the most common factor contributing to bacteremia. In fact, the risk for bacteremia in patients with dialysis catheters is sevenfold that for patients with primary arteriovenous fistulas. Despite efforts to reduce the prevalence of use of hemodialysis catheters, this use increased from 12.7% in 1995 to 22.2% in 1999. In unpublished 1999 data, the CDC identified bacteremia rates per 100 patient months as 0.2 for arteriovenous fistulas, 0.5 for grafts, 5.0 for cuffed catheters, and 8.5 for noncuffed catheters. To reduce the rate of infection, hemodialysis catheters are to be avoided; arteriovenous (AV) fistulas and grafts are the preferred methods of performing hemodialysis. If temporary access is needed for dialysis, a cuffed catheter is preferable to a noncuffed catheter if the catheter is expected to stay in place for longer than 3 weeks. Hemodialysis catheters should be used only for hemodialysis; home care staff should not use the access device for any other purposes (e.g., drawing blood or administering fluids, blood or blood products, or parenteral nutrition) or for nondialysis reasons, except under emergency circumstances (CDC, 2002).

According to the CDC, the causes of the increased rate of infection experienced with central venous catheters used for hemodialysis are not known, but it is thought that manipulations and dressing changes of dialysis catheters by inadequately trained personnel, the duration of catheterization, the mean number of hemodialysis sessions, and cutdown insertion of the catheter may increase the risk of catheter-related infection among hemodialysis patients. Other potential causes of hemodialysis catheter contamination include penetration of organisms from the skin as a result of the pulsating action of the dialysis pump, manipulation of catheter connections by medical personnel with contaminated hands, leakage of contaminated hemodialysis fluid into the blood compartment, and administration of contaminated blood or other solutions through the catheter during the dialysis session. Because of these possible causes of infection, manipulation of the hemodialysis catheter, including dressing changes, should be restricted to staff members trained in hemodialysis catheter care and maintenance (Vanderweghem *et al.*, 1986; CDC, 2002).

Implanted Ports

An implanted venous access device, or port, is tunneled beneath the skin but has a subcutaneous reservoir with a self-sealing septum that is accessed by a noncoring needle punctured through intact skin. An implanted port can be placed centrally or peripherally and can be accessed via the anterior chest wall or on the patient's forearm just below the antecubital fossa. Implanted ports are low maintenance and generally not visible. According to the CDC, implanted ports have the lowest reported rates of catheter-related bloodstream infections among tunneled and nontunneled venous access devices used for long-term vascular access (Pearson, 1996). The rate of infection may be lower because the catheter is placed below the skin level where there is no opening through which microorganisms can be introduced.

PREVENTING CATHETER-RELATED INFECTIONS

Strict adherence to hand hygiene and aseptic technique is the most important activity that can be undertaken by home care staff members to prevent a catheter-related infection. Other measures taken by staff members that may reduce the risk of catheter-related infection include the following:

- selecting an appropriate catheter insertion site
- selecting an appropriate type of catheter
- using barrier precautions during catheter insertion
- replacing peripheral IV access devices at appropriate intervals (given that there are no specific guidelines for routine replacement of central or midline catheters)
- replacing administration sets at appropriate intervals
- replacing IV fluids at appropriate intervals
- maintaining appropriate catheter site care
- avoiding the use of in-line filters for infection control purposes only
- ensuring that only experienced staff members insert and maintain catheters
- using an appropriate flush solution

SELECTING AN APPROPRIATE CATHETER INSERTION SITE

Several factors should be assessed by the home care staff member when determining the site of any peripheral intravenous catheter placement, including the patient's age, condition, and diagnosis; vein size and location; and the type and duration of infusion therapy.

Peripheral Venous Access Site Selection

The vein selected for infusion therapy must be of sufficient size to accommodate the gauge and length of the intravenous catheter to be inserted. Home infusion therapies that should *not* be administered via a peripheral venous catheter include continuous vesicant chemotherapy, parenteral nutrition formulas exceeding 10% dextrose and/or 5% protein, solutions and/or other medications that have a pH less than 5 or greater than 9, and solutions and/or medications that have a serum osmolarity greater than 500 mOsm/L (Infusion Nurses Society, 2000). To promote the longest possible dwell time, the smallest gauge cannula with the shortest length should be selected, to allow adequate blood flow around the catheter and promote proper hemodilution of the infusate. Solutions with a higher osmolarity should be used with a larger peripheral vein.

The site at which a catheter is placed has been shown to influence the subsequent risk of catheter-related infection. In neonate and infant patients, peripheral catheters should be inserted into a scalp, hand, or dorsum of the foot site rather than into a leg or arm or the antecubital fossa. In adults, a peripheral catheter inserted into a lower extremity poses a greater risk of phlebitis than a peripheral catheter inserted into an upper extremity does, and upper extremity sites differ in their risk for phlebitis (Pearson, 1996). In adults, hand-vein insertions have a lower risk of phlebitis than do upper-arm or wrist-vein insertions. Therefore, peripheral intravenous catheters should be inserted in the distal areas of the upper extremities, and subsequent catheter insertions should be made proximal to the previous catheter insertion site. If a medication has infiltrated or extravasated from the vein and the IV catheter cannot be inserted proximal to the previous insertion site, the patient's opposite upper extremity should be used for insertion of a new peripheral IV catheter. Veins at areas of flexion, sclerotic veins, or injured veins should be avoided, unless areas of flexion can be immobilized to reduce the risk of mechanical phlebitis. Veins in the antecubital fossa should not be used for inserting short-line peripheral venous catheters; they should be reserved for the insertion of a midline catheter, a PICC, or a stainless steel needle for the purpose of obtaining a laboratory specimen. Patients who have undergone a mastectomy, an axillary node dissection, or a stroke should not have peripheral venous catheters inserted into the affected arm.

Midline Venous Access and PICC Site Selection

Appropriate veins for the insertion of midline catheters include the basilic and cephalic veins at the antecubital fossa. The site selected for the insertion of midline catheters should be no more than 1 to 2 inches above or below the antecubital fossa. Midline catheters should not be used for routine blood drawing unless there is no other accessible access site. Blood pressure cuffs and tourniquets should not be applied to the arm in which a midline catheter or PICC has been placed. If a medication has infiltrated or extravasated from the vein, the patient's opposite extremity should be used for inser-

tion of a new midline catheter. Patients who have undergone a mastectomy, an axillary node dissection, or a stroke should not have a midline catheter or PICC inserted into the affected arm. Home infusion therapies that should *not* be administered via a midline catheter include continuous vesicant chemotherapy, parenteral nutrition formulas exceeding 10% dextrose and/or 5% protein, solutions and/or other medications that have a pH less than 5 or greater than 9, and solutions and/or medications that have a serum osmolarity greater than 500 mOsm/L (Infusion Nurses Society, 2000).

SELECTING AN APPROPRIATE TYPE OF CATHETER

Catheters that may be inserted by a home or hospice care nurse include short-line peripheral intravenous catheters, midline intravenous catheters, and PICCs. State practice acts govern the role of the licensed practical nurse (LPN) and licensed vocational nurse (LVN) in intravenous therapy and dictate whether an LPN/LVN can insert a short-line peripheral intravenous catheter. Midline catheters and PICCs should be inserted only by registered nurses (RNs). Catheter selection should be on an individual patient basis with consideration of the insertion site with the lowest relative risk of complications (infectious and noninfectious), the insertion technique, and the anticipated type and duration of home infusion therapy.

The peripheral venous catheter selected should be of the smallest possible gauge to maintain adequate perfusion and of the shortest possible length to administer the prescribed infusion therapy. Stainless steel needles should be used with caution because of the high incidence of infiltration into the subcutaneous tissues that can occur during an infusion—a potentially serious complication if the infused fluid is a vesicant. Stainless steel needles should be used primarily for administering a single dose of a nonvesicant medication or fluid or for obtaining a blood specimen. Stainless steel needles used in lieu of a synthetic catheter for peripheral venous access have the same rate of infectious complications as Teflon® catheters (CDC, 2002).

Catheters made of Teflon®, silicone elastomer, or polyurethane appear to be associated with fewer infectious complications than are catheters made of polyvinyl chloride or polyethylene. Catheter materials can also have surface irregularities that increase the adherence by the microorganisms of certain species (e.g., coagulase-negative staphylococci, *Acinetobacter cal-coaceticus*, and *Pseudomonas aeruginosa*) to the catheter; catheters made of these materials are especially vulnerable to microbial colonization and subsequent infection. Additionally, certain catheter materials are more thrombogenic than others. Thrombus formation inside a catheter lumen may predispose the catheter to colonization and an associated catheter-related infection. This association has led to emphasis on preventing catheter-related thrombus as an additional mechanism for reducing the incidence of catheter-related bloodstream infection.

The type of catheter selected for the insertion of a midline catheter or PICC should be based on the staff member's knowledge of and compliance with the techniques required for insertion, potential complications, the prescribed therapy, and the manufacturer's guidelines. The length of the catheter should be appropriate to the size of the patient, so that the integrity of the catheter tip does not need to be altered.

CATHETER INSERTION

Good hand hygiene before and attention to aseptic technique during the insertion of any intravenous catheter provide protection against infection. Hands should be disinfected with an antiseptic agent before and after palpating catheter insertion sites and before and after inserting, replacing, accessing, repairing, or dressing an intravascular catheter. The insertion site should not be palpated after the antiseptic is applied, unless aseptic technique is maintained.

The insertion of a PICC carries a greater risk of infection. According to the CDC, the risk of infection depends on the magnitude of barrier protection used during catheter insertion and not on the sterility of the surrounding environment. Therefore, when PICCs are inserted in the home setting, maximal barrier precautions should be used to reduce the chance of catheter contamination and a subsequent catheter-related bloodstream infection. Such maximal sterile barrier precautions include the use of a cap, mask, sterile gown, sterile gloves, and a large sterile sheet (CDC, 2002). As required by the Occupational Safety and Health Administration (OSHA) Bloodborne Pathogen Standard, either clean or sterile gloves may be worn when inserting an intravascular catheter, except when inserting a PICC, for which sterile gloves are worn.

REPLACING IV ACCESS DEVICES

In adults, the CDC recommends that peripheral venous catheters be replaced at least every 72 to 96 hours to reduce the risk for phlebitis (CDC, 2002), whereas the Infusion Nurses Society's Standards of Practice recommend that a peripheral venous catheter (i.e., short-line, not midline) be removed every 72 hours (Infusion Nurses Society, 2000). For pediatric patients, the CDC recommends that peripheral venous catheters remain in until the IV therapy has been completed, unless complications (e.g., phlebitis or infiltration) occur. This extended dwell time for children is permitted because the risk for phlebitis in that age group has not been shown to increase with the duration of catheterization, as is seen with adults. If the patient has limited venous access sites and there is no evidence of phlebitis or infection, peripheral venous catheters may be left in place for longer periods, although the patient and the insertion site should be closely monitored.

The risk and benefits of replacing an IV access device within the recommended time frames to reduce infectious complications should be weighed against the risk of mechanical complications and the availability of alternate sites (CDC, 2002). Peripheral venous catheters in both adult and pediatric patients should be removed if the patient develops signs of phlebitis (i.e., warmth, tenderness, erythema, and palpable venous cord) at the insertion site or if the catheter malfunctions (Maki & Ringer, 1991; Infusion Nurses Society, 2000). When a catheter is replaced, only one catheter should be used for each cannulation attempt. Once the catheter has been inserted, all junctions between the administration set and add-on devices should be secured, to prevent the separation of the system and the risk of infection.

The optimal dwell time for a midline catheter or PICC is not known, nor is the optimal frequency of replacing the needles used to access implanted ports. The Infusion Nurses Society's Standards recommend changing the noncoring needle at least every 7 days (Infusion Nurses Society, 2000). To reduce the risk of infection, midline catheters should not be routinely replaced (Mermel, Parenteau, & Tow, 1995). However, if purulence is observed at the insertion site (of any catheter), the catheter should be removed. The Infusion Nurses Society's Standards of Practice recommend a maximum dwell time of 2 to 4 weeks for midline catheters. Dwell times of longer than 4 weeks for midline catheters should be based on the length of remaining therapy, the patient's peripheral venous access status, the patient's condition, the condition of the vein in which the catheter is placed, and the skin's integrity (Infusion Nurses Society, 2000).

REMOVING IV ACCESS DEVICES

When a midline catheter, PICC, or nontunneled central venous catheter is removed, digital pressure should be applied to the insertion site with a dry, sterile dressing; an antiseptic ointment may be applied to the catheter site to occlude the skin tract and prevent an air embolism; and a sterile occlusive dressing may be applied. If the patient is on an anticoagulant, digital pressure should be applied for an extended period of time to assure that active bleeding has discontinued. The cannula length should be recorded and the catheter inspected to detect any changes in the integrity of the catheter, and appropriate follow-up actions should be taken if damage is noted. If a catheter defect is noted, the manufacturer and the Food and Drug Administration (FDA) should be notified, as should the patient's physician.

REPLACING ADMINISTRATION SETS

Administration sets, including secondary sets and add-on devices, should be replaced no more frequently than at 72 hour intervals, unless a catheter-related infection is suspected or documented (CDC, 2002). The Infusion Nurses Society's Standards recommend changing the tubing on primary administration intermittent sets every 24 hours (Infusion Nurses Society, 2000). The administration set includes the area from the spike of the tubing entering the fluid container to the hub of the vascular device. Add-on devices, such as extension loops, solid catheter caps, injection and access ports, needles or needleless systems, and extension sets, increase the potential for infection as a result of the increased manipulation and/or the risk of separation, which can increase risk of contamination. When an add-on device is used, it should be of a Luer lock configuration and should be changed when the administration set is changed, when the catheter is changed, if contamination occurs, or whenever the integrity of either product is compromised (CDC, 2002).

Tubing used to administer blood, blood products, or lipid emulsions (those combined with amino acids and glucose in a 3-in-1 admixture or infused separately) must be replaced within 24 hours of initiating the infusion because blood, blood products, and lipid emulsions are more likely than other parenteral fluids to support microbial growth if contaminated. If the solution contains only dextrose and amino acids, the administration set does not need to be replaced more frequently than every 72 hours (CDC, 2002).

NEEDLELESS INTRAVASCULAR DEVICES

Needleless intravascular devices and systems were introduced to reduce the number of injuries related to sharps and to limit the risk of staff members acquiring bloodborne infections (OSHA, 2001). In home care, there have been two reported outbreaks of BSIs in patients receiving total parenteral nutrition (TPN) via a central venous catheter using a needleless infusion system (Danzig et al., 1995; Kellerman et al., 1996). When using needless devices, all components of the system need to be compatible to minimize leaks and breaks in the system. To minimize risk of contamination, the needleless port should be accessed only with a sterile device and wiped off with an antiseptic agent. The needleless components should be changed at least as frequently as the administration set, with the cap(s) changed no more frequently than every 72 hours or according to the manufacturer's recommendations (CDC, 2002).

REPLACING IV SOLUTIONS

In the early 1970s, there was a nationwide epidemic of health care–associated BSIs that was traced to the intrinsic contamination of IV fluid during manufacturing and transport by infectious agents present in the system before it was used (Maki et al., 1976). These outbreaks resulted in the CDC recommendation that IV fluids and administration sets be replaced every 24 hours (Maki, Goldmann, & Rhame, 1973). Since that time, studies have shown that endemic BSIs in hospitals due to in-use contamination of IV fluids are rare and that extrinsic contamination, or contamination introduced into the system during use of IV fluids, is infrequent and sporadic. Even with heavily manipulated lines (e.g., central venous catheters) or TPN fluids, the rate of in-use contamination appears to be low (Pearson, 1996). For that reason, the CDC does not recommend a specific frequency with which IV fluids, including non-lipid-containing parenteral nutrition fluids, need to be replaced. Infusions of lipid-containing parenteral nutrition fluids (e.g., 3-in-1 solutions) must be completed within 24 hours of hanging the solution. When lipid emulsions are given alone, the lipid infusion must be completed within 12 hours of hanging the emulsion. If volume considerations require more time, the infusion should be completed within 24 hours. Infusions of blood or other blood products are to be completed within 4 hours of hanging the blood (CDC, 2002).

CATHETER SITE CARE
Skin Preparation

Skin cleansing and antisepsis of the catheter insertion site are among the most important measures for preventing catheter-related infection. Before a peripheral venous catheter, midline catheter, or PICC is inserted, and during dressing changes, clean skin should be disinfected with an appropriate antiseptic. If the skin is visibly dirty when initiating catheter insertion, it must be cleaned with soap and water before the antiseptic solution is applied; otherwise, the antiseptic solution may not be effective. A 2% chlorhexidine-based preparation is preferred, but tincture of iodine, an iodophor, or 70% alcohol may also be used. Single-unit containers or packets are recommended. The selected antiseptic agent should be allowed to remain on the insertion site and to air dry before proceeding with the catheter insertion (CDC, 2002). If 10% povidone-iodine is used to clean the skin, the povidone-iodine should be allowed time to dry and not be wiped off with a 70% isopropyl alcohol preparation pad, because this negates the effect of the povidone-iodine. If the patient is allergic to povidone-iodine, 70% isopropyl alcohol should be used (Infusion Nurses Society, 2000). The antiseptic agent should be applied at the site and wiped outward in a circular motion, except for chlorhexidine, which should be applied in a back and forth motion. Excess antiseptic should not be wiped off. When the skin is prepared for the insertion of a peripheral IV catheter, an area 2 to 4 inches in diameter is generally considered safe and acceptable. When tincture of iodine is used for skin antisepsis before catheter insertion, it should be removed with alcohol, because it may cause skin irritation. The catheter insertion site should not be palpated after the skin has been cleansed with the antiseptic unless the staff member is wearing sterile gloves.

Applying an organic solvent, such as acetone or ether, to "defat" the skin or remove skin lipids has been a common procedure during routine dressing changes. These agents appear neither to add additional protection against skin colonization nor to decrease significantly the incidence of catheter-related infection (Maki & McCormack, 1987). The use of organic solvents can also increase local inflammation and cause patient discomfort. Therefore, organic solvents should not be applied to the skin before catheter insertion or during dressing changes.

If excess hair needs to be removed from the skin before insertion of a catheter, the hair should be removed by clipping with scissors. Shaving with a razor is not recommended because it could cause microabrasions that could damage the skin's integrity and increase colonization and the risk of infection. Removing the hair with a depilatory is not recommended because of the potential for an allergic reaction. Electric razors should not be used unless they are effective, preserve the skin's integrity, and it is possible to change or disinfect the heads of the devices between patient use (Infusion Nurses Society, 2000).

In the past, topical antimicrobial ointments were routinely applied to the catheter site at the time of catheter insertion and during routine dressing changes to reduce microbial contamination. Studies of this means of preventing catheter-related infections have yielded contradictory findings. Therefore, the CDC does not recommend applying topical antimicrobial or antiseptic ointment or cream to the insertion sites of peripheral venous catheters or central venous catheters, *except* for hemodialysis catheters, because of the potential of the ointment or cream to promote fungal infections and antimicrobial resistance. For central venous catheters used in hemodialysis, however, application of povidone-iodine ointment at the catheter insertion site during each dressing change and at the end of each dialysis session is recommended, provided the ointment does not interact with the material of the hemodialysis catheter, per the manufacturer's recommendation (Levin *et al.*, 1991; CDC, 2002).

Midline and Central Venous Catheter Dressing Changes

Dressings should be changed on peripheral midline catheters and tunneled, nontunneled, or implanted central venous catheter and PICC sites no more often than every 7 days until the insertion site has healed. A dressing should also be placed over the noncoring needle placed in a port; the dressing should be changed every week. Otherwise, a dressing is not needed with a port. Once the exit site of a tunneled central venous catheter is well healed, the home care or hospice organization should follow the physician's orders and its policies and procedures regarding whether dressings are needed. If a dressing is needed, either a sterile gauze dressing or a sterile, transparent, semipermeable dressing may be used to cover the catheter site. If the patient is diaphoretic, or if the site is bleeding or oozing, a gauze dressing is preferable to a transparent, semipermeable dressing. The catheter dressing should be changed every 7 days; when it becomes damp, loosened, or soiled; when inspection of the site is necessary; and at each hemodialysis session. Gauze dressings should be changed every 2 days, except in the case of those pediatric patients for whom the risk for dislodging the catheter outweighs the benefit of changing the dressing. If a gauze dressing is used, adhesive material should be placed around all edges to secure the dressing. A nonocclusive type of dressing, such as a self-adhesive bandage, should not be used in lieu of a gauze dressing. Gauze dressings are not recommended when there is a risk of contamination from secretions or external moisture and bacteria. When a transparent dressing is placed over a gauze dressing, it is considered a gauze dressing and should be changed every 48 hours.

The CDC has not made a formal recommendation regarding the use of chlorhexidine-impregnated sponge (e.g., Biopatch™) dressings to reduce the incidence of infection (CDC, 2002); in one multicenter study, however, a chlorhexidine-impregnated sponge dressing placed over the site of short-term arterial and central venous catheters reduced the risk for catheter colonization and catheter-related bloodstream infection, with no adverse systemic effects resulting from use of this device (Maki et al., 2000). Chlorhexidine sponge dressings should not be used in neonates aged less than 7 days or of gestational age less than 26 weeks (Garland et al., 2001).

Catheter site dressings over peripheral short-line IV devices (i.e., nonmidline catheters) should be replaced when the peripheral short-line intravenous catheter is replaced; when the dressing becomes damp, loosened, or soiled; when inspection of the site is necessary; or if the patient is diaphoretic.

Touch contamination of the catheter insertion site should be avoided when a dressing is replaced. The catheter site should be inspected visually and palpated for tenderness only through the intact dressing (if the patient has no signs or symptoms of an infection) by the home care staff member during each home visit and on a daily ongoing basis by the patient or caregiver. If there is tenderness, fever without an obvious source, or symptoms of a local or BSI, the dressing should be removed and the site directly inspected. When the catheter dressing is changed, either sterile gloves or nonsterile clean gloves with no-touch technique may be used, according to the organization's policies and procedures.

Injection Cap Changes

Injection caps should be cleaned with 70% alcohol or povidone-iodine before the venous system is accessed, to minimize the risk of contamination. Whereas the CDC recommends that injection caps should not be changed more frequently than every 72 hours or according to manufacturers' recommendations (CDC, 2002), there are several more specific recommendations that should be considered and implemented. The injection cap on a midline or central venous catheter should be changed when the catheter dressing is changed, anytime the injection cap is removed from the catheter, if residual blood remains in the injection port, or whenever contamination occurs. The Infusion Nurses Society's Standards recommend changing injection caps at least every 7 days (Infusion Nurses Society, 2000). Injection ports on peripheral short-line venous catheters should be changed when the catheter is replaced.

FILTERS

In-line filters may be perceived to reduce the incidence of infusion-related phlebitis, but there are no data to support their efficacy in preventing infections associated with IV access devices and infusion systems. Infusate-related BSIs rarely occur, and filtration in the pharmacy before use is a more practical and less costly strategy for removing most particulates. In-line filters can become blocked, especially with certain solutions (e.g., lipids), and consequently they can give rise to the need for increased catheter manipulations. Therefore, the CDC does not recommend the routine use of in-line filters for infection control purposes (CDC, 2002).

In-line filters should be used to remove particulate matter that could result in an obstruction to the vascular or pulmonary system, however. The FDA issued a safety alert regarding the hazards of precipitation associated with the administration of TPN. The FDA's alert suggests that a filter be used when either central or peripheral nutrition products are infused. A 1.2 micron air-eliminating filter and bacteria/particulate retentive filter should be used for lipid or TPN admixtures, and a 0.2 micron air-eliminating filter and bacteria/particulate retentive filter should be used for non-lipid-containing admixtures (FDA, 1994; Infusion Nurses Society, 2000). The filter should be located as close to the patient as possible and should be changed at the same frequency with which the IV administration set is changed.

FLUSHING THE CATHETER

Solutions used to flush IV access devices are intended to prevent thrombosis rather than infection. Fibrin deposits and thrombi in catheters, however, can serve as central points for microbial colonization of IV access devices. Catheter thrombosis appears to be one of the most important factors associated with infection of central venous catheters and implanted ports. Thus the use of anticoagulants (e.g., heparin) or thrombolytic agents may have a role in the prevention of catheter-related BSIs. Studies suggest that 0.9% saline solution is just as effective as heparin in maintaining catheter patency and reducing phlebitis in peripheral catheters (Pearson, 1996). The routine use of heparin to maintain catheter patency, even at doses as low as 250 to 500 units, has been associated with thrombocytopenia and thromboembolic and hemorrhagic complications.

Indwelling central venous catheters (e.g., Hickman and Broviac catheters, PICCs, ports) should be routinely flushed with an anticoagulant. The lowest possible amount and concentration should be used to maintain catheter patency. Closed-tip (Groshong) or valved (e.g., pressure activated safety valve [PASV]) catheters are flushed with normal saline only and do not require routine flushing with an anticoagulant.

A peripheral venous heparin lock should be routinely flushed with a 0.9% saline solution. A peripheral venous heparin lock in a neonate or infant should be routinely flushed with a preservative-free 0.9% saline solution. Consideration may be given to the use of a heparin flush solution in low doses (1 to 10 units of preservative-free heparin to 1 mL of preservative-free normal saline) in neonates and infants because of their tiny veins and the small-gauge cannula used in their care. If a heparin lock is used for obtaining blood specimens, a dilute heparin flush solution (10 units/mL) should be used for routine

Exhibit 4-2 Risk Factors Associated with the Development of Catheter-Related Infections During TPN Therapy

Catheter site colonization
Method and site of catheter insertion
Experience of staff member inserting catheter
Use of TPN line for purposes other than administration of TPN fluids
Breaks in protocol for aseptic maintenance of the infusion system
Use of triple-lumen catheters

Source: Reprinted with permission from M. L. Pearson, Guideline for the prevention of intravascular-related infections, *American Journal of Infection Control,* pp. 262–293, © 1996, Mosby-Year Book, Inc.

flushing of the heparin lock. If blood has been withdrawn from the catheter, the catheter should be flushed with 0.9% saline in sufficient amounts to remove residual blood from the catheter's lumen(s) before final flushing with the appropriate solution.

The amount of flush solution used is also a consideration in maintaining catheter patency. The flush volume should be equal to two times the volume capacity of the catheter and any add-on devices. For example, if the volume of a peripheral venous catheter and the extension loop is 1.5 mL, the minimum amount of solution needed to flush the catheter is 3 mL. During and after administration of the flush, positive pressure must be maintained to prevent reflux of blood into the catheter lumen. If resistance is met during the attempt to flush the catheter, no further flushing attempts should be made because this could result in a clot dislodging into the vascular system or in catheter rupture.

CULTURING FOR SUSPECTED INFUSION-RELATED INFECTIONS

Primary BSI (infection related directly to the venous access device or fluid) may occur in home infusion therapy patients. In accordance with physician's orders, blood cultures may be obtained from the patient. The IV fluid, venous catheter, and delivery system should also be cultured according to the organization's policies and procedures to determine the cause of the BSI; physician's orders to obtain cultures from the intravenous solution, catheter, and delivery system are not required, however. Before submitting the culture materials, the home care organization may want to verify the reference laboratory's ability to provide this service. If the catheter is suspected as the source of infection, blood cultures should be obtained through the catheter as well as via a peripheral site. Before a cannula is removed for culture, the surrounding skin should be cleaned with 70% isopropyl alcohol and allowed to air dry. If purulent drainage is present, the skin should be cultured before the skin is cleaned. The semiquantitative culturing technique is the recommended method for culturing. The microbiology laboratory should have a procedure for performing and interpreting these types of cultures (Maki, Weise, & Sarafin, 1977). Again, the organization may want to verify the reference laboratory's ability to provide this service before submitting the culture materials.

When an infusate is suspected of being contaminated, the infusion should be discontinued immediately. The IV bag and tubing should be removed at the IV hub, and the entire set should be returned to the pharmacy. A sample of the IV fluid is not sufficient for determining whether the fluid was contaminated. The central pharmacy should record the type of fluid, the additives, and the lot numbers (of the fluid, additives, and tubing) before sending the IV set and fluid to the microbiology laboratory for culture. The microbiology laboratory should have a procedure for culturing IV fluid for suspected contamination. If intrinsic contamination is strongly suspected and/or documented, the FDA and the manufacturer should be notified.

TPN ADMINISTRATION

Catheter-related bloodstream infection is one of the most important complications of total parenteral nutrition (TPN). Because TPN solutions commonly contain dextrose, amino acids, or lipid emulsions, they are more likely than conventional IV fluids to support the growth of certain microbial species if they become contaminated. Three-in-one TPN solutions, which combine glucose, amino acids, lipid emulsion, and additives in single- or multiliter administration bags, however, do not appear to support greater microbial growth than non-lipid-containing TPN fluids and may be changed safely at 24-hour intervals (Goldmann, Martin, & Worthington, 1973). Most infections that occur during the administration of TPN result from contamination of the catheter rather than from contamination of the fluids (Maki, 1976). Risk factors associated with the development of catheter-related infections are listed in Exhibit 4-2. In

addition, rigorous aseptic nursing care has been shown to reduce greatly the incidence of TPN-related infection.

If the patient has a multilumen catheter, one port should be designated for the administration of TPN only (Snydman, Murray, Kornfeld et al., 1982).

PEDIATRIC PATIENTS

As in adults, most catheter-related bloodstream infections in pediatric patients are caused by staphylococci, with Staphylococcus epidermidis being the most common species. Other species of Gram-positive cocci and fungi are the next most frequently isolated pathogens affecting children, with Malassezia furfur being an especially common pathogen in neonates receiving lipid emulsions. Phlebitis, extravasation, and catheter colonization can be associated with the use of peripheral venous access devices in all patients, but extravasation is the most common complication in children (Garland, J., Dunne, W., Havens, P., Hintermyer, M., Bozette, M., Wincek, J., Bromberger, T., Seavers, M., 1992). Central venous catheters (e.g., Hickman or Broviac catheters or implanted ports) have become more commonly used in treating children with chronic medical conditions, especially malignancies. The Broviac catheter, rather than the Hickman catheter, is preferred for children because of its smaller catheter diameter. If a patient is 4 years of age or older and needs long-term (more than 30 days) vascular access, a PICC, tunneled central venous catheter, or implanted port is recommended (Pearson, 1996). For patients younger than 4 years old who need long-term vascular access, an implanted port is recommended, because an external central venous catheter segment may be contiguous with the diaper area and thus may be easily contaminated. Implanted ports have also been shown to have a longer survival time and fewer infectious complications than other tunneled catheters. A single-lumen central venous catheter is recommended unless multiple ports are essential for the management of the patient (Pearson, 1996).

NONVASCULAR ACCESS DEVICES

Nonvascular access devices include epidural, intrathecal, and ventricular catheters that can be used to administer antineoplastic agents, antibiotics, and analgesic agents. A mask and sterile gloves must be worn when nonvascular access device care and maintenance procedures are performed. Before any medication is infused via a nonvascular access device, the site should be aspirated with a syringe. Epidural devices should be aspirated to make sure that spinal fluid and blood is not aspirated, and intrathecal and ventricular devices should be aspirated to make sure that blood is not aspirated and that spinal fluid is present. If problems are identified, the physician should be contacted and no medications should be administered. All medication administered via a nonvascular access device must be preservative free. When a nonvascular access device is attached to an implant pump, the manufacturer's guidelines should be followed regarding aspiration. Alcohol should not be used to clean the exit site or catheter hub before the nonvascular access device is accessed because the alcohol may enter the central nervous system and have neurotoxic effects (Infusion Nurses Society, 2000).

Epidural Catheter, Port, or Pump

An epidural catheter may be used to administer analgesics or low-dose anesthetics. Epidural catheters are placed in the epidural space on either a short-term or a long-term basis. When a permanent catheter is placed, it is tunneled subcutaneously from the lumbar region and exits into the flank area. Epidural devices and administration sets must be clearly labeled to distinguish them from other catheter sets. A mask and sterile gloves must be worn when catheter care and maintenance procedures are performed. Epidural infusions given on a continuous basis should be administered via an electronic infusion device. Before any medication is infused via the epidural catheter, the site should be aspirated with a syringe to make sure that spinal fluid is not aspirated. If spinal fluid is aspirated, the physician should be contacted, and no medications should be administered. Medication infused into the epidural catheter must be preservative free and administered through a 0.2-micron filter without surfactant. Alcohol should not be used to clean the exit site or to clean the injection port before the epidural catheter is accessed because the alcohol may enter the epidural space via the catheter and cause nerve damage (Infusion Nurses Society, 2000).

Intrathecal Catheter, Port, or Pump

Intrathecal catheters are used to administer certain antineoplastic agents, antibiotics, analgesics, and low-dose anesthetic agents. Intrathecal catheters and administration sets must be clearly labeled to distin-guish them from other catheter sets. Intrathecal catheters may be attached to an internal port or pump. Only noncoring needles should be used to access the intrathecal pump or port, and the manufacturer's guidelines for accessing, filling, and refilling should be followed. A mask and sterile gloves must be worn when catheter care and maintenance procedures are performed. Before any medication is infused via the intrathecal catheter, the site should be aspirated with a syringe to make sure that spinal fluid or blood is not aspirated. If spinal fluid or blood is aspirated, the physician should be contacted, and no medications should be administered. When an intrathecal catheter is attached to an implanted pump, the manufacturer's guidelines should be followed regarding aspiration. Medication infused into the intrathecal catheter must be preservative free and administered through a 0.2-micron filter without surfactant. Alcohol should not be used to clean the exit site or to clean the access site port before the intrathecal catheter is accessed because the alcohol may enter the intrathecal space via the catheter and cause nerve damage (Infusion Nurses Society, 2000).

BLOOD STORAGE FOR HOME TRANSFUSIONS
Blood Storage During Transport

Maintaining the appropriate temperature for blood or blood products is essential in controlling bacterial growth and preventing hemolysis when blood is to be administered in the home. When blood and blood products that will be administered in the home are transported, the blood storage and transportation time should be kept to a minimum, and the blood should be transported directly from the blood center to the patient's home for administration. The blood should be transported in a sealed plastic bag that has been placed in an impervious, clean, thermally insulated cooler. The blood should be stored with wet ice or a coolant that maintains a temperature of 1° to 10°C or 33° to 50°F. Fresh-frozen plasma should be stored at 1° to 6°C or 33.0° to 42.8°F. Blood must be protected against direct exposure to ice packs or other coolant sources. Platelets and thawed fresh-frozen plasma should be stored at room temperature, which should not exceed 37°C, in an impervious, clean, thermally insulated cooler without coolants and without exposure to temperature extremes. Temperature-sensitive monitor tags or monitors may be placed on the blood bag to ensure that the blood has been maintained at the proper temperature during transport and before administration (Fridey, Kasparin, & Issitt, 1994).

Blood Storage in the Patient's Home

If more than 1 unit of blood is to be transfused in the patient's home, the unused component(s) should remain in the insulated cooler until it is transfused into the patient. The blood or blood products should not be stored in the patient's refrigerator or freezer, because temperatures may vary. If the ice melts or if the temperature-sensitive monitors do not display a reading within acceptable temperature limits, the blood center should be contacted for further instructions.

INFECTION CONTROL IN PHARMACEUTICAL SERVICES
Pharmacy Sterile Compounding Requirements

The American Society of Health-System Pharmacists (ASHP) and the U.S. Pharmacopoeia (USP) both publish guidelines for sterile compounding (ASHP, 2000; USP, 2003). It is noteworthy that both organizations consider compounding sterile pharmaceuticals for the home setting riskier than compounding pharmaceuticals for hospital use. The reason for designating a higher risk level for pharmaceuticals prepared for home use is that they are generally compounded in larger quantities and are stored over a longer period of time than drugs dispensed in the hospital. A new chapter in the *2004 United States Pharmacopoeia—National Formulary (USP-NF)* entitled "(797) Pharmaceutical Compounding—Sterile Preparations" describes new requirements for the compounding, preparation, and labeling of sterile drug preparations. The Federal Food, Drug and Cosmetic Act recognizes the *USP-NF* as an "official compendia" of drug standards. Under the act, if a drug product that appears in the *USP-NF* fails to meet the standards for strength, quality, purity, preparing, packaging, or labeling contained in the *USP-NF,* the drug may be deemed "misbranded" or "adulterated" by the Food and Drug Administration. *USP-NF* standards in the chapter on compounding sterile preparations contain requirements related to product standards and additional good pharmacy practices.

The *USP-NF* chapter requirements apply to pharmacies and other facilities that prepare or compound sterile preparations and extend to any health care practitioner involved in the preparation and compounding of sterile products, including compounding and preparation by nurses in patient care areas (but not in the home setting). The *USP-NF* chapter addresses the following:

- responsibilities of all compounding personnel
- classification of IV products into three risk levels, with quality assurance practices specific to each level of risk
- verification of compounding accuracy and sterilization
- personnel training and competence assessment in aseptic manipulation skills
- environmental quality and control
- equipment used in the preparation of compounded sterile products
- verification of automated compounding devices for parenteral nutrition
- finished product release checks and tests
- storage and beyond-use (expiration) dating
- maintaining product quality and control once the product leaves the compounding facility
- packing, handling, storage, and transport of compounded sterile products
- patient or caregiver training
- patient monitoring and adverse events reporting
- a quality assurance program

Appendix 4-A contains a summary of the *USP-NF* chapter requirements based on the three risk levels under which sterile drugs are to be compounded.

Because the Federal Food, Drug and Cosmetic Act recognizes the *USP-NF* as an "official compendia" of drug standards, home care organizations accredited by the Joint Commission on Accreditation of Healthcare Organizations (JCAHO) will be required to comply with the requirements. Table 4-1 contains a crosswalk between the *USP-NF* Chapter 797 requirements and the JCAHO *2004–2005 Comprehensive Accreditation Manual for Home Care.*

Additional information regarding the requirements for compounding sterile products may be directed to the USP directly at 800-822-8772, and the *USP-NF* Chapter 797 requirements may be obtained through the USP website at *(http://www.usp.org).*

Table 4-1 Crosswalk of *USP-NF* Chapter 797 Requirements to the JCAHO *2004-2005 Comprehensive Accreditation Manual for Home Care*

USP-NF *Chapter 797 requirement*	*JCAHO home care standard*
Formal written quality assurance program for sterile compounding, including: • selection of indicators • how results are reported and evaluated • identification of follow-up activities if thresholds are exceeded • delineation of responsibilities for each step in the process • annual analysis of plan	IC.1.10 • PI.1.10 • PI.2.10, PI.2.20 • PI.3.10 • LD.4.10 • LD.4.70
Adequate training and instruction of personnel in performing compounding activities, including: • theoretical principles • practical skills	HR.2.30
Competence assessment of personnel performing compounding activities, including: • passing written test • media fill testing, per risk level	HR.3.10
Environmental design of drug preparation rooms	MM.4.20 LD.3.80 EC.8.10
Air quality testing and environmental monitoring of compounding environment	EC.7.10 (testing) EC.9.10 (monitoring)
Routine disinfection of compounding environment	IC.4.10
Temperature testing of drug-storage areas	EC.6.10
Automated compounding device—verification of accuracy, calibration, and maintenance	EC.6.10
Proper attire (gowning, gloves, etc.)	IC.4.10
Proper scrubbing (hand hygiene)	IC.4.10 National Patient Safety Goal #7
Standard compounding procedures (written), including: • quality control check for proper ingredients • visual inspection of final product	MM.4.20
Sterilization of nonsterile drugs	MM.4.20
Expiration dating, per risk level	MM.4.30
End product testing (sterility, potency, pyrogen)	MM.4.20
Packaging and transport	MM.4.40
Redispensing compounded sterile products	MM.4.80
Patient education	PC.6.10
Patient monitoring and adverse reaction reporting	MM.5.10 (reporting) MM.6.10 (monitoring)
Other (nonspecific to above)	LD.1.30

Source: Adapted from *Joint Commission Perspectives*, April 2004, 24 (4).

Medication Storage

If medications are stored in the home health agency or hospice, the temperature of the refrigerator, and if applicable the freezer, should be monitored on a daily basis during normal business hours and documented in a refrigerator temperature control log. The refrigerator's temperature must be in the range of 2° to 8°C or 35° to 46°F, and the freezer's temperature must be less than −20°C or 4°F. A penny placed on a cup of frozen water can serve as a means of checking the freezer's temperature. If during temperature monitoring the penny is found to have sunk to the bottom of the cup, the freezer has lost power and the items inside have thawed. Another option is to utilize a refrigerator temperature alarm that will go off if temperatures are out of the acceptable ranges. If the temperature of the refrigerator or freezer has not been maintained within the required range, the pharmacist or director should be notified and appropriate follow-up actions should be taken.

Storage and Transport of Parenteral Medications

Once parenteral products have been prepared, they should be held in a refrigerator until they are placed in a clean, insulated cooler for delivery. Food or laboratory specimens should not be stored in the same refrigerator as medications.

Medications that have been compounded by the pharmacy, such as IV antibiotics, compounded analgesic suppositories, IV admixtures, and TPN formulas, should be kept refrigerated in the pharmacy prior to transport to the patient's home. During the transport of compounded medications to be administered in the home, medications that require refrigeration should be placed in a sealed plastic bag and then placed in an impervious, clean, thermally insulated cooler that protects the product from damage, leakage, contamination, and degradation. Noncompounded drugs being delivered to the patient's home, such as heparin or saline flushes, should be placed in a container that prevents product contamination during transport and stored in manner that prevents exposure to extremes of temperature. On the outside of the container used to ship compounded sterile products, written instructions should be provided to the patient/family explaining how to safely open the container and how to store the contents once the container is opened.

Medication Storage in the Patient's Home

The length of time that compounded medication or TPN solution may be refrigerated is based on the stability of the compounded medication. When the medication or TPN is refrigerated in the home, it should be stored in a separate area of the refrigerator, if possible. The compounded medication or TPN solution needs to remain refrigerated until it is taken out to warm to room temperature, about 1 hour prior to infusion. If the medication is stored frozen, it should be thawed in the refrigerator—not left out on the patient's kitchen counter for several hours at room temperature and not microwaved. If the medication must be refrigerated and the patient does not have a refrigerator, the home care organization may provide a refrigerator on a temporary basis. Otherwise, the patient must gain access to a refrigerator (e.g., in a neighbor's kitchen). The temperature in the patient's refrigerator does not have to be monitored or checked with a thermometer, but the refrigerator should keep the medications cold. Medications and TPN solutions must not be used beyond their expiration date or beyond-use date, and they must not be used if any container of parenteral fluid has visible turbidity, leaks, cracks, or particulate matter. When new medications are delivered to the patient, they should be rotated in the refrigerator to ensure that the patient uses the older medications first.

Preparation of Parenteral Medication in the Home

Whenever possible, all routine parenteral fluids should be admixed in the pharmacy in a laminar flow hood using aseptic technique (JCAHO, 2004; CDC, 2002). Medications should be prepared in the patient's home only when (1) the stability of the drug is less than 24 hours after reconstitution or (2) the drug dosage may change so frequently that pharmacy preparation is not possible. If a medication must be mixed in the home, appropriate aseptic technique must be used. The staff member should select a clean, low-traffic area for medication preparation and perform hand hygiene before any medication preparation. Medications prepared in the home should be used immediately. If possible, preparing several doses for the patient's later use should be avoided.

Multidose Vials

A number of studies on the bacterial contamination of multidose vials have been conducted and have revealed considerable variation in bacterial contamination rates—from none to 27% (Mattner & Gastmeier, 2004). To prevent contamination, the rubber access diaphragm of a multidose vial must be disinfected with 70% isopropyl alcohol before a sterile device is inserted into the vial, and touch contamination of the device must be avoided. Single-dose vials should be used for parenteral additives or medications whenever possible (CDC, 2002), and the multiple use of preservative-free vials should be avoided (Mattner & Gastmeier, 2004). The leftover content of single-use vials should not be combined for later use. If multidose vials are used, and if recommended by the manufacturer, the multidose vial should be refrigerated after it is opened. Safe practice recommends that multidose vials be thrown out if contamination is suspected or visible and when the manufacturer's expiration date is reached. Anecdotally, it is known that many organizations require that multidose vials be dated and discarded 30 days after opening. The manufacturer's recommendations for both storage and expiration dating should be followed and applies to properly stored, unopened, or unentered containers. There is no recommendation for the arbitrary discard of multidose vials. However, it is anticipated that USP-797 will govern a time frame for beyond-use dating for opened or entered (e.g., needle-punctured) multiple-dose containers (USP, 2005).

Nursing Care and Administration of Parenteral Medications

Insertion and maintenance of IV access devices by inexperienced or incompetent staff members may increase the risk of catheter colonization and catheter-related bloodstream infection (CDC, 2002). Many home care organizations have established a core group of clinicians qualified and responsible for providing care to patients receiving infusion therapy at home. To reduce catheter-related infections and overall costs, only staff members specially trained in or designated with the responsibility for insertion and maintenance of IV access devices should provide infusion therapy for home care and hospice patients. Continuing education should be provided to ensure that knowledge related to parenteral therapy is maintained.

Competency skills should be monitored upon hire prior to performing patient care, on an ongoing basis, and when new drug therapies or equipment are introduced.

Nursing policies and procedures for home infusion therapy should emphasize methods for preventing catheter-related infection and should be based on CDC guidelines, state and federal regulations, and professional organizations' standards of practice (e.g., INS, APIC). Appendix 4-B contains a summary of the CDC's guidelines for the prevention of IV access device–related infections. Patient assessment for signs and symptoms of potential infection should be performed during every visit. This assessment should include evaluation for systemic infection (e.g., fever, chills, and change in mental status) as well as for local site infection (e.g., redness, pain, swelling, and tenderness at the IV insertion site).

When parenteral medications are given in the home, the medication label must be verified before the medication is administered to the patient. Each label should be written according to the state's board of pharmacy requirements, which may include the patient's name (and if possible other patient identifiers), type of IV solution and additives, dose, date and time of compounding, expiration date, prescribed administration regimen, cautionary and accessory labels, and storage requirements. The nurse administering the medication must check the label to ensure that it matches the medication orders for the patient. If the fluid's appearance is questionable or the container's integrity is compromised, the solution or medication should not be administered and returned to the pharmacy.

PATIENT AND CAREGIVER EDUCATION

A study that reviewed the home care infection incidence rates for patients with central venous access devices over a period of 7 years found that most infections were identified 25 days after the patient's admission to home care. This led the author to conclude that most infections occurred from introduction of bacteria through the catheter hub, because by that time in the course of care, patients were managing their infusion care (Gorski, 2004). This supports the importance of patient and caregiver education, specifically hand hygiene and manipulation of catheter tubing and other supplies, such as syringes. It is imperative that the patient or caregiver responsible for administering IV therapy in the home is well trained and competent. Their knowledge and understanding should be verified by a registered nurse on initiation of IV therapy and throughout the course of care through hands-on demonstrations and practice using the actual equipment and supplies the patient or caregiver will be expected to use. This verification should be designed to demonstrate that the patient and caregiver can correctly and consistently perform the following skills:

1. Describe the therapy involved, why the medication is needed, potential medication side effects, goals of therapy, and expected outcomes.
2. Inspect medications and supplies upon delivery to assure that proper temperatures were maintained during shipment and that there is no evidence of defects or deterioration.
3. Handle, store, and monitor all drug products, related supplies, and equipment in the home, including any special requirements.
4. Inspect visually all drugs, devices, and other items the patient or caregiver is required to use immediately prior to administration, to ensure that all items are acceptable for use.
   - Assure that sterile devices are completely sealed with no evidence of loss of package integrity
   - Inspect the fluid for particulate matter, haziness, discoloration, precipitate, or other deviations from normal appearance
   - Check the container for cracks, leaks, or punctures
5. Check medication labels immediately prior to administration, to ensure the correct medication will be given at the right time and dose to the right patient.
6. Clean the in-home preparation area, wash hands, and use proper aseptic and injection technique. Manipulate all containers, equipment, apparatus, devices, and supplies used in conjunction with administration.
7. Institute all precautions and techniques required for medication administration.
8. Perform catheter care and maintenance to maintain the site free from infection and to maintain catheter patency.
9. Observe and report both local and systemic signs and symptoms of infection and phlebitis, adverse drug events, and catheter misplacement.
10. Respond immediately to emergency or critical situations such as catheter breakage or displacement, tubing disconnection, clot formation, flow obstruction, and equipment malfunction.
11. Understand when to seek and how to obtain professional emergency services or professional advice.
12. Handle, contain, and properly dispose of medical waste generated (e.g., needles, devices, dressings, IV tubing), and clean a biohazardous spill.

The patient or caregiver should be able to demonstrate mastery of these skills before he or she is allowed to administer IV medication unsupervised by a registered nurse. The pharmacy that dispenses the compounded medication, as well as the registered nurse, are responsible for ensuring on admission and on an ongoing basis thereafter that the patient has mastered and is capable of and willing to comply with the items in the foregoing list, and that his or her competence has been assessed and documented in the clinical record. Written information should be provided to the patient or caregiver to supplement the verbal instructions provided (USP, 2003).

REFERENCES

American Society of Health-System Pharmacists. (2000). ASHP guidelines on quality assurance for pharmacy-prepared sterile products. *American Journal of Health-System Pharmacy, 57,* 1150–1169.

Andrivet, P., Bacquer, A., Ngoc, C. V., Ferme, C., Letinier, J. Y., Gautier, H., Gallet, C. B., & Brun-Buisson, C. (1994). Lack of clinical benefit from subcutaneous tunnel insertion of central venous catheters in immunocompromised patients. *Clinical Infectious Diseases, 18,* 199–206.

Banerjee, S. N., Emori, T. G., Culver, D. H., Gaynes, R. P., Jarvis, W. R., Horan, T., Edwards, J. R., Tolson, J., Henderson, T., & Martone, W. J. (1991). Secular trends in nosocomial primary bloodstream infections in the United States, 1980–1989. National Nosocomial Infections Surveillance system. Hospital infections. *American Journal of Medicine, 16,* 86S–89S.

Beck-Sagué, C. M., & Jarvis, W. R. (1993). Secular trends in the epidemiology of nosocomial fungal infections in the United States, 1980–1990. *Journal of Infectious Diseases, 167,* 1247–1251.

Bozzetti, F., Mariani, L., Boggio Bertinet, D., Chiavenna, G., Crose, N., DeCicco, M., Gigli, G., Micklewright, A., Moreno Vollares, J., Orban, A., Pertkiewicz, M., Pironi, L., Planas Vilas, M., Prins, F., Thul, T., Espen Han Working Group. (2002). Central venous catheter complications in 447 patients on home parenteral nutrition: an analysis of over 100,000 catheter days. *Clinical Nutrition, 21*(6), 475–485.

Centers for Disease Control and Prevention. (2002). Guidelines for the prevention of intravascular catheter-related infections. Recommendations of the Hospital Infection Control Practices Advisory Committee (HICPAC). *Morbidity and Mortality Weekly Report, 51,* (RR10).

Centers for Disease Control and Prevention. (1995). Recommendations for preventing the spread of vancomycin resistance: Recommendations of the Hospital Infection Control Practices Advisory Committee (HICPAC). *American Journal of Infection Control, 23,* 87–94.

Danzig, L. E., Short, L. J., Collins, K., Mahoney, M., Sepe, S., Bland, L., & Jarvis, W. R. (1995). Bloodstream infections associated with a needleless intravenous infusion system in patients receiving home infusion therapy. *Journal of the American Medical Association, 273,* 1862–1864.

Do, A., Ray, B., Banerjee, S., Illian, A. F., Barnett B., Pham, M., Hendricks, K., & Jarvis W. R. (1999). Bloodstream infection associated with needle-less device use and the importance of infection control practices in the home health care setting. *Journal of Infectious Diseases, 179,* 442-448.

Food and Drug Administration (FDA). (1994). *FDA safety alert: Hazards of precipitation associated with parenteral nutrition.* Rockville, MD: Department of Health and Human Services.

Fridey, J., Kasparin, C., & Issitt, L. (Eds.). (1994). *Out-of-hospital transfusion therapy.* Bethesda, MD: American Association of Blood Banks.

Garland, J. S., Alex, C. P., Mueller, C. D., Otten, D., Shivpuri, C., Harris, M. C., Naples, M., Pellegrini, J., Buck, R. J., McAuliffe, T. L., Goldmann, D. A., Maki, D. G. (2001). A randomized trial comparing povidone-iodine to a chlorhexidine gluconate-impregnated dressing for prevention of central venous catheter infections in neonates. *Pediatrics, 107,* 1431—1436.

Garland, J., Dunne, W., Havens, P., Hintermeyer, M., Bozzette, M., Wincek, J., Bromberger, T., Seavers, M. (1992). Peripheral intravenous catheter complications in critically ill children: a prospective study. *Pediatrics, 89,* 1145–1150.

Goldmann, D. A., Martin, W. T., & Worthington, J. W. (1973). Growth of bacteria and fungi in total parenteral nutrition. *American Journal of Surgery, 126,* 314–318.

Gorski, L. (2004). Central venous access device outcomes in a homecare agency. *Journal of Infusion Nursing, 27(2),* 104–111.

Infusion Nurses Society. (2000). Infusion nursing standards of practice. *Journal of Intravenous Nursing, 23* (suppl.), 6S.

Joint Commission on Accreditation of Healthcare Organizations (JCAHO). 2004. *2004-2005 Comprehensive Accreditation Manual for Home Care.* Oakbrook Terrace, IL: author published.

Joint Commission Perspectives. (2004). Vol. 24, no. 4. Oakbrook Terrace, IL: Author.

Kellerman, S., Shay, D., Howard, J., Goes, C., Feusner, J., Rosenberg, J., Vugia, P., & Jarvis, W. (1996). Bloodstream infections in home infusion patients: The influence of race and needleless intravascular access devices. *Journal of Pediatrics, 129,* 711–717.

Kluger, D. M., & Maki, D. G. (1999). The relative risk of intravascular device related bloodstream infections in adults. In *Abstracts of the 39th Interscience Conference on Antimicrobial Agents and Chemotherapy,* (p. 514). San Francisco, CA: American Society for Microbiology.

Levin, A., Mason, A. J., Jindal, K. K., Fong, I. W., & Goldstein, M. B. (1991). Prevention of hemodialysis subclavian vein catheter infections by topical povidone-iodine. *Kidney International, 40,* 934–938.

Linares, J., Sitges-Serra, A., Garau, J., Perez, J. L., & Martin, R. (1985). Pathogenesis of catheter sepsis: A prospective study with quantitative and semiquantitative cultures of catheter hub and segments. *Journal of Clinical Microbiology, 21,* 357–360.

Maki, D. (1992). Infections due to infusion therapy. In Bennet, J., Brachman, P., eds. *Hospital Infections,* 3rd Ed. Boston, MA: Little Brown and Co.

Maki, D. G. (1982). Infections associated with intravascular lines. In J. S. Remington (Ed.), *Current Clinical Topics in Infectious Diseases* (pp. 309–363). New York: McGraw-Hill.

Maki, D. G. (1976). Sepsis arising from extrinsic contamination of the infusion and measures for control. In I. Phillips, P. D. Meers, & P. F. D'Arcy (Eds.), *Microbiological hazards of infusion therapy* (pp. 99–143). Lancaster, England: MTP.

Maki, D. G., & Mermel, L. (1998). Infections due to infusion therapy. In J. V. Bennett & P. S. Brachman (Eds.), *Hospital Infections* (4th ed.) (pp. 689–724). Philadelphia: Lippincott-Raven Publishers.

Maki, D. G., Goldmann, D. A., & Rhame, F. S. (1973). Infection control in intravenous therapy. *Annals of Internal Medicine, 79,* 867–887.

Maki, D. G., & McCormack, R. N. (1987). Defatting catheter insertion sites in total parenteral nutrition is no value as an infection control measure. *American Journal of Medicine, 83,* 833–840.

Maki, D. G., Mermel, L. A., Klugar, D., *et al.* (2000). The efficacy of a chlorhexidine-impregnated sponge (Biopatch) for the prevention of intravascular catheter-related infection—a prospective randomized controlled multicenter study [abstract]. Presented at the Interscience Conference on Antimicrobial Agents and Chemotherapy. Toronto, Ontario: American Society for Microbiology.

Maki, D. G., Rhame, F. S., Mackel, D. C., & Bennett, J. V. (1976). Nationwide epidemic of septicemia caused by contaminated intravenous products. *American Journal of Medicine, 60,* 471–485.

Maki, D. G., & Ringer, M. (1991). Risk factors for infusion-related phlebitis with small peripheral venous catheters: A randomized controlled trial. *Annals of Internal Medicine, 114,* 845–854.

Maki, D. G., Weise, C., & Sarafin, H. (1977). A semiquantitative culture method for identifying intravenous-catheter-related infection. *New England Journal of Medicine, 9,* 1305–1309.

Mattner, F., & Gastmeier, P. (2004). Bacterial contamination of multidose vials: A prevalence study. *American Journal of Infection Control, 32,* 12–16.

Mermel, L. A., Parenteau, S., & Tow, S. M. (1995). The risk of midline catheterization in hospitalized patients. A prospective study. *Annals of Internal Medicine, 123,* 841–844.

Merrill, S., Peatross, B., Grossman, M., Sullivan, J., & Harker, W. (1994). Peripherally inserted central venous catheters: Low-risk alternatives for ongoing venous access. *Western Journal of Medicine, 160,* 25–30.

Moureau, N., Poole, S., Murdock, M., Gray, S., & Semba, C. (2002). Central venous catheters in home infusion care: Outcome analysis in 50,470 patients. *Journal of Vascular and Interventional Radiology, 13,* 1009–1016.

Occupational Safety and Health Administration (OSHA). (2001). Occupational exposure to bloodborne pathogens; Needlestick and other sharps injuries: Final rule. 29 CFR 1910. *Federal Register, 66,* 5317–5325.

Occupational Safety and Health Administration (OSHA). (1991). Occupational exposure to bloodborne pathogens: Final rule. 29 CFR 1910.1030. *Federal Register, 56,* 64003–64282.

Pearson, M. J. (1996). Guideline for the prevention of intravascular-related infections. *American Journal of Infection Control, 24,* 262–293.

Pittet, D., Tarara, D., & Wenzel, R. P. (1994). Nosocomial bloodstream infection in critically ill patients: Excess length of stay, extra costs, and attributable mortality. *Journal of the American Medical Association, 271,* 1958–1601.

Raad, I., Davis, S., Becker, M., Hohn, D., Houston, D., Umphrey, J., & Bodey, J. (1993). Low infection rate and long durability of nontunneled silastic catheters. A safe and cost-effective alternative for long-term venous access. *Archives of Internal Medicine, 153,* 1791–1796.

Ryder, M. A. (1995). Peripheral access options. *The Surgical Oncology Clinics of North America, (4),* 395–427.

Salzman, M. B., Isenberg, H. D., Shapiro, J. F., Lipsitz, P. J., & Rubin, L. G. (1993). A prospective study of the catheter hub as the portal of entry for microorganisms causing catheter-related sepsis in neonates. *Journal of Infectious Diseases, 167,* 487–490.

Schaberg, D., Culver, D., & Gaynes, R. (1991). Major trends in the microbial etiology of nosocomial infection. *American Journal of Medicine, 91,*
72S–75S.

Skiest, D., Grant, P., & Keiser, P. (1998). Nontunneled central venous
catheters in patients with AIDS are associated with a low infection rate.
*Journal of Acquired Immune Deficiency Syndromes and Human Retrovi-
rology, 17*(1), 220–226.

Snydman, D. R., Murray, S. A., Kornfeld, S. J., Majka, J. A., & Ellis, C. A.
(1982). Total parenteral nutrition-related infections: prospective epidemiologic study using semiquantitative methods. *American Journal of
Medicine, 73,* 695–699.

Snydman, D. R, Pober, B. R., Murray, S. A., Gorbea, H. F., Majka, J. A., &
Perry, L. K. (1982). Predictive value of surveillance skin cultures in total
parenteral nutrition–related infection. Prospective epidemiologic study
using semiquantitative cultures. *Lancet, 2,* 1385–1388.

U.S. Pharmacopeial Convention, Inc. (2003). U.S. Pharmacopeia 27, Chapter <797> Pharmaceutical Compounding—Sterile Preparations.
Rockville, MD: U.S. Pharmacopeial Convention, Inc.: 2350–2370.

U.S. Pharmacopeial Convention, Inc. (2003). First supplement to U.S. Pharmacopeia 27, Chapter <797> Pharmaceutical Compounding—Sterile
Preparations. Rockville, MD: U.S. Pharmacopeial Convention, Inc.:
1–15.

Vanherwegham, J., Dhaene, M., Goldman, M., Stolear, J., Sabot, J.,
Waterlot, Y., Serruys, E., & Thayse, C. (1986). Infections associated with
subclavian dialysis catheters: The key role of nurse training. *Nephron, 42,*
116–119.

Yu, V., Goetz, A., Wagener, M., Smith, P., Rihs, J., Hanchett, J., &
Zuravleff, J. (1986). Staphylococcus aureus nasal carriage and infection
in patients on hemodialysis: Efficacy of antibiotic prophylaxis. *New
England Journal of Medicine, 10,* 91–96.

Summary of the *USP-NF* Chapter <797>

Criteria	Low-risk Level	Medium-risk Level	High-risk Level
Compounding Conditions	1. Compounded entirely under ISO Class 5 (Class 100) conditions 2. Compounding involves only transfer, measuring, and mixing manipulations with closed or sealed systems that are performed promptly and attentively. 3. Manipulations are limited to aseptically opening ampuls, penetrating sterile stoppers on vials with sterile needles and syringes and transferring sterile liquids into sterile administration devices and packages of sterile products.	1. All conditions listed under low-risk level. 2. Multiple individual or small doses of sterile products are combined or pooled to prepare a compounded sterile product that will be administered either to multiple patients or to one patient on multiple conditions. 3. Compounding process includes complex aseptic manipulations other than single volume transfer. 4. Compounding process requires unusually long duration. 5. The sterile compounded sterile products do not contain broad-spectrum bacteriostatic agents, and are administered over several days.	1. Nonsterile ingredients are incorporated or a nonsterile device is employed before terminal sterilization. 2. Sterile ingredients, components, devices, and mixtures are exposed to air quality inferior to ISO Class 5 (Class 100). 3. Nonsterile preparations are exposed for not more than six (6) hours before being sterilized. 4. Nonsterile preparations are terminally sterilized, but are not tested for bacterial endotoxins. 5. It is assumed that the chemical purity and content strength of ingredients meet their original or compendial specifications in unopened or in opened packages of bulk ingredients.
Quality Assurance Program	Formalized in writing Describes specific monitoring and evaluation activities Reporting and evaluation of results Identification of follow-up activities when thresholds are exceeded Delineation of individual responsibilities for each aspect of the program	Same as low-risk level	Same as low-risk level

Criteria	Low-risk Level	Medium-risk Level	High-risk Level
Quality Assurance Practices	Routine disinfection and quality testing of direct compounding environment Visual confirmation of personnel processes regarding gowning, etc. Review of orders and package of ingredients to assure correct identity and amounts of ingredients Visual inspection of compounded sterile products Media-fill test procedure performed at least annually for each person.	Same as low-risk level	Same as low-risk level
Outcome Monitoring	Yes	Yes	Yes
Reports/Documents	Written policies and procedures Adverse event reporting Complaint procedures Periodic review of quality control documents	Same as low-risk level	Same as low-risk level
Patient and Caregiver Training	Formalized program includes: Understanding of the therapy provided Handling and storage of the compounded sterile product Appropriate administration techniques Use and maintenance of any infusion device involved Use of printed material Appropriate follow-up	Same as low-risk level	Same as low-risk level
Maintaining Product and Quality Control once the Compounded Sterile Product leaves the Pharmacy	Packaging, handling and transport: Written policies and procedures including the packaging, handling, and transport of chemotoxic/hazardous compounded sterile medications Use and storage: Written policies and procedures Administration: Written policies and procedures dealing with issues as handwashing, aseptic technique, site care, etc. Education and training: Written policies and procedures dealing with proper education of patients and caregivers ensuring all of the above.	Same as low-risk level	Same as low-risk level
Storage and Beyond-Use Dating	Specific labeling requirements Specific beyond-use dating policies, procedures and requirements Policies regarding storage	Same as low-risk level	Same as low-risk level

Criteria	Low-risk Level	Medium-risk Level	High-risk Level
Storage and Beyond-Use Dating for Completed Compounded Sterile Products	In the absence of sterility testing, storage periods (prior to administration) are not to exceed the following: Room temperature: ≤48 hours 2°–8°: ≤14 days ≤20°: ≤45 days	Room temperature: ≤30 hours 2°–8°: ≤7 days ≤20°: ≤45 days	Room temperature: ≤24 hours 2°–8°: ≤3 days ≤20°: ≤45 days
Finished Product-Release Checks and Tests	Written policies and procedures address: Physical inspections Compounding accuracy checks Sterility testing Pyrogen testing Potency testing	Same as low-risk level	Same as low-risk level
Compounded Sterile Products Work Environment	Appropriate solid surfaces Limited (but necessary) furniture fixtures, etc. Anteroom Buffer zone	Same as low-risk level	Same as low-risk level
Equipment	Written policies address: Calibration Routine maintenance Personnel training	Same as low-risk level	Same as low-risk level
Components	Written policies and procedures address: Sterile components	Same as low-risk level	Same as low-risk level
Processing: Aseptic Technique	Written policies and procedures address: Specific training and performance evaluation Critical operations are carried out in a direct compounding common area	Same as low-risk level	Same as low-risk level
Environmental Control	Written policies and procedures address: Cleaning and sanitizing the workspaces (direct compounding common area) Personnel and gowning Standard operating procedures	Same as low-risk level	Same as low-risk level
Verification Procedures: Sterility Testing	Not required	Not required	Recommended
Verification Procedures: Environmental Monitoring	Certification of laminar airflow workbenches and barrier isolates every six (6) months Certification of the buffer room/zone and anteroom/zone every six (6) months Bacterial monitoring using an appropriate manner every 6 months	Same as low-risk level	Same as low-risk level
Verification Procedures: Personnel Training and Education	Initially and annually thereafter	Same as low-risk level	Same as low-risk level

Source: Adapted from U.S. Pharmacopoeia. (2003). 2004 United States Pharmacopoeia—National Formulary *(USP-NF)*. USP Tests and Assays Chapter <797>, Pharmaceutical Compounding, Sterile Preparations. *www.usp.org.*

Summary of the CDC's Guidelines for the Prevention of IV Access Device-Related Infections

Device	Replacement and Relocation of Device	Replacement of Catheter Site Dressing	Replacement of Administration Sets	Hang Time for Parenteral Fluids	Insertion Technique
Peripheral venous catheters	In adults, replace catheter and rotate site every 48 to 72 hours. Replace catheter at a different site within 24 hours. In adults, replace heparin locks every 96 hours. In pediatric patients, no recommendation for removal of catheters inserted under emergency conditions.	Replace dressing when catheter is replaced or when dressing becomes damp, loosened, or soiled. Replace dressings more frequently in diaphoretic patients. In patients who have large, bulky dressings that prevent palpation or direct visualization of catheter insertion site, remove dressing daily, visually inspect catheter site, and apply new dressing.	Replace IV tubing, including piggyback tubing and stopcocks, no more frequently than at 72-hour intervals unless clinically indicated. Replace tubing used to administer blood, blood products, or lipid emulsions within 24 hours of initiating infusion. No recommendation for replacement of tubing used for intermittent infusions. Consider short extension tubing connected to device as portion of device. Replace such extension tubing when device is changed.	No recommendation for hang time of IV fluids, including non–lipid-containing parenteral nutrition fluids. Complete infusion of lipid-containing parenteral nutrition fluids (e.g., 3-in-1 solutions) within 24 hours of hanging. When lipid emulsions are given alone, complete infusion within 12 hours of hanging.	Clean
Midline catheters	No recommendation for frequency of catheter replacement.	No recommendation for frequency of routine replacement of catheter site dressings. Replace dressing when catheter is replaced; when dressing becomes damp, loosened, or soiled; or when inspection of site is necessary. Replace dressings more frequently in diaphoretic patients.	Replace IV tubing, including piggyback tubing and stopcocks, no more frequently than at 72-hour intervals. Replace tubing used to administer blood, blood products, or lipid emulsions within 24 hours of initiating infusion.	No recommendation for hang time of IV fluids, including non–lipid-containing parenteral nutrition fluids. Complete infusions of lipid-containing parenteral nutrition fluids (e.g., 3-in-1 solutions) within 24 hours of hanging. When lipid emulsions are given alone, complete infusion within 12 hours of hanging.	Sterile

	Catheter replacement	Dressing	IV tubing replacement	Hang time / fluids	Barrier precautions
PICCs	No recommendation for frequency of catheter replacement.	No recommendation for frequency of routine replacement of catheter site dressing. Replace dressing when catheter is replaced; when dressing becomes damp, loosened, or soiled; or when inspection of site is necessary.	Replace IV tubing, including piggyback tubing and stopcocks, no more frequently than at 72-hour intervals. Replace tubing used to administer blood products or lipid emulsions within 24 hours of initiating infusion.	No recommendation for hang time of IV fluids, including non–lipid-containing parenteral nutrition fluids. Complete infusion of lipid-containing parenteral nutrition fluids (e.g., 3-in-1 solutions) within 24 hours of hanging. When lipid emulsions are given alone, complete infusion within 12 hours of hanging.	Sterile
Central venous catheters (includes nontunneled, tunneled, and totally implanted devices)	Do not routinely replace nontunneled (percutaneously inserted) catheters either by rotating insertion site or use of guidewire. No recommendation for frequency of replacement of tunneled catheters, totally implantable devices (i.e., ports), or needles used to access them.	No recommendation for routine replacement of catheter site dressings. Replace dressing when catheter is replaced; when dressing becomes damp, loosened, or soiled; or when inspection of site is necessary.	Replace IV tubing, including piggyback tubing and stopcocks, no more frequently than at 72-hour intervals. Replace tubing used to administer blood, blood products, or lipid emulsions within 24 hours of initiating infusion.	No recommendation for hang time of IV fluids, including non–lipid-containing parenteral nutrition fluids. Complete infusion of lipid-containing parenteral nutrition fluids (e.g., 3-in-1 solutions) within 24 hours of hanging. When lipid emulsions are given alone, complete infusion within 12 hours of hanging.	Sterile (in acute care or outpatient settings; not suitable for home environment)

Source: Adapted with permission from M. L. Pearson, Guideline for the prevention of intravascular device-related infections, *American Journal of Infection Control,* 1996, 24, pp. 262–293,

CHAPTER 5

Infection Control in Pediatrics, Pets, and Preparation of Food

INFECTION CONTROL IN CARING FOR PEDIATRIC PATIENTS

Keeping a child's environment clean and orderly is important for his or her health, safety, and emotional well-being. One of the most important steps in reducing the number of infectious agents, and therefore the spread of disease, is the thorough cleaning of surfaces that could pose a risk to children or staff members. Surfaces considered most likely to be contaminated are those with which children are likely to have contact. These may include toys that children put in their mouths, crib rails, and diaper changing areas. Routine cleaning with soap and water is the most useful method for removing infectious agents from surfaces. Surfaces that infants and young toddlers are likely to touch or mouth, such as crib rails, should be washed with soap and water and disinfected with a nontoxic disinfectant, such as a bleach solution, on a regular basis and when visibly soiled. Disinfectants containing phenol should not be used for cleaning toys or other items with which an infant may have contact because phenol is a neurotoxin that can be adsorbed through the skin (CDC, 2003a).

Diapering a Child

Two diaper changing methods may be used to minimize the risk of transmitting infection. One method involves the use of gloves, and the other does not. Gloves should be worn when the person changing the diaper has severe dermatitis or hand abrasions with open sores or when the child has severe diaper rash or dermatitis. The recommended procedure outlined in Exhibit 5-1

contains steps to be included when gloves are used. The use of gloves is a matter of personal preference; some staff members prefer to avoid the potential for direct contact with fecal matter. Regardless, hand hygiene with soap and water should be performed after

---

Exhibit 5-1 Changing a Diaper

1. Place the needed supplies (diapers, wipes, ointment) within reach, and if necessary a change of clothes for the child.
2. Place the child on the diapering surface.
3. Remove the child's clothes and soiled diaper.
4. Clean the child's bottom with a premoistened disposable towelette. If the child is female, wipe from front to back.
5. Place the soiled towelette inside the disposable diaper or in a trash receptacle if cloth diapers are used.
6. Place the disposable diaper in a trash receptacle, or place the soiled reusable diaper in the designated diaper pail.
7. If you are wearing gloves, remove and dispose of the gloves in a trash receptacle.
8. Wipe your hands with a premoistened towelette.
9. Diaper and dress the child.
10. Return the child to a safe area. Never leave a child alone on the diapering surface.
11. Clean and disinfect the diapering area.
12. Wash your hands with soap and running water.

Source: Adapted from *The ABC's of Safe and Healthy Child Care,* Centers for Disease Control and Prevention, 1996.

changing a diaper, as proteinaceous material may be present. The hand hygiene guidelines also require using soap and water after using the restroom.

Cleaning and Disinfecting Diaper Changing Areas

Diaper changing areas should be used only for changing diapers. Diaper changing surfaces should be smooth, nonabsorbent, and easy to clean. They should have a raised edge, a low "fence" around the area, or a buckle to prevent the child from falling off. Areas with which children come in close contact during play, such as couches and floor areas, should not be used to change diapers. Diaper changing areas should be cleaned and disinfected on a regular basis and when soiled, as follows:

1. Wipe the surface with a premoistened disposable towelette.
2. Dry the surface with a paper towel.
3. Thoroughly wet the surface with a commercially prepared disinfectant spray or bleach and water solution.
4. Allow the disinfectant to air dry; do not wipe off.

Cleaning and Disinfecting Clothing and Linen

Clothing soiled with bulk fecal material should be washed after the stool is emptied into the toilet, which should be done slowly to avoid splashing. Children's sheets, pillowcases, blankets, and crib mattress pads should be washed weekly and when soiled or wet. If the crib sheet and mattress pad become wet, the crib mattress should be cleaned and disinfected.

Cleaning and Disinfecting "Potty Training" Equipment

If a potty chair is used for toilet training, it should be used in a bathroom area only and, if possible, out of the child's direct reach of the toilet. After the child uses the potty chair, the chair should be emptied into the toilet, with care being taken not to splash or touch the water in the toilet. It should then be rinsed with water and the water poured into the toilet. The chair is not to be rinsed under the faucet of a sink used for food preparation. Finally, the chair should be cleaned and disinfected.

Washing and Disinfecting Toys

If a child has a communicable disease and is on transmission-based precautions, and there are other children in the home, toys should be cleaned and disinfected on a regular basis. Toys that are brought into the home by rehabilitation staff members should be cleaned and disinfected in between patient use as well. Toys that are used by toddlers and older children and that are not placed in the mouth, such as blocks, dolls, tricycles, and trucks, should be cleaned with soap and water on a regular basis or when obviously soiled; for these toys no disinfection is required. To hand wash and disinfect a hard plastic toy or pacifier, the following steps should be taken:

1. Scrub the toy in warm, soapy water. If necessary, use a brush to reach into crevices.
2. Rinse under running hot tap water.
3. Immerse in a mild bleach solution and allow to soak in the solution for a minimum of 10 minutes.
4. Remove from the bleach solution and rinse well in cool water.
5. Air dry.

Alternatively, hard plastic toys can be washed in a dishwasher or in the hot cycle of a washing machine. Items that can be washed in a dishwasher or the hot water cycle of a washing machine do not have to be disinfected, because these machines use water that is hot enough for a long enough period of time to kill most infectious agents. Machine washing in a cold cycle is acceptable if laundry chemicals for cold-water washing are used in the proper concentration (CDC, 2003a). Water-retaining bath toys have been associated with an outbreak of *Pseudomonas aeruginosa* in a pediatric oncology ward (Buttery, Alabaster, Heine, *et al.,* 1998); therefore, these toys should not be shared among other home care patients.

Preparing Infants' Bottles

Two different methods can be used to clean infant bottles, nipples, and bottle collars. Most infant bottles and nipples need only to be cleaned with hot soap and water. The aseptic sterilization method is required only when ordered by the physician and noted on the patient's plan of care.

If the bottles, nipples, and bottle collars are to be cleaned with soap and water, the following method should be followed:

1. Rinse the bottles, nipples, and bottle collars under hot running water.

2. Squeeze a small amount of liquid detergent into each bottle.
3. Scrub the inside of the bottle with a brush, ideally a brush designed for scrubbing infant bottles.
4. Rinse under running hot water.
5. Place the bottles upside down on a clean towel to dry, or place them on a rack designed for air drying infant bottles.
6. Place a small amount of liquid detergent on a sponge, towel, or (ideally) a brush designed for cleaning infant bottle nipples and collars.
7. Rinse the nipples and bottle collars under running hot water, and allow them to air dry.

Bottles, nipples, and bottle collars washed in the hot water cycle of a dishwasher do not need additional disinfection.

If the physician recommends that the bottles be sterilized, the following procedure may be followed:

1. Place all bottles, nipples, and bottle collars in a deep pan.
2. Cover with tap water and boil for 10 minutes.
3. Remove the bottles, nipples, and bottle collars with tongs, and place them on a clean towel with the open ends facing down.

If disposable bottle liners are used, only the nipples and bottle collars need to be sterilized, because the manufacturer sterilizes the plastic bottle liners.

Preparing Infant Formula

Staff should always perform hand hygiene before preparing an infant's formula. The formula should be prepared in bottles that have been either washed in hot water and soap or aseptically sterilized. Unless otherwise noted in the plan of care, the formula may be prepared using bottles that have been cleaned with soap and water. If concentrated liquid or powdered formula is to be used, the following method of preparation is recommended:

1. Boil the water to be used for mixing for at least 5 minutes, and let it cool.
2. Mix the boiled water with the concentrated liquid or powdered formula according to the instructions on the formula label.
3. If applicable, place a disposable bottle liner inside the plastic bottle.
4. Place the nipple on the bottle, and cover it with the bottle collar. If plastic covers are available,

place a cover over the nipple and snap it onto the collar.
5. Cover the formula, and store it in the refrigerator.

Terminal Sterilization

Another technique that can be used to prepare infant formula is called terminal sterilization; this sterilization technique is used only for concentrated formulas (i.e., premixed formulas that are not diluted with water). The steps are as follows:

1. Prepare the formula in clean bottles according to the instructions on the label.
2. Place the nipples upside down on the bottle tops and cover with disks, or put the nipples on upright and cover the nipples with nipple covers.
3. Loosely screw the bottle collars onto the bottles.
4. Using a rack in a large pot or sterilizer, place the bottles in 2 inches of water.
5. Bring the water to a boil, cover, and boil briskly for 10 minutes.
6. Remove the pot or sterilizer from the heat, and let it stand until cool (about 1 hour) before removing the lid.
7. Tighten the bottle collars, and if possible, cover with plastic bottle covers.
8. Place the bottles in the refrigerator.

Infant Formula Storage

Formula made from ready-to-use or concentrated liquid should be used within 48 hours, and formula made from powder should be used within 24 hours. The staff member may prepare enough formula for one feeding or for 24 hours. If the formula is made for one feeding, it should be cooled before the infant is fed. If the infant does not drink all the formula or expressed breast milk in the bottle, the leftover amount should not be returned to the refrigerator for use at the next feeding. It should be poured down the drain, and the bottle and nipple should be rinsed out with hot water and stored until they are washed. When the infant is old enough to eat solid food, the infant food should be poured into a small bowl; the infant should not be fed directly from the infant food jar.

If the staff member accompanies the child out of the home for an extended period of time (e.g., to attend a physician's office visit), an extra bottle of formula or expressed breast milk may need to be taken along. The formula or expressed breast milk should not be left out at room temperature or above 40°F for more than 2 hours. If a longer time before feeding is anticipated, the bottle should be stored on ice or placed in a container with an ice pack. During transport in the summer months, the bottle should be stored in the air-conditioned portion of the vehicle, if possible, to delay melting of the ice.

Human Milk Storage

Expressed breast milk should be placed in a container marked with the date and a notation of any medications taken by the mother. Human milk can be stored in the following ways:

- at room temperature (from 66° to 72°F, or 19° to 22°C) for up to 10 hours
- in a refrigerator (from 32° to 39°F, or 0° to 4°C) for up to 8 days
- in a freezer compartment inside a refrigerator (variable temperature due to the door opening frequently) for up to 2 weeks
- in a freezer compartment with a separate door (variable temperature due to the door opening frequently) for up to 3 to 4 months
- in a separate deep freeze (0°F, or −19°C) for up to 6 months or longer (La Leche League International, 2002)

Thawing Frozen Milk

Frozen milk should be thawed in the refrigerator or by submersion of the container in warm water. Breast milk should never be thawed in a microwave oven, in a pan of boiling water, or by allowing it to stand at room temperature. If milk has been frozen and thawed, it can be refrigerated for up to 24 hours for later use. It should not be refrozen. It is not known whether milk that is left in the bottle after a feeding can be safely kept until the next feeding or if it should be discarded (La Leche League International, 2002). Once the milk has thawed, the container should be shaken gently to blend any fat that has separated.

ANIMAL-ASSISTED ACTIVITIES AND ANIMAL-ASSISTED THERAPY

Many home care programs, especially those that provide hospice services, have established programs that incorporate access to animals as a way to improve the quality of their patients' lives. In programs involving animal-assisted activities and animal-assisted therapy,

a home care or hospice staff member or volunteer brings an animal, such as a dog, cat, or rabbit, to visit the patient at his or her place of residence.

Animal-Assisted Activities

Animal-assisted activities (AAA) provide motivational, educational, recreational, and/or therapeutic benefits to enhance the patient's quality of life. AAA are delivered in a variety of environments by specially trained professionals, paraprofessionals, or volunteers, in association with animals that meet specific criteria. Basically, AAAs are casual "meet and greet" activities that involve pets visiting people. Specific treatment goals are not planned for each visit, volunteers and treatment providers are not required to document the sessions, and the visits can be as long or as short as needed (Delta Society, 2003). An example of an AAA is a visit by a hospice volunteer and his dog to the hospice patients in a contracted nursing home once a month. Although the facility staff is involved in the visits, the hospice team does not set treatment goals for the interactions with the animal.

Animal-Assisted Therapy

Animal-assisted therapy (AAT) is designed to promote improvement in physical, social, emotional, and/or cognitive functioning. Specific goals and objectives for each patient are established. The treatment process is performed by a professional with specialized expertise and incorporated into their scope of services. The patient's progress with regard to the established goals and objectives are measured and documented at each session. For example, if a patient recovering from a stroke has difficulty controlling fine motor skills, an occupational therapist may have the patient manipulate buckles, clasps on leashes, collars, and animal carriers. The patient may also open containers of treats for the dog and feed small pieces of the treats to the dog. The goals of animal-assisted therapy can be any of the following:

- **Physical health**
  Improve fine motor skills
  Improve wheelchair skills
  Improve standing balance
- **Mental health**
  Increase verbal interactions between group members

Increase attention skills (i.e., paying attention or staying on task)

Develop leisure/recreation skills

Increase self-esteem

Reduce anxiety

Reduce loneliness

- **Educational**

Increase vocabulary

Improve long- or short-term memory

Improve knowledge of concepts (e.g., size, color, etc.)

- **Motivational**

Improve willingness to be involved in a group activity

Improve interactions with others

Improve interactions with staff

Increase exercise (Delta Society, 2003)

Difference Between Animal-Assisted Activities and Animal-Assisted Therapy

Although AAAs and AAT may seem similar, AAT is a more formal process and must be characterized by all three of the following criteria:

1. *AAT is directed by professionals as a normal part of their practice* (i.e., physician, occupational therapist, physical therapist, certified therapeutic recreation specialist, nurse, social worker, speech therapist, mental health professional, etc.). For example, a social worker must use the animal in the context of social work. If this same social worker were to visit a group of children on an informal basis, the activity would be considered an AAA.
2. *AAT is goal-directed.* There is a specific end in mind, such as improvement of social skills, range of motion, verbal skills, or attention span. Any visit with an animal may result in the achievement of one or more of these goals. Unless the goals have been identified and defined before the session, the session would not be considered AAT.
3. *AAT is documented.* Each session is documented in the patient's medical record, with the activity and progress noted (Delta Society, 2003).

In the past, anecdotal reports and observations supported the psychological and physical benefits of animal-assisted therapy to patients. More recently, one study found statistical evidence that animal-assisted therapy, even just one 30-minute session per week, was effective in reducing loneliness of residents in long-term care facilities to a statistically significant degree (Banks & Banks, 2002).

Transmission of Zoonotic Diseases

Of the 1400 or so recognized human pathogens, 61% are classified as zoonotic, or naturally communicable between animals and people. Diseases that can cross species barriers and infect humans (e.g., avian flu, monkeypox) are well documented in wild populations of dogs, cats, rodents, turtles, birds and nonhuman primates and in some domesticated companion animals. However, these cases do not necessarily involve healthy, vaccinated, well-cared-for and groomed animals as transmitters of disease. In health care settings, dogs and cats are most commonly encountered animals; however, other animals such as fish, birds, rabbits, reptiles, nonhuman primates, and rodents can serve as sources of zoonotic pathogens that can be transmitted to both the patient and the home or hospice care staff member. For that reason, animals that should not be used for animal-assisted activities or therapy include reptiles, nonhuman primates, rodents, exotic species, wild/domestic animals, and animals less than 1 year old because of their unpredictable behavior (e.g., biting) and problems with elimination control (CDC, 2003a). Animals can also be carriers of antibiotic-resistant bacteria vancomycin-resistant enterococcus (VRE). VRE has been isolated from pets (Devriese *et al,* 1996), and a cat in a geriatric care center was found to be colonized with methcillin-resistant staphaureus (Scott, Thomson et al., 1988). MRSA is an important cause of nosocomial and community-acquired infections worldwide. Dogs and other pets living in close contact with human MRSA carriers can become colonized with MRSA. Van Duijkeren, Wolfhagen, Box, Heck, Wennet, and Fluit reported the first human-to-dog transmission of MRSA in the Netherlands (CDC, 2004). Table 5-1 provides examples of diseases that can be carried by animals and transmitted to humans.

With common sense and some precautions, the benefits of AAAs and AAT usually outweigh the risks. To prevent the transmission of zoonotic diseases, several simple precautions are advised in handling pets or other animals. The most important is to minimize contact with animal saliva, dander, urine, and feces. The

Table 5-1 Examples of Diseases Associated with Zoonotic Transmission

Infectious disease	Cats	Dogs	Fish	Birds	Rabbits	Reptiles[a]	Primates	Rodents[a]
Virus								
Lymphocytic choriomeningitis								+[b]
Rabies	+	+						
Bacteria								
Campylobacteriosis	+	+				+	+	+
Capnocytophaga canimorsus infection	+	+						
Cat scratch disease (Bartonella henselae)	+							
Leptospirosis	+						+	+
Mycobacteriosis			+	+				
Pasteurellosis	+	+			+			
Plague	+			+			+	+
Psittacosis				+				
Q fever (Coxiella burnetti)	+							
Rat bite fever (Spirrillum minus, Streptobacillus monliformis)								+
Salmonellosis	+	+		+	+	+	+	+
Tularemia	+				+			+
Yersiniosis					+	+	+	+
Parasites								
Ancylostomiasis	+	+					+	
Cryptosporidiosis	+							
Giardiasis	+	+					+	
Toxocariasis	+	+					+	
Toxoplasmosis	+	+					+	
Fungi								
Blastomycosis		+						
Dermatophytosis		+			+		+	+

[a]Reptiles include lizards, snakes, and turtles. Rodents include hamsters, mice, and rats.
[b]The + symbol indicates that the pathogen associated with the infection has been isolated from animals and is considered to pose potential risk to humans.

Source: Centers for Disease Control and Prevention. (2003a). *Guidelines for environmental infection control in health-care facilities.* Recommendations of the CDC and the Healthcare Infection Control Practices Advisory Committee (HICPAC). Animals in health-care facilities. Retrieved 1/23/05 from *www.cdc.gov/ncidod/hip/enviro/Enviro_guide_03.pdf.*

following additional guidelines should be followed when an AAA or AAT program is established:

- Animals should have documented proof of current immunizations as recommended by the American Veterinary Medical Association and be on flea, tick, and worm control programs. A veterinarian should evaluate animals with skin rashes. If a fungus or ringworm caused the animal's rash, the animal should be temporarily treated and removed from the program until all lesions are healed.
- Animals must be healthy and free of any signs or symptoms of infection at the time of each visit.

- Animals must be clean and well groomed. To mitigate allergic responses to the animal, bathe the animal within 24 hours of a visit to minimize shedding of animal dander, brush and groom the animal before a visit to remove loose hair or use a therapy animal cape, and clip or blunt the nails at the time of the visit to minimize the potential for injury.
- Animals should be checked for aggression and tolerance with various patients, and their behavior should be monitored.
- All animals should be kept on a leash and be friendly toward children.

- A home care or hospice staff member or volunteer should always be present with the animal, especially when children play with it. Rough play with cats and dogs should be avoided to prevent scratches and bites. Animals should be trained and controlled by persons trained in providing activities or therapies safely and who know the animal's health status and behavior traits. If an incident of biting or scratching by an animal occurs during an AAA or AAT, the scratch, bite, or other break in the skin should be cleaned promptly and the incident should be reported promptly to the appropriate authorities (e.g., infection control staff, the animal program coordinator, local animal control personnel, or the physician). The animal should not be used again for these programs.

At the end of the animal-assisted activity or therapy session, the area should undergo routine cleaning and all those having any animal contact should perform hand hygiene by washing their hands with soap and water, especially if the hands are visibly soiled or contaminated with proteinaceous material, or with an alcohol-based hand rub when the hands are not visibly soiled or contaminated (CDC, 2003a).

PREPARING THE PATIENT'S MEALS
Overview of Foodborne Illnesses

In the United States, an estimated 76 million persons contract foodborne and other acute diarrheal illnesses each year (CDC, 2004a). In addition, foodborne illnesses result in 325,000 hospitalizations and 5200 deaths each year. Known pathogens account for an estimated 14 million illnesses, 60,000 hospitalizations, and 1800 deaths annually (CDC, 2003b). Three pathogens, *Salmonella, Listeria,* and *Toxoplasma,* are responsible for 1500 deaths each year—more than 75% of those caused by known pathogens—whereas unknown agents account for the remaining 62 million illnesses, 265,000 hospitalizations, and 3200 deaths. Overall, foodborne diseases appear to cause more illnesses but fewer deaths than previously estimated (Mead & Slutsker *et al.,* 1999).

When a group of people develop the same illness after ingesting the same food, this is considered a foodborne disease outbreak. Most cases of foodborne disease are single cases not associated with a recognized outbreak. Not all outbreaks or diseases are equally likely to be reported to a public health agency because most cases of foodborne disease are sporadic, and often individuals who develop gastrointestinal symptoms think they have the "stomach flu." More than 250 different diseases can be caused by contaminated food or drink.

The great majority of food items that cause foodborne illnesses are raw or undercooked foods of animal origin, such as meat, unpasteurized milk, eggs, cheese, fish, and shellfish. Harmful bacteria also are commonly present in or on soil, pets, insects, rodents, sneezes, coughs, and unwashed hands. These bacteria can cause problems if they come in contact with food and are allowed to grow. Bacteria can grow rapidly on protein-rich foods such as eggs, milk, and meat, which are usually considered perishable.

Foodborne illness is caused by bacteria or by the toxic substances they produce. For example, *Escherichia coli* 0157:H7 is one of hundreds of strains of the bacterium *E. coli.* Although most strains are harmless and live in the intestines of healthy humans and animals, *E. coli* 0157:H7 produces a powerful toxin and can cause severe illness. A list of foodborne illnesses caused by bacterial sources of contamination is presented in Table 5-2.

The CDC reports that about 85% of all foodborne illnesses are avoidable if appropriate steps are taken and if food is handled properly. Home care staff members can help reduce the hazards of foodborne illness in the patient's home by observing the simple principles of food safety discussed in the next sections.

Shopping for the Patient

If the plan of care includes food shopping for the patient, the following guidelines apply:

- Buy the cold food last, and get it to the patient's home as quickly as possible.
- If other errands need to be performed for the patient, do the grocery shopping last. Never leave perishable food in a hot car.
- Check expiration dates. Buy food only if the "sell-by" or "use-by" date has not expired.
- Buy food in good condition. Make sure that refrigerated food is cold to the touch and that frozen food is rock hard. Canned goods should be free of dents, cracks, or bulging lids, any of which can indicate a serious food poisoning threat.

Table 5-2 Foodborne Illnesses (Bacterial)

Etiology	Incubation period	Signs and symptoms	Duration of illness
Bacillus anthracis	2 days to weeks	Nausea, vomiting, malaise, bloody diarrhea, acute abdominal pain.	Weeks
Bacillus cereus (diarrheal toxin)	10–16 hrs	Abdominal cramps, watery diarrhea, nausea.	24–48 hrs
Bacillus cereus (preformed enterotoxin)	1–6 hrs	Sudden onset of severe nausea and vomiting: diarrhea may be present.	24 hrs
Brucella abortus, B. melitensis, and *B. suis*	7–21 days	Fever, chills, sweating, weakness, headache, muscle and joint pain, diarrhea, bloody stools during acute phase.	Weeks
Campylobacter jejuni	2–5 days	Diarrhea, cramps, fever, and vomiting; diarrhea may be bloody.	2–10 days
Clostridium botulinum children and adults (preformed toxin)	12–72 hrs	Vomiting, diarrhea, blurred vision, diplopia, dysphagia, and descending muscle weakness.	Variable (from days to months). Can be complicated by respiratory failure and death.
Clostridium botulinum infants	3–30 days	In infants <12 months, lethargy, weakness, poor feeding, constipation, hypotonia, poor head control, poor gag and suck.	Variable
Clostridium perfringens toxin	8–16 hrs	Watery diarrhea, nausea, abdominal cramps; fever is rare.	24–48 hrs
Enterohemorrhagic *E. coli* (EHEC), including *E. coli* O157:H7 and other shigatoxin-producing *E. coli* (STEC)	1–8 days	Severe diarrhea that is often bloody, abdominal pain and vomiting. Usually, little or no fever is present. Most common in children <4 years.	5–10 days
Enterotoxigenic *E. coli* (ETEC)	1–3 days	Watery diarrhea, abdominal cramps, some vomiting.	3–>7 days

Please call the state health department for more information on specific foodborne illnesses. These telephone numbers are available at *http://www2.cdc.gov/mmwr/international/relres.html*.

Source: Centers for Disease Control and Prevention. (2001). *Diagnosis and management of foodborne illnesses: A primer for* Physicians Morbidity and Mortality Weekly. Recommendations and reports.

Associated foods	Laboratory testing	Treatment
Insufficiently cooked contaminated meat.	Blood.	Penicillin is first choice for naturally acquired gastrointestinal anthrax. Ciprofloxacin is second option.
Meats, stews, gravies, vanilla sauce.	Testing not necessary, self-limiting (consider testing food and stool for toxin in outbreaks).	Supportive care, self-limiting.
Improperly refrigerated, cooked or fried rice, meats.	Normally a clinical diagnosis. Clinical laboratories do not routinely identify this organism. If indicated, send stool and food specimens to reference laboratory for culture and toxin identification.	Supportive care.
Raw milk, goat cheese made from unpasteurized milk, contaminated meats.	Blood culture and positive serology.	Acute: Rifampin and doxycycline daily for ≥6 weeks. Infections with complications require combination therapy with rifampin, tetracycline and an aminoglycoside.
Raw and undercooked poultry, unpasteurized milk, contaminated water.	Routine stool culture; *Campylobacter* requires special media and incubation at 42°C to grow.	Supportive care. For severe cases, antibiotics such as erythromycin and quinolones may be indicated early in the diarrheal disease. Guillain-Barrè syndrome can be a sequala.
Home-canned foods with a low acid content, improperly canned commercial foods, home-canned or fermented fish, herb-infused oils, baked potatoes in aluminum foil, cheese sauce, bottled garlic, foods held warm for extended periods of time (e.g., in a warm oven).	Stool, serum, and food can be tested for toxin. Stool and food can also be cultured for the organism. These tests can be performed at some state health department laboratories and the CDC.	Supportive care. Botulinum antitoxin is helpful if given early in the course of the illness.
Honey, home-canned vegetables and fruits.	Stool, serum, and food can be tested for toxin. Stool and food can also be cultured for the organism. These tests can be performed at some state health department laboratories and the CDC.	Supportive care. Botulism immuneglobulin can be obtained from the Infant Botulism Prevention Program, Health and Human Services, California. Botulinum antitoxin is generally not recommended for infants.
Meats, poultry, gravy, dried or precooked foods.	Stools can be tested for enterotoxin and cultured for the organism. Because *Clostridium perfringens* can normally be found in stool, quantitative cultures must be done.	Supportive care. Antibiotics not indicated.
Undercooked beef, unpasteurized milk and juice, raw fruits and vegetables (e.g., sprouts), salami, salad dressing, and contaminated water.	Stool culture; *E. coli* O157:H7 requires special media to grow. If *E. coli* O157:H7 is suspected, specific testing must be requested. Shiga toxin testing may be done using commercial kits; positive isolates should be forwarded to public health laboratories for confirmation and serotyping.	Supportive care, monitor renal function, hemoglobin, and platelets closely. Studies indicate that antibiotics may be harmful. *E. coli* O157:H7 infection is also associated with hemolytic uremic syndrome, which can cause lifelong complications.
Water or food contaminated with human feces.	Stool culture. ETEC requires special laboratory techniques for identification. If suspected, must request specific testing.	Supportive care. Antibiotics are rarely needed except in severe cases. Recommended antibiotics include TMP-SMX and quinolones.

(continues)

Table 5-2 Foodborne Illnesses (Bacterial)—*continued*

Etiology	Incubation period	Signs and symptoms	Duration of illness
Listeria monocytogenes	9–48 hrs for gastrointestinal symptoms, 2–6 weeks for invasive disease. At birth and infancy	Fever, muscle aches, and nausea or diarrhea. Pregnant women may have mild flu-like illness, and infection can lead to premature delivery or stillbirth. Elderly or immunocompromised patients may have bacteremia or meningitis. Infants infected from mother at risk for sepsis or meningitis.	Variable
Salmonella spp.	1–3 days	Diarrhea, fever, abdominal cramps, vomiting. *S. typhi* and *S. paratyphi* produce typhoid with insidious onset characterized by fever, headache, constipation, malaise, chills, and myalgia; diarrhea is uncommon, and vomiting is usually not severe.	4–7 days
Shigella spp.	24–48 hrs	Abdominal cramps, fever, and diarrhea. Stools may contain blood and mucus.	4–7 days
Staphylococcus aureus (preformed enterotoxin)	1–6 hrs	Sudden onset of severe nausea and vomiting. Abdominal cramps. Diarrhea and fever may be present.	24–48 hrs
Vibrio cholerae (toxin)	24–72 hrs	Profuse watery diarrhea and vomiting, which can lead to severe dehydration and death within hours.	3–7 days. Causes life-threatening dehydration.
Vibrio parahaemolyticus	2–48 hrs	Watery diarrhea, abdominal cramps, nausea, vomiting.	2–5 days
Vibrio vulnificus	1–7 days	Vomiting, diarrhea, abdominal pain, bacteremia, and wound infections. Most common in the immunocompromised or in patients with chronic liver disease (presenting with bullous skin lesions).	2–8 days; can be fatal in patients with liver disease and the immunocompromised.
Yersinia enterocolytica and *Y. pseudotuberculosis*	24–48 hrs	Appendicitis-like symptoms (diarrhea and vomiting, fever, and abdominal pain) occur primarily in older children and young adults. May have a scarlitiniform rash with *Y. pseudotuberculosis*.	1–3 weeks

Associated foods	Laboratory testing	Treatment
Fresh soft cheeses, unpasteurized milk, inadequate pasteurized milk, ready-to-eat deli meats, hot dogs.	Blood or cerebrospinal fluid cultures. Asymptomatic fecal carriage occurs; therefore, stool culture usually not helpful. Antibody to listerolysin O may be helpful to identify outbreak retrospectively.	Supportive care and antibiotics; Intravenous ampicillin, penicillin, or TMP-SMX are recommended for invasive disease.
Contaminated eggs, poultry, unpasteurized milk or juice, cheese, contaminated raw fruits and vegetables (alfalfa sprouts, melons). *S. typhi* epidemics are often related to fecal contamination of water supplies or street-vended foods.	Routine stool cultures.	Supportive care. Other than for *S. typhi*, antibiotics are not indicated unless there is extra-intestinal spread, or the risk of extra-intestinal spread, or the infection. Consider ampicillin, gentamicin, TMP-SMX, or quinolones if indicated. A vaccine exists for *S. typhi*.
Food or water contaminated with fecal material. Usually person-to-person spread, fecal-oral transmission. Ready-to-eat foods touched by infected food workers, raw vegetables, egg salads.	Routine stool cultures.	Supportive care. TMP/SMX recommended in the U.S. if organism is susceptible; nalidixic acid or other quinolones maybe indicated if organism is resistant, especially in developing countries.
Unrefrigerated or improperly refrigerated meats, potato and egg salads, cream pastries.	Normally a clinical diagnosis. Stool, vomitus, and food can be tested for toxin and cultured if indicated.	Supportive care.
Contaminated water, fish, shellfish, street-vended food.	Stool culture; *Vibrio cholerae* requires special media to grow. If *V. cholerae* is suspected, must request specific testing.	Supportive care with aggressive oral and intravenous rehydration. In cases of confirmed cholera, tetracycline or doxycycline is recommended for adults, and TMP-SMX for children (<8 years).
Undercooked or raw seafood, such as fish, shellfish.	Stool cultures. *Vibrio parahaemolyticus* requires special media to grow. If *V. parahaemolyticus* is suspected, must request specific testing.	Supportive care. Antibiotics are recommended in severe cases: tetracycline, doxycycline, gentamicin, and cefotaxime.
Undercooked or raw shellfish, especially oysters; other contaminated seafood; open wounds exposed to sea water.	Stool, wound, or blood cultures. *Vibrio vulnificus* requires special media to grow. If *V. vulnificus* is suspected, must request specific testing.	Supportive care and antibiotics; tetracycline, doxycycline, and ceftazidime are recommended.
Undercooked pork, unpasteurized milk, contaminated water. Infection has occurred in infants whose caregivers handled chitterlings, tofu.	Stool, vomitus, or blood culture. *Yersinia* requires special media to grow. If suspected, must request specific testing. Serology is available in research and reference laboratories.	Supportive care, usually self-limiting. If septicemia or other invasive disease occurs, antibiotic therapy with gentamicin or cefotaxime (doxycycline and ciprofloxacin also effective).

Food Storage in the Patient's Home

The following are recommended guidelines for storing food in the patient's home:

- Keep the food safe and refrigerated. If indicated in the plan of care, regularly clean the refrigerator's inside surfaces with hot soapy water.
- Suggest that the patient keep the refrigerator as cold as possible without freezing the milk or lettuce. The refrigerator should be set at 40°F or cooler, and the freezer should be set at 0°F. Freeze fresh meat, poultry, and fish immediately if the patient will not consume them within a few days. If milk spoils in 1 week, the refrigerator is too warm.
- Keep all foods wrapped or in covered containers, and make sure the containers are shut tightly.
- Place leftovers in small containers for quick cooling.
- Remove stuffing from poultry or other stuffed meats, and refrigerate the meat and stuffing in separate containers.
- Do not leave leftovers out of the refrigerator for extended periods of time.
- Keep frozen foods in their original wrapping.
- When in doubt, throw it out.

Preparing the Patient's Food

Most foodborne illnesses are caused by the mishandling of food. Cross-contamination can occur when bacteria from one source are transferred to another source. Sponges and kitchen towels used for cleaning can harbor bacteria and lead to cross-contamination. Kitchen towels, sponges, and cloths used in meal preparation and cleaning should be washed often. Sponges should be placed in the dishwasher during every load and should be replaced every few weeks. Cross-contamination can also occur in unexpected places, such as the refrigerator door handle, sink faucet handle, stove knobs, microwave oven handle, highchair, and appliance handles. Grooves in cutting boards can harbor bacteria. Vegetables and salad ingredients should not be cut on a cutting board used for raw meat unless the board has been washed with hot soapy water and disinfected. After contact with meat, poultry, or dairy products, cutting boards can be disinfected with a solution of 2 teaspoons liquid bleach in 1 quart water and rinsed thoroughly or wiped off with a disinfectant-saturated cloth. Blenders and can openers also should

be washed by hand or in the dishwasher each time they are used. The same utensils should not be used to prepare more than one food. For example, one knife should be used to cut up chicken and another one to dice the potatoes. Figure 5-1 shows how cross-contamination can occur.

The following guidelines should be followed for preparing the patient's food:

- Wash hands with running water and soap for 15 seconds before handling food.
- Keep all food preparation items clean.
- Do not leave food between 40° and 140°F for more than 2 hours, and do not thaw foods between 40° and 140°F.
- Do not eat or taste any food before it is cooked.
- Wear non-latex examination gloves if there are any cuts or sores on the hands.
- Keep raw meat, poultry, and fish and their juices, away from other food.
- Marinade meats in the refrigerator and discard any leftover marinade.

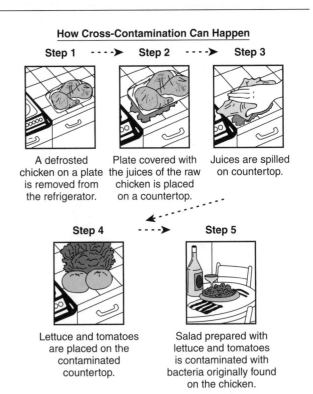

Figure 5-1 Cross-contamination happens when bacteria from one source are transferred to another source, usually inadvertently and unknowingly.

Courtesy of Reckitt & Coleman, Inc., Wayne, New Jersey.

- Thaw food in the microwave or refrigerator, not on the kitchen counter, because bacteria can grow on the outside of food before the inside thaws. An alternative is to cook the food while it is still frozen.
- Check poultry and seafood for stale odors before cooking.
- Wash all fresh fruits and vegetables with cold water.
- Turn your face away, or cover your mouth and nose with a tissue, if you sneeze or cough when preparing food. Then perform hand hygiene again.
- Keep uncooked meats separate from vegetables and from cooked and ready-to-eat foods.
- Stuff a turkey or chicken just before roasting it.
- Do not use cracked eggs.

Cooking and Serving the Patient's Food

These guidelines are recommended for cooking and serving food for the patient:

- Bring sauces, soups, and gravies to a boil. Heat leftovers thoroughly to 165°F.
- Never partially cook meats or casseroles on one day and finish cooking them on another.
- Use a meat thermometer, if the patient has one, to check that the meat is cooked all the way through. Beef, veal, and lamb should reach 160°F, pork should reach 160° to 170°F, and poultry should reach 165° to 180°F.
- Roast meat and poultry at an oven temperature of 325°F or higher.
- Check that the food is cooked enough or is done. Red meat will be brown or gray inside, poultry juices will be clear, and fish will flake with a fork.
- Cook eggs until the yolk and white are firm and no longer runny. Scrambled eggs should have a firm texture.
- If a large quantity of food is cooked for the patient to use later, divide large portions into small, shallow containers for refrigeration. This ensures safe, rapid cooling.
- Never leave food that needs to be refrigerated out for more than 2 hours.
- Use clean dishes and utensils to serve the food, not the dishes used to prepare it.
- Serve grilled food on a clean plate, not one that held raw meat, poultry, or fish.

Microwaving the Patient's Food

Microwaving can leave cold spots in food, where bacteria can survive. The following guidelines will prevent cold spots and ensure that microwaved food is thoroughly cooked:

- Cover the food with a lid or plastic wrap so that steam can aid thorough cooking. Vent the wrap so that it does not touch the food.
- Stir and rotate the food for even cooking. If the microwave does not have a turntable, rotate the dish by hand once or twice during cooking.
- If the microwave cooking instructions require that the food stand for a certain amount of time before eating, make sure that the stand time is observed, because this time is needed to complete cooking.
- Insert an oven temperature probe or a meat thermometer into the food at several spots to check that the food is done.
- If the microwave defrost setting is used to thaw food, cook the food immediately after defrosting.

What If the Patient's Power Goes Out?

If the power goes out and will be coming back on fairly soon, food will last longer if the refrigerator door is kept shut as much as possible. If the power will be off for an extended period, the food should be taken to another freezer, or some other method should be sought to keep the food frozen. Otherwise, it will need to be thrown out. Without power, the refrigerator section should keep food cool for 4 to 6 hours, depending on the kitchen temperature. A full, well-functioning freezer unit or upright or chest freezer should keep food frozen for 2 days. A half-full freezer should keep food frozen for 1 day. After the power comes back on, food that still contains ice crystals or that feels refrigerator-cold can be refrozen. Any thawed food that has risen to room temperature and remained there for 2 hours or more should be discarded. Any food or drink with a strange color or odor must be discarded immediately (USDA, 2004).

Immunocompromised Patients

Persons at high risk for infection should avoid soft cheeses such as feta, brie, camembert; blue-veined cheeses; and Mexican-style cheeses. Hard cheeses, processed cheeses, cream cheese, cottage cheese, and yogurt do not need to be avoided. Cold cuts should be thoroughly reheated before eating. Fruit that the patient will eat raw should be peeled after washing (CDC, 2003c).

Health Department Warnings

If the health department issues a warning to boil water, the water should be maintained at a rolling boil for 1 minute to kill *Cryptosporidium parvum* and other or-

ganisms. After the boiled water cools, it should be placed in a clean bottle or pitcher with a lid and stored in the refrigerator. This water should be used for drinking, cooking, or making ice. Water bottles and ice trays should be cleaned with soap and water before use. The inside of the bottle or tray should not be touched after cleaning (CDC, 2004b).

REFERENCES

Banks, M., & Banks, W. (2002). The effects of animal-assisted therapy on loneliness in an elderly population in long-term care facilities. *The Journals of Gerontology Series A: Biological Sciences and Medical Sciences, 57,* M428–M432.

Buttery, J. P., Alabaster, S. J., Heine, R. G., Scott, S. M., Crutchfield, R. A., Garland, S. M. (1998). Multiresistant *Pseudomonas aeruginosa* outbreak in a pediatric oncology ward related to bath toys. *Pediatr Infect Dis J., 17*(6), 509–513.

Centers for Disease Control and Prevention. (2004a). Preliminary FoodNet data on the incidence of infection with pathogens transmitted commonly through food—Selected sites, United States, 2003. April 30, 2004, *53*(16), 338–343.

Centers for Disease Control and Prevention. (2004b). Water quality. June 1, 2004. Retrieved 1/25/05, from *www.bt.cdc.gov/disasters/floods/water.asp.*

Centers for Disease Control and Prevention. (2003a). Guidelines for environmental infection control in health-care facilities. Recommendations of CDC and the Healthcare Infection Control Practices Advisory Committee (HICPAC). Animals in health-care facilities. Retrieved 7/1/04, from *www.cdc.gov/ncidod/hip/enviro/Enviro_guide_03.pdf.*

Centers for Disease Control and Prevention. (2003b). December 2003. Foodborne illness. Retrieved 1/23/05, from *www.cdc.gov/ncidod/dbmd/diseaseinfo/foodborneinfections_t.htm.*

Centers for Disease Control and Prevention. (2003c). September 2003. Foodborne illness. Retrieved 1/23/05, from *www.cdc.gov/ncidod/dbmd/diseaseinfo/foodborneinfections_g.htm.*

Centers for Disease Control and Prevention. (2001). *Diagnosis and management of foodborne illnesses: A primer for* Physicians Morbidity and Mortality Weekly. Recommendations and reports. January 26, 2001 / 50(RR02); 1–69.

Guidelines for preventing opportunistic infections among hematopoietic stem cell transplant recipients. Recommendations of the CDC, the Infectious Disease Society of America, and the American Society of Blood and Marrow Transplantation. *Morbidity and Mortality Weekly Report.* Recommendations and Reports. 2004;53(18): 383–406.

Delta Society. (2003). About animal-assisted activities & animal-assisted therapy. Retrieved 1/23/05, from *http://www.deltasociety.org/aboutaaat.htm.*

Devriese, L. A., Ieven, M., Goosossens, H., Vandamme, P., Pot, B., Hommez, J., Haesebrouk, F. *et al.* (1996). Presence of vancomycin-resistant enterococci in farm and pet animals. *Antimicrobic Agents and Chemotherapy 40*(10):2285–2287.

Duncan, S. (2000). APIC State of the Art Report: The implications of service animals in health care settings. *American Journal of Infection Control, 28,* 170–180.

La Leche League International. (2002). Human milk storage. Retrieved 1/23/05, from *www.lalecheleague.org/FAQ/milkstorage.html.*

Mead, P., Slutsker, L., Dietz, V., McCaig, L., Bresee, J., Shapiro, C., Griffin, P., Tauxe, R. (1999). Food-related illness and death in the United States. *Emerging Infectious Diseases, 5*(5), 607–625. Retrieved 1/23/05, from *www.cdc.gov/ncidod/eid/vol5no5/pdf/mead.pdf.*

Scott, G., Thomson, R., Malone-Lee J., Ridgeway G. (1988). Cross-infection between animals and man: Possible feline transmission of *Staphylococcus aureus* infection in humans? *Journal of Hospital Infection 12,* 29–34.

United States Department of Agriculture (USDA). (2004). Food Safety and Inspection Service. Focus on freezing. Retrieved 1/23/05, from *www.fsis.usda.gov/fact_sheets/Focus_On_Freezing/index.asp.*

van Dujikeren, E., Wolfhagen, M., Box, A., Heck, M., Wennet, W., Fluit, A. (December 2004). Human-to-dog transmission of methicillian-resistant *Staphylococcus aureus. Emerging Infectious Diseases.* Retrieved 1/23/05, from *http://www.cdc.sou/ncidod/EID/vollono12/04-0387.htm.*

CHAPTER 6

Personal Protective Equipment and Staff Supplies

USE OF PERSONAL PROTECTIVE EQUIPMENT

The Occupational Safety and Health Administration (OSHA) codified universal precautions to protect health care workers against the risk of bloodborne disease with the Occupational Exposure to Bloodborne Pathogen regulations (OSHA, 1991). These regulations prescribe the use of personal protective equipment (PPE) when blood and other potentially infectious materials are handled. There are many model exposure control plans available on the World Wide Web, many from state health departments and others from proprietary sources. As outlined in Chapter 13, OSHA also has revised its regulations related to the selection of equipment to prevent needlestick injuries. Consideration of these regulations should be included in the formulation of a bloodborne pathogen exposure control plan (OSHA, 2001). The Needlestick Safety and Prevention Act requires that an employer consider means to prevent sharp and needlestick injuries within the context of a bloodborne pathogen exposure control plan. Such consideration includes identification of new medical procedures as well as devices that may reduce the risk of worker injury. All health care providers, including home and hospice care organizations, must solicit from nonmanagement employees responsible for provision of patient care input regarding the identification, evaluation, and selection of safer medical devices for sharp injury prevention. This input should be documented. As outlined in Chapter 13, it is required that sharps injuries be documented in a log, with information including type of device, location of the incident, and description of the event.

NEEDLESTICK PREVENTION EQUIPMENT DESIGN

Home and hospice care staff members, caregivers, and patients are at risk of needlestick injuries in the home. Although OSHA cannot regulate the types of sharps purchased and used in the home by patients and family members and subsequently used by home care staff members (OSHA, 2000), it does require that home and hospice care organizations purchase safe medical devices for use by staff (OSHA, 2001). In a study of a blood exposure in home and hospice care, the authors found a rate of 2.8 blood contacts per 1000 procedures and 0.6 percutaneous injuries (Beltrami, McArthur *et al.,* 2000). When comparing this to the results of a study of health care workers in other settings, the researchers concluded that the risk for exposure to bloodborne pathogens in home care is of real concern. Thus, identifying and obtaining safer devices is very important in home and hospice care.

GLOVES

Since the inception of universal/Standard Precautions, the use of gloves as a protective barrier has increased dramatically. Even so, microbial contamination and the transmission of infection have been reported while a health care worker was wearing gloves. It is recognized that wearing gloves creates a warm, moist environment that may support the growth of microorganisms. In addition, gloves frequently develop microscopic holes. Therefore, after gloves are removed, hand hygiene should be performed (CDC, 2002). Gloves should never be considered a substitute for hand hygiene; rather, they should be used as an adjunct to it.

Types of Gloves

Disposable gloves are made from different types of materials, such as natural rubber (e.g., latex) or synthetic materials (e.g., vinyl). Clean, nonsterile, intact disposable gloves of appropriate size and quality for the home care procedure to be performed should be available for each staff member. Should a home or hospice care staff member exhibit an allergy to standard powdered latex gloves, other types of gloves not containing latex must be made available to that individual by the home or hospice care organization. Generally, nonsterile examination gloves are worn, but sterile gloves should be worn when a procedure requires aseptic technique, such as during the insertion of an indwelling urinary catheter.

When to Wear Gloves

OSHA (1991) mandates that gloves be worn when there is a reasonable likelihood of hand contact with blood or other potentially infectious material, mucus membranes, or nonintact skin as well as when vascular access procedures are being performed and contaminated items or surfaces are being handled. The term *reasonable likelihood* is open to interpretation and may result in varying policies and procedures among different home or hospice care organizations. The home or hospice care organization's bloodborne pathogen exposure control plan should outline the situations in which staff members are required to wear gloves. Generally, staff members should wear gloves when:

- handling blood and other potentially infectious materials that are visibly contaminated with blood
- when having contact with mucus membranes
- handling or touching contaminated items or surfaces
- performing any invasive procedure, including venous access procedures and heelsticks or fingersticks
- performing wound care
- staff members' hands are chapped, cut, scratched, or abraded
- contamination is likely with uncooperative or combative patients
- touching the patient's abraded or nonintact skin
- providing care for a patient with active bleeding
- handling any drainage collection appliance
- taking a rectal temperature

- obtaining or handling laboratory specimens
- there is the possibility of exposure to blood or body fluids

Gloves are not necessary when routine injections are given as long as hand contact with blood or other potentially infectious material is not anticipated. If bleeding is anticipated and the staff member is required to clean the site after the injection, gloves must be worn. Additionally, if the patient's skin is abraded, gloves must be worn (OSHA, 1992b).

If a home care organization provides maternal and child services in which staff members will be teaching new mothers about breastfeeding and observing or coaching return breastfeeding demonstrations, gloves do not need to be worn because breast milk is not included in OSHA's definition of potentially infectious material. OSHA has determined that gloves should be worn if contact with breast milk will be frequent, such as in milk banking (OSHA, 1992a).

When Gloves Should Be Changed or Removed

Gloves should be changed between tasks and procedures on the same patient, after contact with material that may contain a high concentration of microorganisms (e.g., during changing and cleaning of an incontinent patient's bed or removing an old dressing), and after contact with infective material that may have high concentrations of bacteria or virus. In addition, gloves should be removed and changed when the integrity of the gloves is in doubt (e.g., if the gloves are torn or punctured) and between patient care procedures as soon as safety permits. Gloves should be removed as soon after the task is completed to avoid cross-contamination. Hands should not touch potentially contaminated environmental surfaces or items in the patient's room after the gloves are removed, and hand hygiene should be performed to prevent the transfer of microorganisms to others and the environment. Disposable, single-use gloves should not be washed or decontaminated for reuse.

Latex Allergies

Many home and hospice care staff members are allergic to latex gloves. The signs and symptoms of an allergic reaction to latex gloves and other natural rubber products may include skin rash; hives; nasal, eye, or sinus symptoms; asthma; and (rarely) shock. These allergic reactions are mainly due to the proteins that fasten to the powder used in some latex gloves that can cause reactions through contact or breathing. Table 6-1 contains lists of items commonly used in home care that contain latex. Options with traditional latex include extra-thin gloves (which allow for more sensitivity in palpation), gloves with texture for handling breakable items, and powder-free gloves to reduce allergic reactions. Nylon or cotton glove liners are available, but because hands perspire when in gloves, the protective factor can be lost.

Preventing Allergic Reactions to Latex in the Workplace

Latex allergy may be prevented if the home or hospice care organization adopts policies to protect staff members from undue latex exposure. The goal is to reduce exposure to allergy-causing proteins (antigens). The National Institute for Occupational Safety and Health (NIOSH) recommends that home and hospice care organizations take the following steps to protect staff members from latex exposure and allergy (NIOSH, 1997):

- Provide staff members with nonlatex gloves to use when there is little potential for contact with infectious materials.
- If latex gloves are chosen for barrier protection, provide reduced-protein, powder-free gloves.
- Provide staff members with educational programs and training materials about latex allergy.
- Periodically screen high-risk staff members for latex allergy symptoms. Detecting symptoms early and removing symptomatic staff members from

latex exposure are essential for preventing long-term health effects.
- Evaluate current prevention strategies whenever a worker is diagnosed with latex allergy.

Staff members with ongoing exposure to latex should take the following steps to protect themselves (NIOSH, 1997):

- Use nonlatex gloves for activities that are not likely to involve contact with infectious materials.
- Choose powder-free latex gloves with reduced protein content.
- Avoid using oil-based creams or lotions when wearing latex gloves unless they have been shown to reduce latex-related problems.
- Recognize the symptoms of latex allergy: skin rashes; hives; flushing; itching; nasal, eye, or sinus symptoms; asthma; and shock.
- Avoid direct contact with latex gloves and products if symptoms of latex allergy develop until a physician experienced in treating latex allergy can be seen.

Consult a physician regarding the following precautions:

- avoiding contact with latex gloves and products
- avoiding areas where powder from the latex gloves worn by others might be inhaled
- telling the home care organization's management about the latex allergy
- wearing a medical alert bracelet
- taking advantage of all latex allergy education and training provided by the home care organization

Table 6-1 Products Containing Latex

Medical equipment	Personal protective equipment	Office supplies	Medical supplies
Blood pressure cuffs	Gloves	Adhesive tape	Condom-style urinary collection device
Breathing circuits	Goggles	Erasers	Enema tubing tips
Stethoscopes	Rubber aprons	Rubber bands	Injection ports
	Surgical masks		IV tubing
	Gowns		Oral and nasal airways
			Rubber tops of multidose vials
			Syringes
			Tourniquets
			Urinary catheters
			Wound drains

Source: Reprinted from *Preventing allergic reactions to natural rubber latex in the workplace.* The Centers for Disease Control and Prevention, National Institute for Occupational Safety and Health Alert, Atlanta, GA, June 1997.

MASKS, RESPIRATORY PROTECTION, EYE PROTECTION, AND FACE SHIELDS

Face masks, goggles, and face shields can be used alone or in combination to prevent exposure to bloodborne pathogens and other infectious agents that may be encountered during patient care activities. The type of mask selected depends on the purpose of the mask. In some instances, masks and other facial protection are worn to prevent exposure of mucus membrane (i.e., mouth, nose, eyes) to bloodborne pathogens. Such an exposure might occur during tracheal suctioning. In other situations, a mask is worn to prevent exposure to an infectious agent that is droplet spread (refer to Chapter 8). To protect home and hospice care staff from droplet-spread infections, there are two types of masks available for use in health care settings: surgical masks and procedure or isolation masks. The Food and Drug Administration (FDA) requires that surgical masks be fluid-resistant. Home and hospice care organizations should select the masks most suitable to the needs of their staff.

The next level of respiratory protection is referred to as respiratory protection. Respirators, rather than masks, are recommended to provide protection from airborne pathogens such as active pulmonary tuberculosis. The CDC (CDC, 2004) recommends the use of a NIOSH-approved N95 respiratory protective device when caring for patients with airborne infections. In addition to tuberculosis, illnesses in this category include severe acute respiratory syndrome (SARS), smallpox, and viral hemorrhagic fevers (CDC, 2004). There is no data to recommend the use of an N95 respirator for other airborne infections such as chickenpox and measles.

When to Wear a Mask

The staff member should wear a surgical face mask and goggles or a face shield when home or hospice care procedures are likely to generate splashes or sprays of blood or other body fluids, as outlined by OSHA (OSHA, 1991) and for compliance with Standard Precautions (CDC, 2004). For protection against droplet-borne illnesses such as influenza or pertussis, the home care staff can use surgical masks when working within 3 feet of the infected patient or family member (CDC, 2005). The home or hospice care staff member should wear a NIOSH-approved N95 respiratory protective device when entering the home of a patient (or family/household member) with suspected or confirmed active pulmonary tuberculosis, until the patient is no longer infectious. N95 respirators are also recommended for the care of patients with smallpox, SARS, and viral hemorrhagic fevers while in the contagious state (CDC, 2004).

N95 respiratory protective devices classified as disposable may be reused by the same home care staff member as long as they remain functional (CDC, 1994). The manufacturer's guidelines should be followed for inspecting, cleaning, and maintaining respirators, to ensure that the N95 respiratory protective device continues to function properly. Masks and eye protection should be put on before gloving and taken off after removal of contaminated gloves.

Gowns

Gowns appropriate to the activity and amount of fluid likely to be encountered should be worn when splashing of clothing or skin with blood or other potentially infectious material is likely to occur during patient care activities. Gowns should be worn when direct contact with the patient's body fluids and soiling of clothing are likely. If the patient is cared for using Contact Precautions, gowns should be worn for patient care activities (e.g., bathing the patient) that could lead to the contamination of the home or hospice care staff member's clothing.

Gowns should be made of or lined with impervious material, should protect all areas of exposed skin, and should prevent soiling of clothing during home or hospice care procedures. If a garment becomes soiled with blood or other potentially infectious material, it should be removed immediately or as soon as feasible, and the hands should be washed to prevent the spread of microorganisms. Gowns made of single-layer polyolefin films offer the most protection but are uncomfortable because the fabric does not breathe. Reinforced gowns made of a combination material that includes polyolefin film offer the next-best level of protection. Cotton and cotton-polyester blends offer the least protection because they have limited fluid protection.

Donning and Removing Personal Protective Equipment

Nurses and other home care and hospice staff are frequently concerned about the correct order in which to put on PPE as well as how to remove it in the best manner, to avoid contamination of their hands as well as the environment. To address this concern, the CDC has published two helpful figures outlining donning, and removal of PPE (Figures 6-1 and 6-2). These instructive illustrations can be used to train staff on the

SEQUENCE FOR DONNING PERSONAL PROTECTIVE EQUIPMENT (PPE)

The type of PPE used will vary based on the level of precautions required; e.g., Standard and Contact, Droplet or Airborne Infection Isolation.

1. GOWN
- Fully cover torso from neck to knees, arms to end of wrists, and wrap around the back
- Fasten in back of neck and waist

2. MASK OR RESPIRATOR
- Secure ties or elastic bands at middle of head and neck
- Fit flexible band to nose bridge
- Fit snug to face and below chin
- Fit-check respirator

3. GOGGLES OR FACE SHIELD
- Place over face and eyes and adjust to fit

4. GLOVES
- Extend to cover wrist of isolation gown

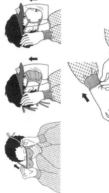

USE SAFE WORK PRACTICES TO PROTECT YOURSELF AND LIMIT THE SPREAD OF CONTAMINATION
- Keep hands away from face
- Limit surfaces touched
- Change gloves when torn or heavily contaminated
- Perform hand hygiene

SECUENCIA PARA PONERSE EL EQUIPO DE PROTECCIÓN PERSONAL (PPE)

El tipo de PPE que se debe utilizar depende del nivel de precaución que sea necesario; por ejemplo, equipo Estándar y de Contacto o de Aislamiento de infecciones transportadas por gotas o por aire.

1. BATA
- Cubra con la bata todo el torso desde el cuello hasta las rodillas, los brazos hasta la muñeca y dóblela alrededor de la espalda
- Átesela por detrás a la altura del cuello y la cintura

2. MÁSCARA O RESPIRADOR
- Asegúrese los cordones o la banda elástica en la mitad de la cabeza y en el cuello
- Ajústese la banda flexible en el puente de la nariz
- Acomódesela en la cara y por debajo del mentón
- Verifique el ajuste del respirador

3. GAFAS PROTECTORAS O CARETAS
- Colóquesela sobre la cara y los ojos y ajústela

4. GUANTES
- Extienda los guantes para que cubran la parte del puño en la bata de aislamiento

UTILICE PRÁCTICAS DE TRABAJO SEGURAS PARA PROTEGERSE USTED MISMO Y LIMITAR LA PROPAGACIÓN DE LA CONTAMINACIÓN
- Mantenga las manos alejadas de la cara
- Limite el contacto con superficies
- Cambie los guantes si se rompen o están demasiado contaminados
- Realice la higiene de las manos

Figure 6-1 Donning Personal Protective Equipment

SEQUENCE FOR REMOVING PERSONAL PROTECTIVE EQUIPMENT (PPE)

Except for respirator, remove PPE at doorway or in anteroom. Remove respirator after leaving patient room and closing door.

1. GLOVES
- Outside of gloves is contaminated!
- Grasp outside of glove with opposite gloved hand; peel off
- Hold removed glove in gloved hand
- Slide fingers of ungloved hand under remaining glove at wrist
- Peel glove off over first glove
- Discard gloves in waste container

2. GOGGLES OR FACE SHIELD
- Outside of goggles or face shield is contaminated!
- To remove, handle by head band or ear pieces
- Place in designated receptacle for reprocessing or in waste container

3. GOWN
- Gown front and sleeves are contaminated!
- Unfasten ties
- Pull away from neck and shoulders, touching inside of gown only
- Turn gown inside out
- Fold or roll into a bundle and discard

4. MASK OR RESPIRATOR
- Front of mask/respirator is contaminated — DO NOT TOUCH!
- Grasp bottom, then top ties or elastics and remove
- Discard in waste container

PERFORM HAND HYGIENE IMMEDIATELY AFTER REMOVING ALL PPE

SECUENCIA PARA QUITARSE EL EQUIPO DE PROTECCIÓN PERSONAL (PPE)

Con la excepción del respirador, quítese el PPE en la entrada de la puerta o en la antesala. Quítese el respirador después de salir de la habitación del paciente y de cerrar la puerta.

1. GUANTES
- ¡El exterior de los guantes está contaminado!
- Agarre la parte exterior del guante con la mano opuesta en la que todavía tiene puesto el guante y quíteselo
- Sostenga el guante que se quitó con la mano enguantada
- Deslice los dedos de la mano sin guante por debajo del otro guante que no se ha quitado todavía a la altura de la muñeca
- Quítese el guante de manera que acabe cubriendo el primer guante
- Arroje los guantes en el recipiente de deshechos

2. GAFAS PROTECTORAS O CARETA
- ¡El exterior de las gafas protectoras o de la careta está contaminado!
- Para quitárselas, tómelas por la parte de la banda de la cabeza o de las piezas de las orejas
- Colóquelas en el recipiente designado para reprocesar materiales o de materiales de deshecho

3. BATA
- ¡La parte delantera de la bata y las mangas están contaminadas!
- Desate los cordones
- Tocando solamente el interior de la bata, pásela por encima del cuello y de los hombros
- Voltee la bata al revés
- Dóblela o enróllela y deséchela

4. MÁSCARA O RESPIRADOR
- La parte delantera de la máscara o respirador está contaminada — ¡NO LA TOQUE!
- Primero agarre la parte de abajo, luego los cordones o banda elástica de arriba y por último quítese la máscara o respirador
- Arrójela en el recipiente de deshechos

EFECTÚE LA HIGIENE DE LAS MANOS INMEDIATAMENTE DESPUÉS DE QUITARSE CUALQUIER EQUIPO DE PROTECCIÓN PERSONAL

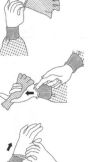
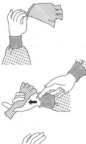
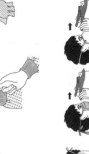
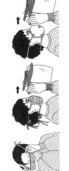
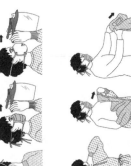
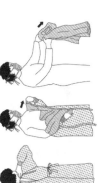
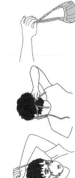
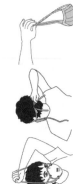
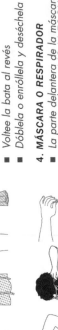
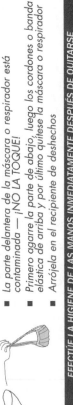

Figure 6-2 Removing Personal Protective Equipment

use of PPEs and can be incorporated into organizational procedures.

RESUSCITATION EQUIPMENT

One-way valve pocket masks, resuscitation bags, or other ventilation devices should be made available to minimize the risk of unprotected mouth-to-mouth resuscitation. Each staff member should have one-way valve resuscitation equipment in his or her possession during home visits to use in the resuscitation of patients. Disposable airway devices are preferred and should not be used on more than one patient.

PATIENT TRANSPORT OUTSIDE THE HOME

Patients infected with virulent or epidemiologically important organisms (e.g., SARS or pulmonary tuberculosis) should leave their homes only for essential purposes, such as dialysis, physician office visits, or emergency department visits, to reduce the opportunities for transmission of microorganisms. When the patient must leave the home, it is important that he or she wears a barrier (e.g., a surgical mask or a dressing over a wound) to reduce the potential spread of infection to susceptible persons with whom the patient may come in contact. The patient also should be instructed about precautions he or she can take to prevent the spread of infection. When staff are aware, the physician office and/or emergency department personnel should be notified of the patient's impending arrival and any precautions that they must take to reduce the risk of transmission of microorganisms.

STAFF MEMBER ACCESS TO PERSONAL PROTECTIVE EQUIPMENT

If staff members take a supply bag with them into the patient's home when they visit, it is not necessary that each individual member have every type of personal protective equipment. What is most important is that the equipment is available to the staff member in the home. For example, for a private-duty home care case involving 24-hour coverage by registered nurses, licensed practical nurses, or licensed vocational nurses for a ventilator-dependent patient, the home care organization may place in the home a box of nonsterile gloves, goggles, gowns, resuscitation equipment, and any other supplies for use by staff. As another example,

each staff member does not need to be issued his or her own N95 respiratory protective device to bring to every home visit. As long as the staff member is provided with an N95 respiratory protective device that is seal-checked before making a home visit for which such respiratory protection is necessary, that is sufficient.

Many organizations provide each staff member an "OSHA kit," or "PPE kit," which contains all the personal protective equipment that may be needed during a home visit. The type of personal protective equipment provided to each staff member will vary based on the likelihood of exposure to blood and other potentially infectious body fluids. The risk of occupational exposure is greater for a nurse or a home health aide, for instance, than it is for a social worker or a hospice chaplain. If a professional or nonprofessional staff member is expected to perform cardiopulmonary resuscitation (CPR) in the event of cardiopulmonary arrest, he or she should have a one-way valve resuscitation mask on his or her person or have access to one in the home. If the staff member is not required to perform CPR according to the home or hospice care organization's policies and procedures, a resuscitation mask does not have to be in the home or issued to the staff member. As long as the staff member has immediate access to the necessary supplies during the course of care, that is sufficient.

TRAINING

OSHA requires that home and hospice care organizations educate staff members on the location and use of personal protective equipment upon hire and on an annual basis. Refer to Chapter 13, Exhibit 13-5 for required training elements. Table 6-2 provides guidelines as to whether gloves and other personal protective equipment should be worn when various home care tasks are performed.

NURSING SUPPLY BAG

A nursing supply bag is not required, although most home and hospice care organization staff members who provide intermittent home care services use one. Ideally, the bag should be constructed of a washable fabric and have multiple compartments for the storage of supplies. If the inside or outside of the bag becomes significantly soiled, the bag should be washed in hot soapy water, rinsed, and dried in a dryer or hung to air

Table 6-2 Staff Member Barrier Requirements

Task	Gloves	Gown or plastic apron	Mask	Goggles	One-way valve resuscitation mask
Giving a bath	Optional	If soiling is likely			
Blood glucose monitoring	Required				
Changing visibly soiled linens	Required	Required			
Cleaning blood/body fluid spills	Required	If soiling is likely	If splashing is likely	If splashing is likely	
Cleaning incontinent patient	Required	If soiling is likely			
Performing CPR					Required
Inserting peripheral short-line or midline catheter	Required				
Inserting peripherally inserted central catheter	Required				
Ostomy care	Required				
Tracheostomy care	Required	If soiling is likely likely	If splashing is likely	If splashing is likely	
Wound care	Required	Optional		If splashing from irrigation	

Note: The type of personal protective equipment needed for a task is based on three criteria: volume of blood or fluids expected, length of time for which exposure is expected, and conditions of the exposure such as temperature, humidity, and the possibility of unpredictable situations. This information is intended to serve as a guideline only and may not identify all equipment necessary to take care of a home care patient. Each home care situation should be assessed to determine the minimum type of personal protective equipment required. Personal protective equipment generally is not required for patient assessments, feeding the patient, assisting with ambulation, or taking vital signs unless the patient requires transmission-based precautions.

dry. On a regular basis and when soiled, the internal contents should be removed, and the inside of the bag should be cleaned with a disinfectant wipe.

"Bag Technique"

There has been ongoing debate regarding "bag technique" and whether a barrier placed under supply bags is required. First, it should be recognized that the nursing supply bag is a noncritical item. Although it may contain some critical or semicritical items, the bag itself does not come into contact with the patient. Thus, there is no scientific rationale for barrier placement, and studies have not shown that a barrier placed under a nursing bag in the home is effective against preventing the transmission of infections; therefore, such a barrier is not required.

The supply bag should be placed on a clean, dry surface away from small children and pets. If the patient's home environment is heavily infested with insects or rodents, the bag should not be brought in. The supplies that will be needed for the home visit can be taken out of the bag and placed in a disposable container, such as a brown paper bag or a plastic bag, or they can be carried in a "fanny pack." When the visit is over, the reusable, noncritical supplies can be cleaned and then carried back to the vehicle to be placed inside the nursing bag. The disposable bag that was used to carry the supplies into the patient's home should be discarded.

As a good infection control measure, staff members should perform hand hygiene before reaching into the bag to obtain any necessary supplies. Reaching into the bag generally signifies the beginning of patient care activities, and the hands should always be washed before patient care is provided. When noncritical equipment is taken out of the nursing supply bag and used in patient care, it should be cleaned, if necessary, before it is returned to the bag. Chapter 9 provides additional information about how and when medical equipment such as blood pressure cuffs and stethoscopes should be cleaned. If the patient has equipment in the home that can be used in patient care (e.g., a thermometer), it is preferable that the patient's equipment be used in lieu of the equipment from the nursing supply bag. Before reaching into the bag again to obtain additional supplies, the staff member must make certain that gloves that were used to provide patient care are removed. Otherwise, the equipment can become contaminated. Inside the supply bag, semicritical items should be kept covered and critical items should be contained in sterile wrappers that will prevent contamination.

Bag Contents

Not every staff member must be issued a supply bag, but all staff members should have access to the needed supplies in the home. Most important is that the personal protective equipment and supplies needed to provide patient care are available to the staff when they are needed. As mentioned earlier, home care organizations that provide private-duty services or hospices that provide continuous care may store gloves, gowns, a CPR mask, and hand hygiene supplies in a box kept in the patient's home for staff members' use. Intermittent rehabilitation staff members may use a fanny pack to carry antiseptic hand rub for hand hygiene, other needed supplies, and personal protective equipment.

INFECTION CONTROL SUPPLIES

Infection control supplies should be available for home care staff members who are providing direct patient care and for admission staff. Frequently, when a patient is referred to a home care organization, only partial information is received from the referral source, and the admitting staff member may need personal protective equipment, such as a mask, that was not anticipated. Infection control supplies may be kept in a supply bag that either is carried from patient home to patient home or is left in the patient's home for staff members' use. Staff members who visit patients but do not provide direct, hands-on patient care, such as social workers, chaplains, and dietitians, do not need to have in their possession a full complement of infection control supplies. Minimally, the supplies should include an antiseptic hand rub, a mask, gloves, and a one-way valve resuscitation mask (if the home or hospice care organization requires staff members to be certified in basic life support). If a patient is on airborne, droplet, or Contact Precautions, additional personal protective equipment such as a gown and a mask or an N95 respiratory protective device (for airborne precaution) should be provided to the staff member or made available in the home.

Exhibit 6-1 lists infection control supplies that should be available to both staff who provide direct patient care and staff who go to the patient's home to screen the patient for admission to the home care program.

Exhibit 6-1 Supplies to Be Made Available as Needed to Staff Providing Direct Patient Care and Admission Staff

- Antimicrobial soap
- Antiseptic hand rub product
- Hand-drying supplies
- Lotion or cream
- One-way valve resuscitation mask (only if staff are required to be CPR certified)
- Nonsterile examination gloves
- Impermeable gown
- Surgical mask
- Goggles
- Blood spill kit
- Sharps container
- Impervious red container or container labeled as biohazardous to carry laboratory samples
- Red plastic bag or bag labeled as biohazardous
- Sterile gloves for procedures requiring sterile technique
- 70% ethyl alcohol wipes or other disinfectant
- N95 respirator

REFERENCES

Beltrami, E., McArthur, M., McGeer, A., Armstrong-Evans, M., Lyons, D., Chamberland, M., & Cardo, D. (2000). The nature and frequency of blood contacts among home healthcare workers. *Infection Control and Hospital Epidemiology, 21*(12), 765–770.

Centers for Disease Control and Prevention. (2002). Guideline for hand hygiene in health-care settings: Recommendations of the Healthcare Infection Control Practices Advisory Committee and the HICPAC/SHEA/APIC/IDSA Hand Hygiene Task Force. *Morbidity and Mortality Weekly Report, 51*(RR16), 1–44.

Centers for Disease Control and Prevention. (1994). Guidelines for preventing the transmission of *Mycobacterium tuberculosis* in health-care facilities. *Morbidity and Mortality Weekly Report, 43*(RR13), 1–125.

Centers for Disease Control and Prevention. (2005). Guideline for isolation precautions: Preventing transmission of infectious agents in healthcare settings. (Retrieved on June 15, 2004, from http://www.cdc.gov/nc.dod/hip/hicpac).

National Institute for Occupational Safety and Health. (1997). Preventing allergic reactions to natural rubber latex in the workplace. *National Institute for Occupational Safety and Health Alert,* No. 97-135. Retrieved 9/5/04, from *http://www.cdc.gov/niosh/latexalt.html.*

Occupational Safety and Health Administration. (2001). Occupational exposure to bloodborne pathogens; Needlestick and other sharps injuries, Final rule. 29 CFR 1910. Retrieved 9/5/04, from *www.OSHA.gov.*

Occupational Safety and Health Administration. (2000). Standards interpretation: The BBP standard applicability to home health care service workers. Retrieved 9/5/04, from *http://www.osha.gov/pls/oshaweb/owadisp.show_document?p_table=INTERPRETATIONS&p_id523454.*

Occupational Safety and Health Administration. (1992a, December 14). Breast milk does not constitute occupational exposure as defined by standard. *OSHA Standards Interpretation and Compliance Letters.* Retrieved 9/5/04, from *http://www.osha-slc.gov/OshDoc/Interp_data/I19921214A.html.*

Occupational Safety and Health Administration. (1992b, September 1). Using gloves in administering routine injections. *OSHA Standards Interpretation and Compliance Letters.* Retrieved 9/5/04, from *http://www.osha-slc.gov/OshDoc/Interp_data/I19920901A.html.*

Occupational Safety and Health Administration. (1991). Occupational exposure to bloodborne pathogens: Final rule. 29 CFR 1910, 1030. *Federal Register, 56,* 64003–64282.

CHAPTER 7

Multidrug-Resistant Organisms

Chapter 8 discusses the CDC's 2004 *Draft Guideline for Isolation Precautions: Preventing Transmission of Infectious Agents in Healthcare Settings* with respect to the overall approach to using isolation precautions in home care. This chapter will address some of the isolation issues related to the care of patients with MDROs in the home as well as the administrative considerations.

Various microorganisms, including bacteria and mycobacteria, viruses, fungi, and prions, can cause infections in humans. As discussed in Chapter 2, these organisms can cause a variety of conditions, including colonization, active infection, chronic infection, and latent infection. A wide variety of vaccines have been developed to protect humans from infection (e.g., hepatitis B vaccine, pneumococcal vaccine). When vaccine protection is not available or feasible, infections may require treatment with antimicrobial agents to limit their effect on the infected host. There are antimicrobials to treat viral infections such as hepatitis C (e.g., antiviral agents), fungal infections such as aspergillosis (e.g., antifungal agents), and the largest class, antibiotics, to treat bacterial infection. The term *multidrug-resistant organisms (MDRO)* refers to bacteria that have developed resistance to antibiotics.

MDROs have been recognized since the earliest development of antibiotics. In 1928, Dr. Alexander Fleming, a Scottish physician, discovered that a product of mold, *Penicillium,* could stop bacterial growth and determined that this naturally occurring agent might be used to treat bacterial infections. Eventually, the antibiotic penicillin was introduced for common use in 1943, and within four years physicians and scientists recognized that the bacteria were able to overcome the effects of penicillin and exhibit resistance. Since then many antibiotics have been introduced for the treatment of infections, and many reports of resistance have resulted.

MDROs are defined as bacteria that are resistant to one or more classes of antibiotics (Institute of Medicine, 1998). The names given to common MDROs, such as methcillin-resistant *Staph aureus* (MRSA) and vancomycin-resistant enterococcus (VRE), may seem to imply that these bacteria are resistant to one specific drug. This is not so, however. The drug name is used to simplify the identification of the resistant organism; these bacteria are actually resistant to all but one or two of the antibiotics commercially available for their potential treatment. For example, although *Staph aureus* has been treated with a variety of drugs in the penicillin class, methcillin is the drug used to designate the resistance to this class.

BASIC SCIENCE: BUGS VERSUS DRUGS

There are many types of bacteria (see Chapter 2, Table 2-2) that can cause many types of human infections. Microbiologists have developed methods to

---

The CDC's 2004 Draft Guideline for Isolation Precautions was published in the CDC website for public review in June 2004. Much of the information in the draft Isolation Guideline was used to develop Chapters 7 and 8 of this text. However, at the time of publication, the Isolation Guideline was still undergoing internal CDC review. The final Guideline will be available on the CDC website in 2005.

identify these microorganisms by their genus and species. There are two additional identification categories that describe bacteria, according to how their cellular wall reacts to a particular stain called Gram's stain. Thus, we refer to bacteria as Gram positive or Gram negative and by their genus and species name. For example, the genus *Staphylococci* are Gram positive organisms that occur in various species, such as *Staphylococcus aureus* and *Staphylococcus epidermidis*. *Pseudomonads* are a genus of Gram negative bacteria with species such as *Pseudomonas aeruginosa* and *Pseudomonas cepacia* (now called *Burkholderia cepacia*).

Scientists and pharmaceutical researchers have developed many types of antibiotics to treat the various genera and species of Gram positive and Gram negative bacteria. In addition to penicillins, other classes of antibiotics include aminoglycocides (e.g., gentamicin and tobramicin), cephalosporins (e.g., cefuroxime, ceftriaxone), monobactams (e.g., imipenem), quinolones (e.g., ciprofloxacin), and many others, including vancomycin (Williams & Peterson, 2000).

When a physician orders a clinical culture (e.g., blood, urine, sputum) from a home care patient and the nurse brings the specimen to the laboratory, the microbiology section of the lab performs culture and sensitivity testing. Preparing the culture involves a number of methods, including Gram staining, that allow the microbiologist to determine the genus and species of all the bacteria found within the specimen. A positive blood culture usually yields only a single bacteria (e.g., *Streptococcus pneumonia*), whereas a wound culture may yield several genera and species of bacteria—especially a wound, such as a sacral pressure ulcer, that is prone to contamination. Once each species of bacteria is identified individually and isolated into a pure culture (a culture containing only one species), antibiotic testing called susceptibility testing is performed.

There are a couple of methods that laboratories can use to perform susceptibility testing, including disk diffusion and broth dilution to determine the minimal inhibitory concentration (MIC) (Rosen-Kotelainen, 2000). In disk diffusion, various tablets—or disks—containing a known quantity of antibiotic are placed in a Petri dish already inoculated with the bacteria. The microbiologist incubates the dish and then, about 24 to 48 hours later, observes and measures which antibiotics prevented the growth of the bacteria around the disk (Figure 7-1). The microbiologist measures the

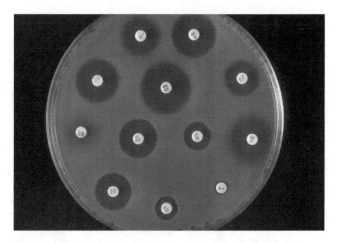

Figure 7-1 Disk diffusion antibiotic susceptibility testing

growth of the bacteria and determines the zone of inhibition. If the bacteria grow all the way up to and around the disk, they are determined to be resistant to that drug.

Through MIC testing, the microbiologist can determine what amount of the antibiotic will inhibit the growth of the bacteria by placing increasing concentrations of antibiotics in a series of mini–test tubes or broth dilutions. This is called *in vitro* testing, referring to testing in the laboratory. (*In vivo* means "in the body.") There are national standards for interpreting MIC results; these standards provide criteria to determine if the bacteria are susceptible or resistant to the antibiotics tested (NCCLS, 2002). When the culture and sensitivity report comes back to the patient's physician and medical record, it lists the bacteria that were found and the susceptibility results (i.e., susceptible or resistant) for a group or panel of selected antibiotics. There are standard panels for Gram negative organisms that are different from the drug panels for Gram positive organisms (see Table 7-1). The physician should use the susceptibility results to determine the best antibiotic for the treatment of the patient's infection. The results may also identify an MDRO.

HOW ARE MDROs ACQUIRED OR DEVELOPED?

Patients may acquire infection or colonization with an MDRO in two ways. Most commonly, the organism is transmitted to a portal of entry via the hands or by

Table 7-1 Sample antibiotic panels for susceptibility testing

Gram-negative organisms	Gram-positive organisms
Ampicillin	Amoxicillin
Cefazolin	Cefazolin
Cefepime	Ciprofloxacin
Ceftazidime	Clindamicin
Ceftriaxone	Cloxicillin
Ciprofloxacin	Erythromycin
Gentamicin	Oxacillin
Imipenem	Penicillin
Nitrofurantoin	Rifampin
Ofloxacin	Tetracycline
Piperacillin	TMP/SMX
TMP/SMX	Vancomycin
Tobramycin	

fomites from another environmental source. This occurs frequently in hospitals, and if the transmission is widespread, there may be an outbreak of a specific MDRO. Although direct or indirect transmission is the most common means of acquiring an MDRO, there is another risk. Bacteria may develop resistance *in vivo* while colonizing or infecting a patient through one of several biologic mechanisms. This less-common risk explains why various new MDROs are emerging, such as was reported when VRSA (vancomycin-resistant *Staph aureus*) was identified in 2002. VRSA had not been recognized before and was detected in two home care patients (CDC, 2002a; CDC, 2002b, Chang, 2003).

Bacteria, like other living organisms, have DNA. In some bacteria, the DNA can spontaneously mutate to cause the bacteria to become resistant to an antibiotic. This is a natural defense mechanism. This resistance in the DNA can also spread to another bacterium through sexual conjugation. Thus, bacteria in the same environment (either within a human or within an environmental reservoir) can share resistance through the transfer of DNA. A third mechanism of resistance is through a different type of DNA called a plasmid. Plasmids can transfer antibiotic resistance from one bacterium to another and from one strain to another (Williams & Peterson, 2000).

There are many thousands of bacterial species that infect and colonize human beings, and there are hundreds of antibiotics that are used to treat infections. As bacteria are exposed to the various antibiotics, they can

develop resistance through one of the mechanisms described in the previous paragraphs. This resistance can be identified when a microbiologist analyzes the MIC results and recognizes that a bacterium that is usually sensitive to a specific antibiotic has become resistant *in vitro*. *In vitro* resistance is interpreted to indicate that the bacteria is also resistant *in vivo* and therefore that the specific antibiotic will not be effective in treatment of the infection.

EPIDEMIOLOGY OF MDROs

Health care has observed the development of MDROs for many decades. MRSA was first seen in the United States in 1968, and many other MDROs have been identified since then. Initially, MDROs were seen in severely ill, hospitalized patients and most frequently in intensive care units (ICUs). These patients were at greatest risk for MDROs for a variety of reasons, including the following:

1. ICU patients typically are treated with a variety of antibiotics, which tends to suppress normal flora and to allow MDROs to proliferate.
2. The prolonged presence of invasive medical devices, such as Foley catheters, central venous lines, and endotracheal tubes, allows contamination and colonization of these devices and providing a portal of entry for invading bacteria.
3. Prolonged lengths of stay in the ICU and hospital facilitate exposure to other ICU patients with MDROs and, occasionally, exposure to environmental sources of MDROs.

In the 1980s, Gram negative MDROs such as *Klebsiella* and *Pseudomonas* were common problems in ICU patients. These resistant organisms frequently caused outbreaks of nosocomial infection and were the focus of much attention and effort by hospital infection control programs. In the 1990s, however, MRSA and VRE became more commonly recognized in hospital patients, both in ICUs and in other medical/surgical settings. VRE was first recognized in a U.S. hospital in 1989, and within 10 years, 15% of the enterococcus isolated in hospitalized patients was vancomycin-resistant. MRSA has also increased dramatically, especially in critical care patients, in whom more than 50% of the *Staph aureus* found is MRSA (French, 2004).

Critically ill patients eventually leave the ICU for medical/surgical units and then in time are discharged to skilled nursing facilities, rehabilitation hospitals, long-term acute-care hospitals, or home. Thus, an increased prevalence of MDROs outside of acute-care hospitals in other types of residential care settings and in the community has been recognized (Chambers, 2001). MDROs can be transmitted from one resident to another in long-term care, just as they can be in acute-care hospitals. Studies seem to indicate that transmission is less frequent in these settings than in the hospital, however (Strausbaugh, Crossley *et al.*, 1996).

In home and hospice care, many patients are known to be colonized or infected with MDROs, although there are probably numerous other home care or hospice patients that are unrecognized. Even so, there have been no reports as of this writing of any MDROs spreading from one patient to another in home care. This may be explained by the lack of recognition of individual cases of spread, given the infrequency with which cultures are ordered for patients in home care. In 2002, however, there were two cases of vancomycin-resistant *S. aureus* (VRSA) identified and reported in two individual patients, both of whom were receiving home care (CDC 2002a; CDC 2002b; Chang *et al.*, 2003). Both patients had multiple risk factors, including chronic illnesses such as diabetes, end stage renal disease, and peripheral vascular disease, for which they were receiving ongoing medical care. Both had received many courses of antibiotic therapy that included vancomycin. One patient was also receiving chronic hemodialysis. The CDC investigated both of these cases, due to the significant concern over a newly recognized and feared MDRO: VRSA. The investigators obtained cultures from many other patients, including other dialysis patients in the same dialysis center as well as other home care patients within the two agencies providing care for the infected patients. No additional cases of VRSA were identified.

In both instances, it appears that the VRSA developed as a result of transfer of resistance from one bacterial strain to another. Both patients had cultures positive for VRE prior to the recognition of VRSA. Scientists postulate that the genetic material causing resistance to vancomycin was transferred *in vivo* from the enterococcus to the *S. aureus*. When subsequent cultures were obtained, the VRSA was identified. In the dialysis patient, the VRSA initially was isolated from a central venous catheter exit site. The patient had previously been culture positive for MRSA as well as VRE. In addition to the catheter exit site, VRSA was cultured from a chronic foot ulcer, from which VRE and *Klebsiella oxytoca* were also identified. The other patient also had a chronic foot ulcer that was culture positive for VRSA.

IDENTIFYING PATIENTS WITH MDROs

In both cases of VRSA, cultures were obtained in the course of medical care to identify the causes of infection in order to select the appropriate antibiotic for treatment. Although it is unknown how long either of the patients had VRSA, there was no evidence of transmission to other patients or to family/household members or home care staff. This may not have been the case if these patients had been hospitalized; VRSA might have spread more easily to other high-risk patients via the hands of health care workers.

This raises the potential benefit of identifying patients with MDROs more proactively using surveillance cultures, rather than depending upon clinical cultures (cultures ordered by their physicians to treat an acute episode of infection). There is considerable controversy regarding the need and benefit of performing surveillance cultures to identify and control MDROs. So far, the experience with this approach has been in hospitals, although some suggest that surveillance culturing should be applied in all health care settings (Muto, Jernigan, Ostrowsky *et al.*, 2003). To institute the use of surveillance cultures, the infection control program develops criteria for screening new patients at the time of admission, to determine if they are infected or colonized with an MDRO. For example, a patient transferring from a hospital known to have a high prevalence of MRSA would be cultured upon admission to another hospital. Patients undergoing chronic hemodialysis might also routinely be cultured if admitted to the hospital, as might other chronically ill patients such as diabetics with peripheral vascular disease and ulcers who experience frequent hospitalizations.

Although this approach may seem prudent, it may or may not be practical. It requires significant staff time to select and obtain cultures from newly admitted patients; there is considerable expense related to the processing and interpretation of surveillance cultures, which are not reimbursed by insurance carriers; and depending upon the selection of sites for culture and the number and quality of cultures, it may not identify every MDRO in every patient. Then, there is the issue of ongoing surveillance cultures for patients remaining in a hospital, nursing home, residential setting, or home care. Thus, this approach is fraught with controversial issues and problems and is not guaranteed to lead to the successful identification and control of MDROs.

The 2004 CDC Draft Guideline for Isolation Precautions (CDC, 2004) includes discussion of this approach but does not recommend its implementation. Rather, the Guideline takes a more universal, practical approach, prescribing that all providers in all settings, including home care and hospice, comply with the consistent application of Standard Precautions. This approach not only protects the home care and hospice staff member from potential exposure to blood-borne pathogens, but the barrier precautions and hand hygiene required by the Standard Precautions also reduce the risk of transferring MDROs—whether they are recognized or not.

In home care and hospice, most MDRO patients are identified at the time of admission through information provided by the hospital from which the patient was discharged. This information is provided upon referral to the home care or hospice organization so that staff can consider how the MDRO will affect patient scheduling, equipment use, or application of barrier precautions. Unless the patient is receiving hospice care in a facility for pain and symptom management or respite, placement is not an issue in home care. Even though the use of Standard Precautions should be customary in all home care and hospice organizations, many home care and hospice providers have toiled with how and when to apply Contact Precautions in the home for patients who are infected or colonized with MDROs.

In order to improve ongoing management of MDROs, home care and hospice organizations should consider the proactive approach outlined in the Draft CDC Guideline on Isolation Precautions (CDC, 2004). The Guideline recommends that health care organizations become more active in assuring the appropriate use of antibiotics (which is not under the direct control of the home care or hospice organization) and the prevention and control of MDROs through establishment of administrative policies and procedures. Such policies include: 1) making the control of MDROs an organizational priority; 2) selecting specific MDROs as target organisms for prevention, control, and surveillance, based upon previous experience as well as current epidemiology of MDROs; 3) conducting ongoing

surveillance and monitoring of target MDROs; 4) providing education on MDROs for all health care staff including initial orientation and ongoing training; and 5) implementing appropriate use of isolation precautions and patient placement.

Home care and hospice organizations should review the recommendations to determine which should be adopted in their practice, recognizing that hospitals and residential settings have more experience and challenges with MDROs. Initially, if the home care or hospice organization does not have an established surveillance system for MDROs or does not know its actual experience (e.g., the actual number of patients with MDROs, by type, in a past time period), efforts should be made to establish a surveillance system. Although it may be possible to review records to determine the organization's past experience with MDROs, it may be preferable to develop and implement a concurrent data collection system.

Such a system may be as simple as establishing a line listing of all patients either admitted with infection or colonization with an MDRO or identified during home or hospice care. As outlined in Chapter 11 on surveillance, a line listing is a simple list of patients, including a patient identifier and other demographic data elements, along with information about their infection (in this case, their MDRO) (see Table 7-2).

From this information, the home care or hospice organization can develop a quarterly report of MDROs in order to monitor and track its experience. For example, monitoring can identify which hospitals most often refer patients with MDROs and what organisms they have. An organizational prevalence rate of MDROs

---

Table 7-2 MDRO Line Listing Data Elements

1. Patient identifier (name or record number)
2. Age
3. Gender
4. Diagnostic code (or indication of type of patient, such as home care or hospice, and type of care being provided)
5. Date of admission to home care or hospice
6. Referral source
7. Admitted with MDRO or identified/acquired after admission
8. Date of initial diagnosis with MDRO (if identified or acquired during home or hospice care)
9. MDRO (e.g., MRSA, VRE)
10. Site(s) of colonization or infection

can be calculated by taking the number of MDRO patients over the total number of patients cared for during the specified time period, times 100. This will provide the percent of MDRO patients for that reporting period (e.g., 8 MDRO patients of 150 total patients = 5.3% MDRO patients). Similarly, the rate of a specific organism can be calculated. If 4 of the 8 MDROs are MRSA, the prevalence rate of MRSA is 50%.

This data can be accumulated over months and years to better understand and describe the organization's experience with MDROs. If the rate of MDROs increases, the organization can potentially identify the reason (e.g., increased number of referrals from a specific source). Although cultures are much less frequently obtained in home care and hospice patients, the organization should be particularly aware of newly identified patients with MDROs, especially if this information was not provided (or recognized) by the referral source. There should be continuous awareness of the potential for transmission of a MDRO from one patient to another and, if suspected or recognized, the incident should be investigated to identify a potential cause and to address any procedures that may need improvement. However, there has not been transmission of any MDRO in home care or hospice reported to date.

MANAGING PATIENTS WITH MDROs IN HOME CARE

Since the publication of the earlier guidelines for prevention and control of MRSA (Boyce, Jackson, Pugliese, 1994) and VRE (CDC, 1995), there has been confusion and inconsistency regarding the application of the recommendations in home care. This is largely based upon the fact that these publications were focused on hospital care and did not provide specific direction for home care. Thus, nurses in these settings had to read, interpret, and adapt the recommendations to their specific setting and patient population, making the best clinical judgments they could with minimal guidance and little or no scientific evidence.

As discussed in Chapter 8 on isolation, the Draft Guideline for Isolation Precautions (CDC, 2004) focuses on the consistent application of Standard Precautions. The Isolation Guideline also provides discussion and evidence related to the management of MDROs in all health care settings. The guiding principle in determining a home care or hospice organization's approach to MDRO control is that the organization must determine the actual risk to the patient population and the specific strategies appropriate for preventing transmission.

As a first step, the home care or hospice organization should determine its policy regarding the identification and control of MDROs. There is no standard approach for all home care or hospice providers. Because there have been no reports of MDRO transmission in home care, however, it may be less necessary for home care or hospice organizations to implement a rigorous program for identification and control than it is for high-risk settings such as ICUs. High-risk settings need to be more aggressive in surveillance and control measures such as patient placement issues and the use of barrier precautions.

There are several factors that should be considered in the development of these policies and procedures in home care and hospice. First, an agency should consider its past experience and referral patterns with patients known to be infected or colonized with MDROs. If the agency provides high-tech care, including home infusion therapy, it may frequently accept and care for more complicated high-risk patients. These are the patients most likely to have MDROs. In contrast, an agency that provides more personal care and assistance may not provide care to many patients with MDROs, or even know that they have them. The home care or hospice organization's leadership should look at past and current experience to determine the likelihood of patients with MDROs, and if possible, it should describe the frequency and types of MDROs it has experienced in the past. Through this exercise, clinical leadership can determine the extent of the need for extra efforts and use of control strategies beyond Standard Precautions.

If past experience is minimal, the organization may determine that it will be vigilant in observing any new experiences or trends in MDROs. Referring hospitals may be helpful in providing information about what MDROs are prevalent. This information can be requested from the infection control practitioner within those hospitals. The agency should not ask for specific patient information, but it can ask the infection control practitioner about its experience with MDROs in the past 2 to 3 years (i.e., the frequency of MDROs and the types of patients most often identified with them). Based on this information, the agency can determine its potential for admitting and caring for MDRO patients.

The type of MDRO, usually either MRSA or VRE, may vary by geographic location or even by hospital.

If the agency has experienced many patients with MDROs in the past or anticipates an increase in admissions with MDROs, it may want to review the Isolation Guideline and revise its current practices through revised policies and procedures. Some organizations have been stringent in caring for any patient known to have an MDRO and have applied Contact Precautions for every visit. Others have examined these patients on

a case-by-case basis and have made decisions depending upon the patient's condition. Still other agencies have continued to use Standard Precautions for all patients, including those known to have MDROs.

The 2004 Draft Guideline for Isolation Precautions provides guidance for formulating agency policies and procedures as well as for managing individual patients. As stated earlier, the Isolation Guideline focuses on Standard Precautions for all patients (see Table 7-3). Based upon the circumstances within

Table 7-3 Management of MDROs in Home Care and Hospice

Administrative Measures	Staff Education	Surveillance	Infection Control Measures	Environmental Measures
Make prevention and control of MDROs an organizational priority, as appropriate to past experience and local epidemiology. Implement systems to: • Identify patients with MDROs on admission to home care and hospice • Communicate the presence of an MDRO on transfer or discharge to another care setting • Assure that the presence of an MDRO is communicated to staff providing patient care in the home.	Address MDROs in orientation and ongoing education for all staff, including paraprofessionals. Emphasize compliance with Standard Precautions and hand hygiene. Educate staff on criteria for implementation of additional precautions (e.g., Contact Precautions).	Initiate and maintain a line listing or log of patients known to be colonized or infected with MDROs receiving home care or hospice services. Analyze the surveillance data periodically (e.g., quarterly) to identify patterns or trends in organisms or common referral sources. Identify, when possible, patients who become colonized or infected with an MDRO while receiving home care or hospice services. If a *home care-acquired* MDRO is identified: • Consult with an infection control professional or health care epidemiologist with expertise and knowledge of the prevention and control of MDROs to assist in assessment and planning activities. • Implement appropriate measures to control the transmission of MDROs.	Observe Standard Precautions during all patient care activities, assuming that any patient could be colonized or infected with an MDRO. Perform hand hygiene when indicated. Implement Contact Precautions under circumstances that would normally indicate their use, such as during the care of patients with draining wounds or uncontrolled secretions/excretions. Dedicate reusable patient care items (e.g., blood pressure cuff and thermometer) or disposable patient care items (e.g., stethoscope) to patients known to be colonized or infected with an MDRO. Minimize equipment taken into the home, such as nursing bags that are carried in and out of the home. If visibly soiled, clean and disinfect any equipment removed from the home and intended for use with other patients.	No special or terminal cleaning of patient's room or home setting is required.

Source: Copyright © 2005, Emily Rhinehart and Mary Friedman.

home care or hospice, as well as the lack of evidence for transmission of MDROs in home care, the routine use of Contact Precautions is probably not necessary in home care. This statement assumes that Standard Precautions are applied appropriately and hand hygiene is adequate. The circumstances in home care and hospice are the chief rationale for this approach. Home care and hospice patients are cared for in their own environment, which does not include or put other patients at risk. Although there are exceptions to this, such as two burn patients recovering at home together, having one patient in the home is still the general norm. In the case of two elderly patients who both have diabetes and stasis ulcers, it is likely that transmission would occur normally through the sharing of bed linens, towels, and so on, rather than being associated with home care per se.

If a home care or hospice patient with an MDRO is simply colonized with the organism and has no specific risk factors for transmission, gowns and gloves should be used as prescribed by Standard Precautions. However, if there are additional circumstances that may increase the risk for transmission of an MDRO, the home care or hospice organization will need to determine if Contact Precautions may be necessary. That said, these are patients for whom Contact Precautions would likely be implemented even if they were not known to be colonized or infected with an MDRO. Examples may include patients with draining wounds whose drainage is difficult to contain with routine dressing changes, patients with poorly controlled respiratory secretions that increase the likelihood of environmental contamination, or patients with uncontrolled incontinence or diarrhea. In these circumstances, contamination of the environment as well as staff members' clothing may be more likely. Implementation of Contact Precautions would then be necessary.

Whether the organization determines Standard Precautions are adequate or implements Contact Precautions for a specific patient, other strategies to prevent transmission of MDROs can also be considered.

If there is significant potential that the home care environment is contaminated with an MDRO, there may be concern for transmission by inanimate objects that may routinely be taken from one home to another. This would include blood pressure cuffs, stethoscopes, and other noncritical items, including the nursing bag. If the nurse feels there is considerable risk that the environment is contaminated, he or she may decide to dedicate reusable or disposable patient equipment to this patient's use and leave the blood pressure cuff, etc. in the home. In addition, the care plan can direct each nurse to minimize the equipment taken into the home—pens, phones, etc.—leaving the nursing bag in the car and taking only what is needed into the home for the visit. In this way, inanimate objects that may become contaminated are not subsequently taken to other patients' homes. An additional strategy to improve the margin of safety is to schedule the visit to an MDRO patient as the final visit of the day. Thus, if clothing or inanimate objects become contaminated, they will not be taken into another patient's home. That said, it is unlikely that inanimate objects that are not directly used on the patient would pose a risk to another patient (e.g., pens and pencils as compared to stethoscopes and blood pressure cuffs).

There should be no need for additional environmental cleaning or controls (e.g., containment of wound irrigation supplies) beyond what would be normal.

EDUCATION OF HOME CARE AND HOSPICE STAFF

Whether or not MDROs are a major concern, home care and hospice organizations must continuously educate their staff on the principles and application of Standard Precautions. When appropriate, information about specific patients with MDROs as well as the agency's experience and policies for managing MDROs should be included.

REFERENCES

Boyce, J., Jackson, M. M., Pugliese, G. (1994). Methicillin-resistant *Staphylococcus aureus:* A briefing for acute care hospitals and nursing facilities. *Infection Control and Hospital Epidemiology, 15,* 105–113.

Centers for Disease Control and Prevention. (2004). Draft guideline for isolation precautions: Preventing transmission of infectious agents in health-care settings. (Retrieved June 15, 2004, from http://www.cdc.gov/ncidod/hip/isoguide.htm).

Centers for Disease Control and Prevention. (2002a). *Staphylococcus aureus* resistant to vancomycin—United States. *Morbidity and Mortality Weekly Report, 51*(26), 565–567.

Centers for Disease Control and Prevention. (2002b). Public health dispatch: Vancomycin-resistant *Staphylococcus aureus*—Pennsylvania. *Morbidity and Mortality Weekly Report, 51*(40), 902.

Centers for Disease Control and Prevention. (1995). Recommendations for preventing the spread of vancomycin resistance. *Morbidity and Mortality Weekly Report, 44*(RR12), 1–13.

Chambers, H. (2001). The changing epidemiology of *Staphylococcus aureus? Emerging Infectious Diseases.* Retrieved 10/7/04, from http://www.cdc.gov/ncidod/eid/vol7no2/chambers.htm.

Chang, S., Sievert, D., Hageman, J., Boulton, M., Tenover, F., Downes, F., Shah, S., Rudrik, J., Pupp, G., Brown, W., Cardo, D., Fridkin, S. (2003). Infection with vancomycin-resistant *Staphylococcus aureus* containing the vanA resistance gene. *New England Journal of Medicine*, 348, 1342–1347.

French, G. (2004). Antimicrobial resistance in hospital flora and nosocomial infections. In G. Mayhall (Ed.), *Hospital Epidemiology and Infection Control* (pp. 1613–1636). Philadelphia: Lippincott Williams and Wilkins.

Institute of Medicine. (1998). Antimicrobial resistance: Issues and options. Workshop report. In P. F. Harrison, & J. Lederberg (Eds.), Washington DC: National Academy Press.

Muto, C. A., Jernigan, J. A., Ostrowsky, B. E., Richet, H. M., Jarvis W. R., Boyce, J. M., & Farr, B. M. (2003). SHEA guideline for preventing nosocomial transmission of multidrug-resistant strains of *Staphylococcus aureus* and enterococcus. *Infection Control and Hospital Epidemiology, 24*(5), 362–386.

National Committee for Clinical Laboratory Standards. (2002). Performance standards for antimicrobial susceptibility testing: Twelfth informational supplement. Document M100-S12. Wayne, PA: NCCLS.

Rosen-Kotelainen, H. (2000). Laboratory diagnostics. In R. Olmsted (Ed.), *APIC text of infection control and epidemiology: Principles and practice* (pp. 67–26–28). Washington, DC: Association for Professionals in Infection Control and Epidemiology, Inc.

Strausbaugh, L., Crossley, K., Nurse, B., & Thrupp, L. (1996). Antimicrobial resistance in long-term care facilities. *Infection Control and Hospital Epidemiology, 17*(2), 129–140.

Williams, D., & Peterson, P. (2000). Antimicrobial use and the development of resistance. In R. Olmsted (Ed.), *APIC text of infection control and epidemiology: Principles and practice* (pp. 61–1–7.). Washington, DC: Association for Professionals in Infection Control and Epidemiology, Inc.

CHAPTER 8

Isolation Precautions in Home Care

Isolation precautions, including Standard Precautions and the use of appropriate personal protective equipment such as gowns, gloves, masks, and goggles have two primary goals in home care: (1) to protect home care and hospice staff from potential exposure to infectious agents, including bloodborne pathogens and (2) to prevent transmission of microorganisms from an infected or colonized patient to other patients via home care or hospice staff or patient care equipment. Until the recent publication of the Centers for Disease Control and Prevention's *Draft Guideline for Isolation Precautions: Preventing Transmission of Infectious Agents in Healthcare Settings** (CDC, 2004a; hereafter referred to as the Isolation Guideline), most home care and hospice organizations' policies and procedures for isolation precautions were based on the 1996 publication, "Guideline for Isolation in Hospitals" (Garner, 1996). The recommendations presented in this guideline required significant interpretation and adaptation to customize them for suitable home care or hospice practice. This has led to a wide variation in practice and to organizations implementing more precautions than necessary (Friedman & Rhinehart, 2000). Because most published studies of transmission of infectious diseases and organisms related to health care delivery are based on hospital care, evidence regarding transmission risks and effective prevention

strategies outside acute care is scarce. The 2004 Draft Isolation Guideline attempts to provide practical information about precautions in non-acute care settings, including the prevention and control of multidrug-resistant organisms (MDROs). Refer to Chapter 7 for a discussion of the prevention control and management of MDROs in home care.

The application of isolation precautions to prevent transmission of infectious agents is based on the principles discussed in Chapter 2. Any tactic or procedure incorporated into an isolation policy should be scientifically based and should consider the agent, the host, and the environment (see Figure 2-1, p. 8). In addition to the recommendations provided in the Isolation Guideline, the chain of infection (see Figure 2-2, p. 8) should also be considered in developing and applying policies and procedures for home care and hospice precautions. Home care and hospice staff should be educated about the chain of infection, and these principles should be incorporated into the decision making that may be required during the course of care since not every individual situation can be addressed in a policy or procedure. As demonstrated in the chain of transmission, precautions must be based on the mode of transmission of the infection, the portal of exit from the infected or colonized patient, and the portal of entry for the susceptible

---

*The CDC 2004 *Draft Guideline for Isolation Precautions: Preventing Transmission of Infectious Agents in Healthcare Settings* was published in the CDC website for public review in June 2004. Much of the information in the draft Isolation Guideline was used to develop Chapters 7 and 8 of this text. However, at the time of publication, the Isolation Guideline was still undergoing internal CDC review. The final Guideline will be available on the CDC website in 2005 (www.cdc.gov).

host (another patient or a home care or hospice staff member). Other factors, including the length of time the patient is contagious and the type of care that is being provided, should also be considered. Actions should not be arbitrary, and rituals should be avoided. Scientific knowledge and principles should be applied in assessing the risk of transmission and in taking steps to interrupt the transmission and thus to reduce the risk.

ISOLATION GUIDELINES

Since it began publishing guidance about preventing the transmission of infectious agents in hospitals in 1970, the CDC has always based its recommendations on scientific principles. The 1983 Isolation Guideline introduced the approach of isolation categories based on the mode of transmission ("category-specific isolation"). In the late 1980s, a new category, called "Universal Precautions," was introduced in response to the risk of transmission of bloodborne pathogens, including Hepatitis B and human immunosuppressive virus (HIV), to health care workers. The concepts of Universal Precautions and Body Substance Isolation were incorporated into the 1996 Isolation Guideline as "Standard Precautions" (Garner, 1996). The 2004 Draft Isolation Guideline reaffirms the use of Standard Precautions in all health care settings as the principal strategy for preventing transmission of infectious agents. It also addresses the prevention and control of MDROs.

A new term and type of precaution found in the 2004 Draft Isolation Guideline (CDC, 2004a) is "Respiratory Hygiene/Cough Etiquette." This category was developed in response to increased risk of transmission of respiratory viruses such as SARS (Sudden Acute Respiratory Syndrome) and influenza. Epidemiologic studies of the SARS outbreaks in Canada and Asia demonstrated a failure to implement basic control measures with patients, visitors, and health care personnel having signs and symptoms of respiratory tract infection (McDonald, Simor, Su et al., 2004). Although this type of precaution may be more applicable to hospice care provided in a facility in which patients and families gather and potentially transmit these illnesses, home care and hospice staff should be knowledgeable of the components of Respiratory Hygiene/Cough Etiquette in order to teach this behavior to patients, family members, and caregivers.

The basic control measures included in Respiratory Hygiene/Cough Etiquette are covering of the mouth/nose with a tissue when coughing and hand hygiene after contact with respiratory secretions. Implementation of Respiratory Hygiene/Cough Etiquette in hospice care facilities involves educating staff, patients, and visitors as well as posting signs to remind and alert those admitted for care and treatment to follow these simple rules of etiquette while in the facility. Some hospitals are also providing masks for symptomatic patients and visitors to wear while in the facility, in order to prevent droplet transmission.

STANDARD PRECAUTIONS

Standard Precautions should be utilized with all patients regardless of their diagnosis or presumed infection status; they are the primary method of preventing transmission of infectious agents in home care. Standard Precautions apply to all contact with blood; body fluids, secretions, and excretions (except sweat), regardless of whether they contain visible blood; nonintact skin; and mucus membranes. Standard Precautions are designed to reduce the risk of transmission of microorganisms from both recognized and unrecognized sources of infection (CDC, 2004a). Table 8-1 provides recommendations for implementing Standard Precautions. Chapter 6 provides additional information about the use of personal protective equipment.

TRANSMISSION-BASED PRECAUTIONS

When Standard Precautions are not sufficient to interrupt transmission of communicable disease, additional strategies, transmission-based precautions, should be employed (CDC, 2004a). The three types of transmission-based precautions are Airborne Isolation, Droplet Precautions, and Contact Precautions. An additional category, called "Protective Environment" (PE), is also referred to the in Draft Isolation Guideline (CDC, 2004). This category is based on a guideline that was developed to direct the care of hospitalized patients who have undergone bone marrow transplants (CDC, 2000a); it is not relevant to home care. This category of isolation precautions is specifically designed to protect severely immunosuppressed patients from such airborne environmental pathogens as *Aspergillus sp.* and other filamentous molds and fungi that can cause serious infections in this at-risk population. PE strategies

Table 8-1 Standard Precautions (from the 2004 Draft Isolation Guideline)

Component	Recommendations
Hand hygiene	After touching blood, body fluids, secretions, excretions, contaminated items; immediately after removing gloves; between patient contacts
Personal protective equipment (PPE)	
• Gloves	For touching blood, body fluids, secretions, excretions, contaminated items; for touching mucous membranes and nonintact skin
• Mask, eye protection, face shield	During procedures and patient-care activities, likely to generate splashes or sprays of blood, body fluids, secretions
• Gown	During procedures and patient-care activities, when contact with clothing/exposed skin with blood/body fluids, secretions, and excretions is anticipated
Soiled patient-care equipment	Handle in a manner that prevents transfer of microorganisms to others and to the environment; wear gloves if visibly contaminated; perform hand hygiene.
Environmental control	Develop procedures for routine care, cleaning, and disinfection of environmental surfaces, especially frequently touched surfaces in patient-care areas.
Textiles and laundry	Handle in a manner that prevents transfer of microorganisms to others and to the environment.
Needles and other sharps	Do not recap, bend, break, or hand-manipulate used needles; if recapping is required, use a one-handed scoop technique only; use safety features when available; place used sharps in puncture-resistant container.
Patient resuscitation	Use mouthpiece, resuscitation bag, other ventilation devices to prevent contact with mouth and oral secretions.
Patient placement	Prioritize single-patient room if patient is at increased risk of transmission, is likely to contaminate the environment, does not maintain appropriate hygiene, or is at increased risk of acquiring infection or developing adverse outcome following infection.
Respiratory Hygiene/Cough Etiquette (source containment of infectious respiratory secretions in symptomatic patients, beginning at initial point of encounter, e.g., triage and reception areas)	Instruct symptomatic persons to cover mouth/nose when sneezing/coughing; use tissues and dispose in no-touch receptacle; observe hand hygiene after soiling of hands with respiratory secretions; wear surgical mask if tolerated or maintain spatial separation, >3 feet if possible.

Source: CDC Draft Guideline on Isolation Precautions: Preventing Transmission of Infectious Agents in Healthcare Settings. (Retrieved June 15, 2004 from *http://www.cdc.gov/ncidod/hip/isoguide.htm.*

are applied within hospitals in specially designed units with laminar air flow and HEPA (high-efficiency particulate air) filtration.

Airborne Isolation

Selected strategies for Airborne Isolation may be used occasionally in home care or hospice, but with modifications since the home environment does not include negative pressure rooms. A modified approach to Airborne Isolation should be used for patients known to be or suspected of being infected with an agent transmitted by the airborne route—that is, via tiny respiratory secretions known as airborne droplet nuclei. These small particles (5 μm or smaller) can remain suspended in the air and can be dispersed widely by air currents within a room or

over a long distance. Diseases transmitted by airborne droplet nuclei include active pulmonary or laryngeal tuberculosis that has not been adequately treated, chickenpox, measles, smallpox, certain viral hemorrhagic fevers (VHFs), and probably SARS, under certain circumstances. Home care and hospice staff may need to consider the use of masks, respirators, and other strategies to protect themselves if there is a family member or other resident in the home of a patient who is known to have or suspected of having one of these illnesses.

In hospitals and other residential care settings, Airborne Isolation requires that the infected patient be placed in a single room with negative air pressure and adequate air exchanges (AIA, 2001). Because this is usually not possible in the home, the home care and hospice staff must evaluate the situation, educate the patient the family and household members about how the infectious agent may be transmitted to others, and determine how to most effectively avoid exposure and potential transmission.

Home care or hospice staff members should wear an N-95 respirator upon entering a home in which a patient or household member is known to have or suspected of having active or inadequately treated pulmonary or laryngeal TB, draining tuberculin skin lesions, smallpox, viral hemorrhagic fever, or SARS. There is debate and some controversy as to whether an N-95 respirator or surgical mask should be worn upon entry to a home in which a patient or household member is known to have or suspected of having measles, chickenpox, or disseminated herpes zoster (CDC, 2004a).

Prevention of exposure to airborne infections by other household members or visitors should also be considered. Most adults and children are immune to chicken pox and measles due to past infection or immunization. Thus, there are few circumstances where susceptible individuals would be identified. The other airborne infections (i.e., smallpox, viral hemorrhagic fever, or SARS) are less common and more serious, however. Family and household members exposed to an individual with active pulmonary or laryngeal TB are commonly identified, skin tested, and treated (as necessary) by a public health agency. It is very difficult to avoid exposure to TB within a household. Public health providers may recommend that a susceptible individual, especially a child, who has not been exposed be removed from the home while the individual with TB is contagious.

Home care or hospice staff should wear an N-95 respirator when entering the home of a TB patient as long as the individual is considered contagious. The determination of when it is safe to discontinue precautions is based on the provision of appropriate therapy, improvement of signs and symptoms, and the results of three sputum smears for AFB (acid-fast bacilli). Once the three smears, obtained on three separate days, are negative, precautions may be discontinued (CDC, 1994). AFB smears can be obtained and interpreted in a day or two, alleviating the need to obtain negative AFB cultures, which can take several weeks to incubate and interpret.

As outlined in Chapter 13, the CDC has drafted contingency plans in the event of an outbreak or epidemic of smallpox. This plan includes the care of patients in their homes, as appropriate, in order to move them out of hospitals and other residential care settings as soon as it is safe to do so. Thus, home care staff may partic-

ipate in this care under the direction of state or local public health authorities. Both Airborne Isolation and Contact Precautions are recommended during the care of patients with smallpox for the duration of the illness. This duration is approximately 3 to 4 weeks and ends once scabs have crusted and separated (CDC, 2004a).

If patients with SARS are cared for in their homes by home care staff, the staff would likely be supported or directed by public health professionals as well. Should an individual infected with SARS require care at home, the residence should be assessed to ensure the arrangements are suitable and others are not put at risk. Conducting this assessment may be a public health role, but home care staff may be asked to assist. The SARS patient should have a private room in which to sleep and rest, if possible. If there is more than one bathroom, a bathroom should be designated for the sole use by the patient. If the home is a multiple-family dwelling, it is ideal if there is a separate air-handling system for the apartment or dwelling housing the patient (CDC, 2004b).

There should be someone available and identified as the primary caregiver at home to ensure the SARS patient has food and medications and their other personal needs are met. The SARS patient should not leave the home during the illness unless it is absolutely necessary. Should such a necessity arise, public transportation should not be used. The patient should wear a mask, if it is tolerated, during transport by private vehicle. If the patient cannot tolerate a mask, others within the vehicle should wear masks or N-95 respirators. Other household members should remain separate from the SARS patient as much as possible, and the number of residents in the household during the illness should be kept to a minimum. Relocation of those at risk, such as those with underlying chronic illness, should be accomplished, if possible. The caregiver should limit access to the home by unexposed visitors, allowing only those with an essential need to enter the home (CDC, 2004b).

The SARS patient should be instructed to practice Respiratory Hygiene/Cough Etiquette and should be provided with sufficient tissues. Tissues and other waste that may be contaminated with respiratory secretions should be discarded in a lined waste container and then be placed within another container for disposal with household waste. If possible, the SARS patient should wear a surgical mask while in the presence of others. If this is not tolerable, the other individuals present should wear surgical masks when in the presence of the SARS patient. The home care organization should instruct the family and household members on how SARS is transmitted, explain how masks should be used, and provide a sufficient supply of masks. Hand hygiene should be encouraged for the patient, family, and household members as well as for home care staff. Home care staff should use gloves when caring for the patient if contact with respiratory secretions is anticipated. Family members should also be instructed not to share towels, bedding, or eating or drinking utensils with the patient. Laundry can be washed as usual, however, as can dishes, glasses, etc. (CDC, 2004b).

The family or caregiver of the SARS patient should be instructed on the cleaning and disinfection of environmental surfaces that may be contaminated with respiratory secretions. A household disinfectant can be utilized to clean surfaces whenever they are soiled or possibly contaminated, with special attention to surfaces frequently touched by the patient. If possible, the bathroom used by the patient should be cleaned and disinfected daily. The individual carrying out any of these cleaning and disinfecting tasks should be instructed to wear household utility gloves.

VHF, such as Ebola and Lassa fever virus, have rarely been seen in the United States (to date there have been imported cases only). There is potential for the introduction of one of these agents into the United States, due to the significant amount of international travel by citizens of the United States and other countries. VHFs are also potential bioterrorism agents, as cited in a document from the CDC in 2000 (CDC, 2000b). An excellent discussion of VHFs can be found in the consensus statement developed by the Working Group on Civilian Biodefense (Borio *et al.,* 2002). A single case or a few cases of VHF would likely be cared for in an acute-care setting; however, should an outbreak or epidemic of VHF occur, home care organizations could be called upon to provide care. The types of VHFs known to be transmitted from person to person are Ebola, Marburg, Lassa fever, and New World. The others are transmitted via mosquito vectors. It is clear from epidemiologic studies in Africa that these infectious agents are usually transmitted through contact with blood or bloody body fluids. There is some evidence of transmission via the airborne route, however. Therefore, patients with one of these viral infections should be placed on Contact Precautions as well as Airborne Isolation (CDC, 2004a).

Transport of patients with airborne infections during their contagious stage should be avoided. If this is not possible, the Isolation Guideline recommends placing a surgical mask on the patient during transport, if the patient is not in a private vehicle. The staff at the destination (e.g., a physician's office or a dialysis clinic) should be alerted to the patient's status in order to manage the visit and place the patient in an appropriate room. Both home care staff and staff receiving the patient should use the appropriate respiratory protection during transport and care.

Linen and laundry can be washed with soap and water, with no special treatment. Cups and glasses used by the patient should not be shared among family members before being washed. No special treatment of dishes and eating utensils is required. Chapter 9 provides information about handling linen and laundry and cleaning dishes, glasses, cups, and eating utensils.

Droplet Precautions

In addition to Standard Precautions, Droplet Precautions should be used for a patient known or suspected of being infected with microorganisms transmitted by large-particle respiratory droplets (5 mm or larger). Large droplets do not remain suspended in the air and do not travel more than 3 feet from the patient. Droplets may be spread to others who are physically close to the patient (closer than 3 feet) as a result of the patient coughing or sneezing, or during clinical procedures such as suctioning, which generates aerosolized respiratory droplets.

Diseases or conditions that require Droplet Precautions include invasive *Hemophilus influenzae* type b disease (meningitis, pneumonia, epiglottis, and sepsis) and invasive *Neisseria meningitidis* disease (meningitis, pneumonia, and sepsis). Other serious bacterial respiratory infections spread by droplet transmission include diphtheria (pharyngeal), *Mycoplasma pneumoniae* disease, pertussis, pneumonic plague, and streptococcal pharyngitis, pneumonia, or scarlet fever in infants and young children. Serious viral infections spread by droplet transmission include adenovirus, influenza, mumps, parvovirus B19, and rubella. Infants and children with adenoviral infection require both Contact and Droplet Precautions due to the inability of children to continue secretions (CDC, 2004a).

Personal Protective Equipment for Droplet Precautions

In addition to Standard Precautions, home and hospice care staff members and other individuals who will be within 3 feet of a patient diagnosed with or suspected to have one of the above conditions should wear a surgical mask. Staff members should wear a mask when performing procedures such as wound care, bathing, checking vital signs, or auscultating the lungs. A mask does not need to be worn when the staff member will not have close (within 3 feet) physical contact with the patient.

Patient Placement for Droplet Precautions

Whenever possible, patients requiring Droplet Precautions should be placed in a room away from susceptible individuals. When a separate room is not available or when the patient leaves the room, he or she should maintain a distance of at least 3 feet from other family members and visitors at all times to ensure that droplets not be spread. The patient should be instructed to use respiratory hygiene/cough etiquette and not to share personal items such as drinking cups (CDC, 2004a). If a follow-up of exposures with the household is necessary, this is usually managed by a public health department (as would occur with tuberculosis or bacterial meningitis) or by the family's physician (as might occur with streptococcal infections). The family should be instructed about the contagious nature of droplet infection; visits from family members and friends should be discouraged while the patient's or any family member's illness is potentially contagious. Appendix 8-A lists illnesses requiring Droplet Precautions and the duration for which Precautions should be maintained.

Linen and laundry can be washed with soap and water, with no special treatment. Cups and glasses used by the patient should not be shared among family members before being washed. No special treatment of dishes and eating utensils is required. Chapter 9 provides information about handling linen and laundry and cleaning dishes, glasses, cups, and eating utensils.

Droplet Precautions During Patient Transport

If it is medically necessary for an adult patient requiring Droplet Precautions to leave the home while his or her disease is contagious, the patient should wear a surgical mask unless he or she is being transported in a private vehicle. With small children, wearing a mask is not necessary since they do not usually cough with as great a force as adults; in addition, the mask may frighten them or they may refuse to keep the mask on. Every effort should be made to minimize close physical contact between the patient and other persons. The mask should be put on whenever the patient enters a building or closed space where he or she may come in close contact with others. The directions for notifying other health care providers that were described for Airborne Precautions can be followed for Droplet Precautions as well. When the patient is no longer on Droplet Precautions, terminal cleaning of the room where the patient resided is not required. Chapter 9 provides additional information about cleaning environmental surfaces in the home.

Contact Precautions

In addition to Standard Precautions, Contact Precautions should be used to interrupt person-to-person transmission of infectious organisms transmitted by direct or indirect contact when transmission may not be interrupted by Standard Precautions alone. Direct contact involves skin-to-skin contact with the patient, as occurs in the performance of patient care activities that require touching the patient's skin. Indirect contact involves contact with the patient's care items or environmental surfaces in the home that may be contaminated with pathogenic agents. In hospitals and nursing homes, Contact Precautions may be implemented for all or selected patients with MDROs. However, based on experience in home care, Standard Precautions, if practiced consistently, should be adequate for patients with MDROs. Chapter 7 provides a more comprehensive discussion of the management of MDROs in home care.

Diseases or conditions that require Contact Precautions include, but are not limited to, the following:

- enteric infections with a low infectious dose or prolonged environmental survival (e.g., *Clostridium difficile*)
- enterohemorrhagic *Escherichia coli* 0157:H7, shigellosis, hepatitis A, or rotavirus in patients wearing diapers or those who are incontinent
- respiratory syncytial virus, parainfluenza virus, or enteroviral infections in infants and children
- viral or hemorrhagic conjunctivitis
- skin infections that are highly contagious or that may occur on dry skin (cutaneous), including:
  - herpes simplex virus (neonatal or mucocutaneous)
  - impetigo
  - major (noncontained) abscesses, cellulitis, or decubiti
  - pediculosis
  - scabies

- staphylococcal furunculosis in infants and young children
- herpes zoster (disseminated or in the immunocompromised host)

Patients with varicella (chickenpox) and disseminated herpes zoster require both Contact Precautions and Airborne Isolation. Infants and children with adenovirus infection require both Contact and Droplet Precautions (CDC, 2004a).

Linen and laundry can be washed with soap and water, with no special treatment. Cups and glasses used by the patient should not be shared among family members before being cleaned. No special treatment of dishes and eating utensils is required. Chapter 9 presents additional information about cleaning linens, laundry, dishes, glasses, cups, and eating utensils.

Gowns, Gloves, and Handwashing for Contact Precautions

Whereas gloves are worn for specific activities or contacts for Standard Precautions, when a patient requires Contact Precautions, gloves should be worn for all direct patient contact as well as for contact with the patient's immediate environment, patient care items, and equipment. Staff members should change gloves after contact with a patient (e.g., when bathing the patient, making the bed, or changing a dressing) or after contact with inanimate objects that may have high concentrations of microorganisms (e.g., items contaminated with stool). Staff members should remove gloves before leaving the patient care area and immediately use an antiseptic hand rub or wash their hands if soiled, of if the patient has Clostridium difficile-associated diarrhea. Staff members should be careful not to touch potentially contaminated environmental surfaces (e.g., doorknobs, sinks, or commodes) or items in the patient's room after gloves are removed and the hands are washed, to prevent the transfer of microorganisms to the patient's environment or to the next patient visited.

In addition to wearing a gown as outlined under Standard Precautions (see Table 8-1), staff members should wear a clean, nonsterile gown for a patient requiring Contact Precautions when there is substantial contact with the patient (such as would occur with bathing, dressing, or wound care), environmental surfaces, or items in the patient's room or if such contact is anticipated as well as when the patient is incontinent or has diarrhea, an ileostomy, a colostomy, or uncontained wound drainage. The gown should not be worn out of the patient's room or immediate care area. After the gown is removed, the staff member's clothing should not contact potentially contaminated environmental surfaces, to prevent the transmission of microorganisms to the environment or the next patient visited.

Contact Precautions During Patient Transport

Patients requiring Contact Precautions may need to attend physician appointments or may wish to visit sites not related to health care. If possible, the colonized or infected site should be covered. If a visit to another health care provider is necessary (e.g., a trip to a physician's office or emergency department), staff at the location should be informed of the need for Contact Precautions upon the patient's arrival.

Guidelines for Discontinuing Contact Precautions

Guidance for the duration of Contact Precautions is found in Appendix 8-A. Once a patient is no longer on Contact Precautions, terminal cleaning of the room where the patient resided is not required. Chapter 9 provides information about cleaning environmental surfaces in the home. Appendix A from the Isolation Guideline is included to provide an alphabetical listing of diagnosis and conditions along with the appropriate category of precautions as well as duration of use.

INITIAL ASSESSMENT AND IMPLEMENTATION OF PRECAUTIONS

The information guiding the decision to place a home care of hospice patient on transmission-based precautions should be outlined in the home care or hospice organization's patient care policies and procedures and should not depend on a physician's order. The need for precautions may be determined based on the report of the patient's history and current condition from a referral source, the physician's order, or information obtained and/or observations made during the initial assessment or any assessment made during the course of home care.

At the time of admission, the patient may not have a definitive diagnosis of an infectious disease. The patient may be symptomatic, or the diagnosis may be pending laboratory results. In these cases, the appropriate Transmission-based Precautions should be initiated based on the staff member's assessment and professional experience or judgment, pending the results of laboratory tests. If the patient presents with a clinical

Table 8-2 Clinical Syndromes or Conditions Warranting Additional Empiric Precautions to Prevent Transmission of Epidemiologically Important Pathogens Pending Confirmation fo Diagnosis*

Clinical Syndrome or Condition†	Potential Pathogens‡	Empiric Precautions
Diarrhea		
Acute diarrhea with a likely infectious cause in an incontinent or diapered patient	Enteric pathogens§	Standard plus Contact (pediatrics and adult)
Meningitis	Neisseria meningitidis	Droplet for first 24 hrs. of antimicrobial therapy; mask and face protection for intubation
	Enteroviruses	Contact for infants and children
Rash or exanthems, generalized, etiology unknown		
Petechial/ecchymotic with fever	Neisseria meningitidis	Droplet for first 24 hrs. of antimicrobial therapy
Vesicular	Varicella, smallpox, or vaccinia virus	Airborne Isolation plus Contact; Contact if vaccinia
Maculopapular with cough, coryza, and fever	Rubeola (measles) virus	Airborne Isolation
Respiratory infections		
Cough/fever/upper lobe pulmonary infiltrate in an HIV-negative patient or a patient at low risk for human immunodeficiency virus (HIV) infection	M. tuberculosis; severe acute respiratory syndrome virus (SARS-CoV)	Airborne Isolation; add Contact plus eye protection if history of SARS exposure, travel
Cough/fever/pulmonary infiltrate in any lung location in an HIV-infected patient or a patient at high risk for HIV infection	M. tuberculosis	Airborne Isolation
Respiratory infections, particularly bronchiolitis and pneumonia, in infants and young children	Respiratory syncytial virus, parainfluenza virus, adenovirus, influenza virus	Contact plus Droplet; Droplet may be discontinued when adenovirus and influenza have been ruled out
Skin or Wound Infection		
Abscess or draining wound that cannot be covered	Staphylococcus aureus, group A streptococcus	Contact

*Infection control professionals should modify or adapt this table according to local conditions. To ensure that appropriate empiric precautions are implemented always, healthcare organizations must have systems in place to evaluate patients routinely according to these criteria as part of their preadmission and admission care.

† Patients with the syndromes or conditions listed may present with atypical signs or symptoms (e.g., neonates and adults with pertussis may not have paroxysmal or severe cough). The clinician's index of suspicion should be guided by the prevalence of specific conditions in the community, as well as clinical judgment.

‡ The organisms listed under the column "Potential Pathogens" are not intended to represent the complete, or even most likely, diagnoses, but rather possible etiologic agents that require additional precautions beyond Standard Precautions until they can be ruled out.

§ These pathogens include enterohemorrhagic Escherichia coli O157:H7, Shigella spp, hepatitis A virus, and rotavirus.

Source: CDC Draft Guideline on Isolation Precautions: Preventing Transmission of Infectious Agents in Healthcare Settings. (Retrieved June 15, 2004 from http://www.cdc.gov/ncidod/hip/isoguide.htm.

syndrome or condition on admission or at any time throughout the course of care, the patient should be treated as if he or she were contagious and should be placed on the appropriate Transmission-based Precautions. The CDC recommends this empiric use of Transmission-based Precautions to avoid potential exposure or transmission while the confirmation of a diagnosis is pending (CDC, 2004). Table 8-2 describes situations and clinical syndromes or conditions that warrant the empiric use of isolation precautions.

INFORMING OTHERS OF ISOLATION PRECAUTIONS WHILE MAINTAINING PATIENT CONFIDENTIALITY

During the patient's initial assessment, the admitting staff member will determine whether precautions beyond Standard Precautions should be taken. If Transmission-based Precautions need to be implemented, the staff member will initiate the appropriate precautions, include the information in the clinical record and care plan, and inform the supervisory staff and other staff members who will be providing patient care. The clinical managers should ensure that the appropriate personal protective equipment is available to staff members or that a sufficient supply is available in the patient's home for the staff's use.

Isolation signs in the home are not necessary, especially for Standard Precautions. If the home or hospice care organization determines that there is some benefit to the use of signs, however, the signs should be labeled and in such a manner that the general public will not know the patient's diagnosis or the specific clinical condition for which the infection control precautions have been instituted. If isolation signs are used, they should state the type of precautions that are in effect. It is considered a breach in confidentiality for a home care or hospice staff member to require staff that a sign be posted that states particulars such as "possible TB," "TB precautions," "stool precautions," "hepatitis precautions."

PATIENT AND FAMILY EDUCATION RELATED TO ISOLATION PRECAUTIONS

Patient and family education related to isolation precautions is important in preventing the transmission of microorganisms from an infected or colonized patient to other individuals in the home via family members. All patients and families should receive basic education about Standard Precautions. Especially during influenza season, patients and family members should also be taught Respiratory Hygiene/Cough Etiquette. As applicable, the patient and family should receive education about Airborne Isolation, Droplet Precautions, or Contact Precautions. The education should address hand hygiene options, modes of transmission, the length of time the patient's disease will be contagious, when isolation precautions may be discontinued, when to use personal protective equipment, patient placement in the home, and strategies to prevent the transmission of infection when the patient must leave the home.

REFERENCES

AIA Guidelines for design and construction of hospitals and healthcare facilities. (2001). Washington, DC: American Institute of Architects.

Borio, L., Inglesby, T., Peters, C. J., Schmaljohn, A., et al., 2002. Hemorrhagic fever viruses as biological weapons: Medical and public health management. *Journal of the American Medical Association, 287*(18), 2391–2405.

Centers for Disease Control and Prevention (2004a). Draft Guideline for isolation: preventing transmission of infectious agents in healthcare settings. (Retrieved 06/15/04 from *http://www.cdc.gov/ncidod/hip/isoguide.html.*)

Centers for Disease Control and Prevention. (2004b). Severe Acute Respiratory Syndrome; Supplement 1: Infection control in healthcare, home and community settings. Retrieved 10/4/04 from *http://www.cdc.gov/ncidod/sars/guidance/I/pdf/patients_home.pdf.*

Centers for Disease Control and Prevention. (2000a). Guidelines for preventing opportunistic infections among hematopoietic stem cell transplant recipients. Recommendations of the CDC, Infectious Disease Society of America, and the American Society of Blood and Marrow Transplantation. *Morbidity and Mortality Weekly Report, 49*(RR10), 1–125.

Centers for Disease Control and Prevention. (2000b). Biological and chemical terrorism: Strategic plan for preparedness and response. *Morbidity and Mortality Weekly Report, (49)* (RR04), 1–14.

Centers for Disease Control and Prevention. (1994). Guidelines for preventing the transmission of *Mycobacterium tuberculosis* in health-care facilities. *Morbidity and Mortality Weekly Report, 43*(RR13), 1–125.

Friedman, M. M., & Rhinehart, E. 2000. Improving infection control in home care: From ritual to science-based practice. *Home Healthcare Nurse, 18*(2), 99–105.

Garner, J. S. (1996). Guideline for isolation precautions in hospitals. *Infection Control and Hospital Epidemiology, 17,* 53–80.

McDonald, L. C., Simor, A., Su, I., Maloney, S., Ofner, M., Chen, K., Lando, J., McGeer, A., Lee, M., & Jernigan., D. 2004. SARS in healthcare facilities, Toronto and Taiwan. *Emerging Infectious Diseases, 10*(5). (Retrieved 10/5/04 from *http://www.cdc.gov/ncidod/EID/vol10no5/03-0791.htm.*)

APPENDIX 8-A

Type and Duration of Precautions
for Selected Infections and Conditions

| Infection/Condition | Precautions | | |
	Type*	Duration†	Comments
Abscess			
Draining, major	C	DI	No dressing or containment of drainage; until drainage stops or can be contained by dressing
Draining, minor or limited	S		Dressing covers and contains drainage
Acquired human immunodeficiency syndrome (HIV)	S		
Actinomycosis	S		
Adenovirus infection, in infants and young children (also, see gastroenteritis, adenovirus)	D, C	DI	
Amebiasis	S		
Anthrax			Postexposure chemoprophylaxis; consider postexposure vaccine
Cutaneous	S		Contact Precautions if large amount of drainage cannot be contained
Pulmonary	S		
Aerosolizable spore-containing powder	A, C	DE	Until decontamination of environment complete (644)
Antibiotic-associated colitis (see Clostridium difficile)			
Arthropod-borne viral encephalitides (eastern, western, Venezuelan equine encephalomyelitis; St. Louis, California encephalitis; West Nile Virus)	S		Not transmitted from person to person except rarely by transfusion, and for West Nile virus by organ transplant, by breast milk, or transplacentally install screens in windows and doors in endemic areas Use DEET-containing mosquito repellants and clothing to cover extremities

*Type of Precautions: A, Airborne Isolation; C, Contact; D, Droplet; S, Standard; when A, C, and D are specified, also use S.

† Duration of precautions: CN, until off antimicrobial treatment and culture-negative; DI, duration of illness (with wound lesions, DI means until wounds stop draining); DE, until environment completely decontaminated; U, until time specified in hours (hrs.) after initiation of effective therapy; Unknown: criteria for establishing eradication of pathogen has not been determined.

Source: CDC Draft Guideline on Isolation Precautions: Preventing Transmission of Infectious Agents in Healthcare Settings. (Retrieved June 15, 2004 from http://www.cdc.gov/ncidod/hip/isoguide.htm

Infection/Condition	Precautions		
	Type*	Duration†	Comments
Arthropod-borne viral fevers (dengue, yellow fever, Colorado tick fever)	S		Not transmitted from person to person except by transfusion, rarely Install screens in windows and doors in endemic areas Use DEET-containing mosquito repellants and clothing to cover extremities
Ascariasis	S		Not transmitted from person to person
Aspergillosis	S		Contact Precautions and AII if massive soft tissue infection with copious drainage and repeated irrigations required
Avian influenza	A, D, C	14 days after onset of symptoms	AII preferred (D if AII rooms unavailable); N95 respiratory protection (surgical mask if N95 unavailable); eye protection (goggles, face shield within 3 feet of patient); 14 days after onset of symptoms or until an alternative diagnosis is established or until diagnostic test results indicate that the patient is not infected with influenza A H5N1virus. Human-to-human transmission inefficient and rare, but risk of reassortment with human influenza strains and emergence of pandemic strain serious concern.
Babesiosis	S		Not transmitted from person to person except by transfusion, rarely
Blastomycosis, North American, cutaneous or pulmonary	S		Not transmitted from person to person
Botulism	S		Not transmitted from person to person
Bronchiolitis (see respiratory infections in infants and young children)	C	DI	Use mask according to Standard Precautions and until influenza and adenovirus have been ruled out as etiologic agents
Brucellosis (undulant, Malta, Mediterranean fever)	S		Not transmitted from person to person
Campylobacter gastroenteritis (see gastroenteritis)			
Candidiasis, all forms including mucocutaneous	S		
Cat-scratch fever (benign inoculation lymphoreticulosis)	S		Not transmitted from person to person
Cellulitis	S		
Chancroid (soft chancre)	S		
Chickenpox (see varicella)			
Chlamydia trachomatis			
Conjunctivitis	S		
Genital	S		
Respiratory	S		
Cholera (see gastroenteritis)			
Closed-cavity infection			
Open drain in place; limited or minor drainage	S		Contact Precautions if there is copious uncontained drainage
No drain or closed drainage system in place	S		
Clostridium			
C. botulinum	S		Not transmitted from person to person
C. difficile (also see gastroenteritis, *C. difficile*)	C	DI	Assess need to discontinue antibiotics Avoid the use of shared electronic thermometers Ensure consistent environmental cleaning and disinfection

Infection/Condition	*Precautions* *Type**	*Duration†*	*Comments*
C. perfringens			
Food poisoning	S		Not transmitted from person to person
Gas gangrene	S		Not transmitted from person to person
Coccidioidomycosis (valley fever)			
Draining lesions	S		Not transmitted from person to person
Pneumonia	S		Not transmitted from person to person
Colorado tick fever	S		Not transmitted from person to person
Congenital rubella	C	Until 1 yr. of age	Standard Precautions if nasopharyngeal and urine cultures negative after 3 mos. of age
Conjunctivitis			
Acute bacterial	S		
Chlamydia	S		
Gonococcal	S		
Acute viral (acute hemorrhagic)	C	DI	
Corona virus associated with SARS (SARS-CoV) (see severe acute respiratory syndrome)			
Coxsackie virus disease (see enteroviral infection)			
Creutzfeldt-Jakob disease CJD, vCJD	S		Use disposable instruments or special sterilization/disinfection for surfaces, objects contaminated with neural tissue if CJD or vCJD suspected and has not been R/O; no special burial procedures
Croup (see respiratory infections in infants and young children)			
Cryptococcosis	S		Not transmitted from person to person
Cryptosporidiosis (see gastroenteritis)			
Cysticercosis	S		Not transmitted from person to person
Cytomegalovirus infection, neonatal or immunosuppressed	S		No additional precautions for pregnant HCWs
Decubitus ulcer (pressure sore) infected			
Major	C	DI	If no dressing or containment of drainage; until drainage stops or can be contained by dressing
Minor or limited	S		If dressing covers and contains drainage
Dengue fever	S		Not transmitted from person to person
Diarrhea, acute-infective etiology suspected (see gastroenteritis)			
Diphtheria			
Cutaneous	C	CN	Until 2 cultures taken 24 hrs. apart negative
Pharyngeal	D	CN	Until 2 cultures taken 24 hrs. apart negative
Ebola viral hemorrhagic fever (see viral hemorrhagic fevers)			
Echinococcosis (hydatidosis)	S		Not transmitted from person to person
Echovirus (see enteroviral infection)			
Encephalitis or encephalomyelitis (see specific etiologic agents)			
Endometritis	S		
Enterobiasis (pinworm disease, oxyuriasis)	S		
Enterococcus species (see multidrug-resistant organisms if epidemiologically significant or vancomycin resistant)			
Enterocolitis, *C. difficile* (see *C. difficile,* gastroenteritis)			

Infection/Condition	Precautions		
	Type*	Duration†	Comments
Enteroviral infections	S		Use Contact Precautions for diapered or incontinent children for duration of illness and to control institutional outbreaks
Epiglottitis, due to *Haemophilus influenzae* type b	D	U 24 hrs.	
Epstein-Barr virus infection, including infectious mononucleosis	S		
Erythema infectiosum (also see Parvovirus B19)	S		
Escherichia coli gastroenteritis (see gastroenteritis)			
Food poisoning			
Botulism	S		Not transmitted from person to person
C. perfringens or welchii	S		Not transmitted from person to person
Staphylococcal	S		Not transmitted from person to person
Furunculosis, staphylococcal	S		
Infants and young children	C	DI	
Gangrene (gas gangrene)	S		Not transmitted from person to person
Gastroenteritis	S		Use Contact Precautions for diapered or incontinent persons for the duration of illness or to control institutional outbreaks for gastroenteritis caused by all of the agents below
Adenovirus	S		Use Contact Precautions for diapered or incontinent persons for the duration of illness or to control institutional outbreaks
Campylobacter species	S		Use Contact Precautions for diapered or incontinent persons for the duration of illness or to control institutional outbreaks
Cholera	S		Use Contact Precautions for diapered or incontinent persons for the duration of illness or to control institutional outbreaks
C. difficile	C	DI	Assess need to discontinue antibiotics
			Avoid the use of shared electronic thermometers ensure consistent environmental cleaning and disinfection
Cryptosporidium species	S		Use Contact Precautions for diapered or incontinent persons for the duration of illness or to control institutional outbreaks
E. coli			
Enteropathogenic O157:H7 and other shiga toxin-producing strains	S		Use Contact Precautions for diapered or incontinent persons for the duration of illness or to control institutional outbreaks
Other species	S		Use Contact Precautions for diapered or incontinent persons for the duration of illness or to control institutional outbreaks
Giardia lamblia	S		Use Contact Precautions for diapered or incontinent persons for the duration of illness or to control institutional outbreaks
Noroviruses	S		Use Contact Precautions for diapered or incontinent persons for the duration of illness or to control institutional outbreaks. Persons who clean areas heavily contaminated with feces or vomitus should wear masks; ensure consistent environmental cleaning and disinfection

Infection/Condition	Precautions		
	Type*	Duration†	Comments
Rotavirus	C	DI	Ensure consistent environmental cleaning and disinfection; prolonged shedding may occur in the immunocompromised
Salmonella species (including *S. typhi*)	S		Use Contact Precautions for diapered or incontinent persons for the duration of illness or to control institutional outbreaks
Shigella species	S		Use Contact Precautions for diapered or incontinent persons for the duration of illness or to control institutional outbreaks
Vibrio parahaemolyticus	S		Use Contact Precautions for diapered or incontinent persons for the duration of illness or to control institutional outbreaks
Viral (if not covered elsewhere)	S		Use Contact Precautions for diapered or incontinent persons for the duration of illness or to control institutional outbreaks
Yersinia enterocolitica	S		Use Contact Precautions for diapered or incontinent persons for the duration of illness or to control institutional outbreaks
German measles (see rubella; see congenital rubella)			
Giardiasis (see gastroenteritis)			
Gonococcal ophthalmia neonatorum (gonorrheal ophthalmia, acute conjunctivitis of newborn)	S		
Gonorrhea	S		
Granuloma inguinale (Donovanosis, granuloma venereum)	S		
Guillain-Barré syndrome	S		Not an infectious condition
Hand, foot, and mouth disease (see enteroviral infection)			
Hantavirus pulmonary syndrome	S		Not transmitted from person to person
Helicobacter pylori	S		
Hepatitis, viral			
Type A	S		Provide hepatitis A vaccine postexposure as recommended
Diapered or incontinent patients	C		Maintain Contact Precautions in infants and children <3 years of age for duration of hospitalization; for children 3–14 yrs. of age for 2 weeks after onset of symptoms; >14 yrs. of age for 1 week after onset of symptoms
Type B-HbsAg positive; acute or chronic	S		See specific recommendations for care of patients in hemodialysis centers
Type C and other unspecified non-A, non-B	S		See specific recommendations for care of patients in hemodialysis centers
Type D (seen only with hepatitis B)	S		
Type E	S		Use Contact Precautions for diapered or incontinent individuals for the duration of illness
Type G	S		
Herpangina (see enteroviral infection)			
Herpes simplex (*Herpesvirus hominis*)			
Encephalitis	S		
Mucocutaneous, disseminated or primary, severe	C	Until lesions dry and crusted	
Mucocutaneous, recurrent (skin, oral, genital)	S		

Infection/Condition	Precautions		
	Type*	Duration†	Comments
Neonatal	C	Until lesions dry and crusted	Also, for asymptomatic, exposed infants delivered vaginally or by C-section and if mother has active infection and membranes have been ruptured for more than 4 to 6 hrs. until infant surface cultures obtained at 24–36 hrs. of age negative after 48 hrs. incubation
Herpes zoster (varicella-zoster)			
Disseminated disease in any patient Localized disease in immunocompromised patient	A, C	DI	Susceptible HCWs should not enter room if immune caregivers are available; if entry is required, susceptibles must wear nose/mouth protection; once disseminated disease has been ruled out discontinue A, C. Provide exposed susceptibles post-exposure vaccine within 5 days or place unvaccinated exposed susceptibles on administrative leave for 10–21days
Localized in patient with intact immune system with lesions that can be contained/covered	S	DI	Susceptible HCWs should not provide direct patient care when other immune caregivers are available
Histoplasmosis	S		Not transmitted from person to person
Human immunodeficiency virus (HIV)	S		Post-exposure chemoprophylaxis for high-risk blood exposures
Impetigo	C	U 24 hrs.	
Infectious mononucleosis	S		
Influenza	D	5 days except DI in immunocompromised persons	Private room when available or cohort; avoid placement with high-risk patients; keep doors closed; mask patient when transported out of room; chemoprophylaxis/vaccine to control/prevent outbreaks
Avian influenza (see Avian influenza)			
Kawasaki syndrome	S		Not an infectious condition
Lassa fever (see viral hemorrhagic fevers)			
Legionnaires' disease	S		
Leprosy	S		
Leptospirosis	S		
Lice (head [pediculosis], body, pubic)	C	U 24 hrs.	
Listeriosis	S		Person-to-person transmission rare
Lyme disease	S		Not transmitted from person to person
Lymphocytic choriomeningitis	S		Not transmitted from person to person
Lymphogranuloma venereum	S		
Malaria	S		Not transmitted from person to person except through transfusion, rarely; install screens in windows and doors in endemic areas; use DEET-containing mosquito repellants and clothing to cover extremities
Marburg virus disease (see hemorrhagic fevers)			
Measles (rubeola)	A	DI	Susceptible HCWs should not enter room if immune care providers are available; wear nose/mouth protection regardless of immune status; no recommendation for type of protection, i.e., surgical mask or respirator; post-exposure vaccine within 72 hrs. or immune globulin within 6 days

Infection/Condition	Precautions		
	Type*	Duration†	Comments
Melioidosis, all forms	S		Not transmitted from person to person
Meningitis			
Aseptic (nonbacterial or viral; also see enteroviral infections)	S		Contact with infants and young children
Bacterial, gram negative enteric, in neonates	S		
Fungal	S		
Haemophilus influenzae, type b known or suspected	D	U 24 hrs.	
Listeria monocytogenes	S		Not transmitted from person to person
Neisseria meningitidis (meningococcal) known or suspected	D	U 24 hrs.	
Streptococcus pneumoniae	S		
Tuberculosis	S		Concurrent, active pulmonary disease or draining cutaneous lesions necessitate addition of airborne precautions
Other diagnosed bacterial	S		
Meningococcal disease: sepsis, pneumonia, meningitis	D	U 24 hrs.	Postexposure chemoprophylaxis for household contacts, HCWs exposed to respiratory secretions; postexposure vaccine only if outbreak.
Molluscum contagiosum	S		
Monkeypox	A, C	Until lesions crusted	See www.cdc.gov/ncidod/monkeypox for most current recommendations. Pre- and post-exposure smallpox vaccine recommended for exposed HCWs
Mucormycosis	S		
Multidrug-resistant organisms (MDROs), infection or colonization (e.g., MRSA, VRE, VISA, ESBLs)	S/C		MDROs judged by the infection control program, based on local, state, regional, or national recommendations, to be of clinical and epidemiologic significance. Contact Precautions required in settings with evidence of ongoing transmission, acute care settings with increased risk for transmission, or wounds that cannot be contained by dressings; see Recommendations and Appendix B, recommendations for management options; criteria for discontinuing precautions not established. Contact state health department for guidance regarding new or emerging MDRO
Mumps (infectious parotitis)	D	U 9 days	After onset of swelling, susceptible HCWs should not provide care if immune caregivers are available.
Mycobacteria, nontuberculosis (atypical)			
Pulmonary	S		
Wound	S		
Mycoplasma pneumonia	D	DI	
Necrotizing enterocolitis	S		Contact Precautions when cases temporally clustered
Nocardiosis, draining lesions, or other presentations	S		
Norovirus (see gastroenteritis)			
Norwalk agent gastroenteritis (see gastroenteritis)			
Orf	S		
Parainfluenza virus infection, respiratory in infants and young children	C	DI	
Parvovirus B19	D		Maintain precautions for duration of hospitalization when chronic disease occurs in an immunodeficient patient. For patients with transient aplastic crisis or red-cell crisis, maintain precautions for 7 days. Duration of precautions for immunosuppressed patients with persistently positive PCR not defined

Infection/Condition	Precautions		
	Type*	Duration†	Comments
Pediculosis (lice)	C	U 24 hrs. after treatment	
Pertussis (whooping cough)	D	U 5 days	Private room preferred Cohorting an option Post-exposure chemoprophylaxis for household contacts and HCWs with prolonged exposure to respiratory secretions
Pinworm infection	S		
Plague *(Yersinia pestis)*			
Bubonic	S		
Pneumonic	D	U 72 hrs.	Antimicrobial prophylaxis for exposed HCW
Pneumonia			
Adenovirus	D, C	DI	
Bacterial not listed elsewhere (including Gram negative bacterial)	S		
B. cepacia in patients with CF, including respiratory tract colonization	C	Unknown	Avoid exposure to other persons with CF; private room preferred. Criteria for D/C precautions not established. See CF foundation guideline
B. cepacia in patients without CF (see Multidrug-resistant organisms)			
Chlamydia	S		
Fungal	S		
Haemophilus influenzae, type b			
Adults	S		
Infants and children	D	U 24 hrs.	
Legionella spp.	S		
Meningococcal	D	U 24 hrs.	
Multidrug-resistant bacterial (see multidrug-resistant organisms)			
Mycoplasma (primary atypical pneumonia)	D	DI	
Pneumococcal	S		
Pneumocystis carinii	S		Avoid placement in the same room with an immunocompromised patient
Staphylococcus aureus	S		
Streptococcus, group A			
Adults	S		
Infants and young children	D	U 24 hrs.	
Varicella-zoster	A	DI	Contact Precautions if skin lesions present
Viral			
Adults	S		
Infants and young children (see respiratory infectious disease, acute)			
Poliomyelitis	C		
Prion disease (See Creutzfeld-Jacob Disease)			
Psittacosis (ornithosis)	S		Not transmitted from person to person
Q fever	S		
Rabies	S	DI	If patient has bitten another individual or saliva has contaminated an open wound or mucous membrane, wash exposed area thoroughly and administer postexposure prophylaxis

Infection/Condition	Type*	Duration†	Comments
Rat-bite fever (*Streptobacillus moniliformis* disease, *Spirillum minus* disease)	S		
Relapsing fever	S		
Resistant bacterial infection or colonization (see multidrug-resistant organisms)			
Respiratory infectious disease, acute (if not covered elsewhere)			
Adults	S		
Infants and young children	C	DI	
Respiratory syncytial virus infection, in infants, young children, and immunocompromised adults	C	DI	
Reye's syndrome	S		Not an infectious condition
Rheumatic fever	S		Not an infectious condition
Rickettsial fevers, tickborne (Rocky Mountain spotted fever, tickborne typhus fever)	S		Not transmitted from person to person except through transfusion, rarely
Rickettsialpox (vesicular rickettsiosis)	S		
Ringworm (dermatophytosis, dermatomycosis, tinea)	S		
Ritter's disease (staphylococcal scalded skin syndrome)	S		
Rocky Mountain spotted fever	S		Not transmitted from person to person except through transfusion, rarely
Roseola infantum (exanthem subitum; caused by HHV-6)	S		
Rotavirus infection (see gastroenteritis)			
Rubella (German measles) (also see congenital rubella)	D	U 7 days after onset of rash	Susceptible HCWs should not enter room if immune caregivers are available. Wear nose/mouth protection, e.g., surgical mask, regardless of immune status
Rubeola (see measles)			
Severe acute respiratory syndrome (SARS)	A, D, C	DI plus 10 days after resolution of fever, provided respiratory symptoms are absent or improving	AII preferred; D if AII rooms unavailable. N95 or higher respiratory protection; surgical mask if N95 unavailable; eye protection (goggles, face shield); aerosol-producing procedures and "supershedders" highest risk for transmission; vigilant environmental disinfection (see *www.cdc.gov/ncidod/sars*)
Salmonellosis (see gastroenteritis)			
Scabies	C	U 24	
Scalded skin syndrome, staphylococcal (Ritter's disease)	S		Contact Precautions for 24 hours after initiation of effective therapy if outbreak within a unit
Schistosomiasis (bilharziasis)	S		
Shigellosis (see gastroenteritis)			
Smallpox (variola; see vaccinia for management of vaccinated persons)	A, C	DI	Until all scabs have crusted and separated (3–4 weeks). Non-vaccinated HCWs should not provide care when immune HCWs are available; N95 or higher respiratory protection required for susceptible and successfully vaccinated individuals; postexposure vaccine within 4 days of exposure protective.
Sporotrichosis	S		

Infection/Condition	Precautions		
	Type*	Duration†	Comments
Spirillum minus disease (rat-bite fever)	S		
Staphylococcal disease (*S aureus*)			
Skin, wound, or burn			
Major [a]	C	DI	No dressing or dressing does not contain drainage adequately
Minor or limited [b]	S		Dressing covers and contains drainage adequately
Enterocolitis	S		Use Contact Precautions for diapered or incontinent children for duration of illness
Multidrug-resistant (see multidrug-resistant organisms)			
Pneumonia	S		
Scalded skin syndrome	S		
Toxic shock syndrome	S		
Streptobacillus moniliformis disease (rat-bite fever)	S		Not transmitted from person to person
Streptococcal disease (group A streptococcus)			
Skin, wound, or burn			
Major	C	U 24 hrs.	No dressing or dressing does not contain drainage adequately
Minor or limited	S		Dressing covers and contains drainage adequately
Endometritis (puerperal sepsis)	S		
Pharyngitis in infants and young children	D	U 24 hrs.	
Pneumonia in infants and young children	D	U 24 hrs.	
Scarlet fever in infants and young children	D	U 24 hrs.	
Serious invasive disease, e.g., necrotizing fasciitis, toxic shock syndrome	D	U24 hrs.	Contact Precautions for draining wound as above; follow recommendations for antimicrobial prophylaxis in selected conditions
Streptococcal disease (group B streptococcus), neonatal	S		
Streptococcal disease (not group A or B) unless covered elsewhere	S		
Multidrug-resistant (see multidrug-resistant organisms)			
Strongyloidiasis	S		
Syphilis			
Latent (tertiary) and seropositivity without lesions	S		
Skin and mucous membrane, including congenital, primary, secondary	S		
Tapeworm disease			
Hymenolepis nana	S		Not transmitted from person to person
Taenia solium (pork)	S		Not transmitted from person to person
Other	S		Not transmitted from person to person
Tetanus	S		Not transmitted from person to person
Tinea (e.g., fungus infection, dermatophytosis, dermatomycosis, ringworm)	S		
Toxoplasmosis	S		
Toxic shock syndrome (staphylococcal disease, streptococcal disease)	S		
Trachoma, acute	S		

	Precautions		
Infection/Condition	Type*	Duration†	Comments
Trench mouth (Vincent's angina)	S		
Trichinosis	S		
Trichomoniasis	S		
Trichuriasis (whipworm disease)	S		
Tuberculosis *(M. tuberculosis)*			
Extrapulmonary, draining lesion including scrofula)	A, C		Discontinue precautions only when patient is improving clinically and drainage has ceased or there are three consecutive negative cultures of continued drainage. Examine for evidence of active pulmonary tuberculosis
Extrapulmonary, no draining lesion, meningitis	S		Examine for evidence of pulmonary tuberculosis
Pulmonary or laryngeal disease, confirmed	A		Discontinue precautions only when patient on effective therapy is improving clinically and has three consecutive sputum smears negative for acid-fast bacilli collected on separate days
Pulmonary or laryngeal disease, suspected	A		Discontinue precautions only when the likelihood of infectious TB disease is deemed negligible, and either 1) there is another diagnosis that explains the clinical syndrome or 2) the results of three sputum smears for AFB are negative. Each of the three sputum specimens should be collected 8–24 hours apart, and at least one should be an early-morning specimen
Skin-test positive with no evidence of current active disease	S		
Tularemia			BSL 2 laboratory only for processing cultures
Draining lesion	S		Not transmitted from person to person
Pulmonary	S		Not transmitted from person to person
Typhoid (*Salmonella typhi*) fever (see gastroenteritis)			
Typhus, endemic and epidemic	S		Not transmitted from person to person
Urinary tract infection (including pyelonephritis), with or without urinary catheter	S		
Vaccinia (vaccination site, adverse events following vaccination) *			Only vaccinated HCWs have contact with active vaccination sites and care for persons with adverse vaccinia events; if unvaccinated, only HCWs without contraindications to vaccine may provide care
Vaccination site care (including autoinoculated areas)	S		Vaccination recommended for vaccinators; for newly vaccinated HCWs: semi-permeable dressing over gauze until scab separates, with dressing change as fluid accumulates, 3–5 days; gloves, hand hygiene for dressing change; vaccinated HCW or HCW without contraindication to vaccine for dressing changes.
Eczema vaccinatum	C	Until lesions dry and crusted, scabs separated	For contact with virus-containing lesions and exudative material
Fetal vaccinia	C		
Generalized vaccinia	C		
Progressive vaccinia			
Postvaccinia encephalitis	S		
Blepharitis or conjuctivitis	S/C		Use Contact Precautions if there is copious drainage
Iritis or keratitis	S		

Infection/Condition	Type*	Duration†	Comments
		Precautions	
Vaccinia-associated erythema multiforme (Stevens Johnson Syndrome)	S		Not an infectious condition
Secondary bacterial infection (e.g., *S. aureus,* group A beta hemolytic streptococcus)	S/C		Follow organism-specific (strep, staph most frequent) recommendations and consider magnitude of drainage
Varicella	A, C	Until lesions dry and crusted	Susceptible HCWs should not enter room if immune caregivers are available; wear nose/mouth protection regardless of immune status; no recommendation for type of protection, i.e., surgical mask or respirator; in immunocompromised host with varicella pneumonia, prolong duration of precautions after lesions crusted; post-exposure vaccine within 120 hours; VZIG within 96 hours for post-exposure prophylaxis for susceptible exposed persons for whom vaccine is contraindicated, including immunocompromised persons, pregnant women, newborns whose mother's varicella onset is ≤5 days before delivery or within 48 hrs. after delivery
Variola (see smallpox)			
Vibrio parahaemolyticus (see gastroenteritis)			
Vincent's angina (trench mouth)	S		
Viral hemorrhagic fevers due to Lassa, Ebola, Marburg, Crimean-Congo fever viruses	A, C	DI	Add eye protection, double gloves, leg and shoe coverings, and impermeable gowns, according to hemorrhagic fever specific barrier precautions. Notify public health officials immediately if Ebola is suspected (*www.bt.cdc.gov*)
Viral respiratory diseases (not covered elsewhere)			
Adults	S		
Infants and young children (see respiratory infectious disease, acute)			
Whooping cough (see pertussis)			
Wound infections			
Major	C	DI	No dressing or dressing does not contain drainage adequately
Minor or limited	S		Dressing covers and contains drainage adequately
Yersinia enterocolitica gastroenteritis (see gastroenteritis)			
Zoster (varicella-zoster) (see herpes zoster)			
Zygomycosis (phycomycosis, mucormycosis)	S		

CHAPTER 9

Guidelines for Cleaning and Disinfection

Although the epidemiology of infections acquired through the provision of home and hospice care has not been adequately studied, there is evidence that the use of medical devices in the home increases the risk of infection (Danzig *et al.,* 1995; Do *et al.,* 1999, Kellerman *et al.,* 1996). Each home and hospice care organization must identify the devices that are used in the provision of patient care, determine if their use should be one-time only (e.g., needles and syringes); more than one time, but for a single patient (e.g., disposable wound irrigation sets); or for multiple patients after reprocessing (e.g., blood pressure cuffs). For those items that are reusable, the home and hospice care organization must develop a procedure for cleaning and reprocessing them, depending upon their use and the potential risk of transmitting an infectious agent from one patient to another (refer to Chapter 2). Although this may seem an overwhelming task, there are many resources to assist the home and hospice care organization in (1) categorizing the device and its criticality of use (i.e., its potential to contribute to a health care–associated infection) and (2) determining the appropriate steps and materials necessary for reprocessing the device for use by another patient.

This chapter has been compiled using many resources, including the APIC Guideline for Sterilization and Disinfection (Rutala, 1996) and the Guideline for Environmental Infection Control in HealthCare Facilities (CDC, 2003). The chapter's content and guidance also rely heavily on the scheme developed by E. H. Spaulding in 1968. When Dr. Spaulding's approach to categorizing devices according to their use and risk for transmission is understood, the scheme can be applied to determine the necessary level of cleaning and disinfec-

tion, and the development of policies and procedures for reprocessing equipment in an informed, safe manner.

SPAULDING'S SCHEME

Spaulding classifies patient care equipment into three categories (Spaulding, 1968):

Critical items: devices that enter sterile tissue or spaces and thus must be sterile for use (e.g., intravenous therapy catheters and needles, indwelling urinary catheters).

Semicritical items: devices that contact mucus membranes and nonintact skin (e.g., oral suction catheters). These items require intermediate-level disinfection or high-level disinfection.

Noncritical items: equipment that contacts intact skin and thus should be clean for use or undergo low-level disinfection (e.g., stethoscopes, blood pressure cuffs).

The category of equipment and its intended use determine the type and level of cleaning, disinfection, or sterilization necessary to reduce the risk of infection and to render the equipment safe for use. Noncritical, semicritical, and critical items that may be used in the home and hospice care setting include, but are not limited to, those identified in Table 9-1.

DEFINITION OF TERMS

Cleaning is the first step in the reprocessing of any reusable equipment. Cleaning is the physical removal of visible organic material or soil from objects, environmental surfaces, and skin. Cleaning will remove

Table 9-1 Categorization of Home Care Equipment

Noncritical items	Semicritical items	Critical items
Apnea monitor	Oral or rectal thermometers	Dialysate solution
Back support belt	Laryngeal mirror	IV fluids
Bandage scissors	Tub used for soaking nonintact skin	IV catheters and tubing
Bath basin	Oral suction catheter	Irrigation solution
Blood pressure cuff	Respiratory therapy equipment:	Needles
Blood glucose monitor	• Humidifier	Tracheal suction catheter
Bedpan	• Nebulizer and reservoir	Urinary catheter
Cane	• Oral airway	
Commode	• Breathing circuit of mechanical ventilators	
Crutches	• Manual ventilation bag	
Doppler unit	• Nasal cannula	
Hydrotherapy equipment (used for intact skin)		
Infusion pump		
IV pole		
Linen		
Nail clippers		
Pulse oximeter		
Scales		
Shampoo board		
Stethoscope		
Suction collection canister		
Tape measure		
Tympanic or axillary thermometer		
Ultrasonic stimulator		
Urinal		
Walker		
Wheelchair		
Work surfaces		

Source: Friedman, M. (1996). Designing an Infection Control Program to meet JCAHO's Standards. *CARING 15,* 18–25. Used with permission from the National Association for Home Care and Hospice.

most microorganisms but will not destroy them. Thus, depending upon use, some items require additional steps for disinfection or sterilization. Removing all organic matter from the equipment is the most important step in reprocessing. If the equipment is not properly cleaned first, additional steps for disinfection or sterilization will not be effective. Cleaning consists of washing an item with a detergent or disinfectant-detergent and water, rinsing the item, and thoroughly drying it. Items need to be cleaned before they can be disinfected because organic material, such as total parenteral nutrition solution, enteral feeding solution, or blood, may have collected on the surface.

Decontamination is the use of physical or chemical means to remove, inactivate, or destroy pathogens on a surface or item to prevent transmission of infectious agents and render the item or surface safe for handling, use, or disposal (Occupational Safety and Health Administration [OSHA], 1991). The physical act of scrubbing with a detergent or surfactant and rinsing with water removes a large number of microorganisms from soiled or contaminated surfaces. Thus, cleaning is a form of decontamination.

A *germicide* is an agent that destroys microorganisms on both living tissue and inanimate objects, hence the suffix -*cide* to reflect the destruction of microorganisms. There are three types of germicides: antiseptics, disinfectants, and chemical sterilants. An *antiseptic* is a germicide that is used on skin or tissue. Antiseptics should not be used to decontaminate inanimate objects such as devices or environmental surfaces. A *disinfectant* is a germicide used to eliminate pathogenic microorganisms from inanimate objects and surfaces. A *chemical sterilant* is a liquid chemical placed on an inanimate object that destroys all forms of microbial life, including fungal and bacterial spores.

The disinfection process uses specific chemicals that have been tested to determine their effectiveness in killing selected microorganisms, including bacteria, mycobacteria, and viruses. Disinfectants do not ordinarily kill bacterial spores, however. Before an item can be disinfected, it must be cleaned to remove organic matter, because organic matter can neutralize the disinfectant. In addition, without proper cleaning the disinfectant may not be able to penetrate the debris and destroy microorganisms.

In home and hospice care, disinfection is usually accomplished by soaking, spraying, or drenching an item in a liquid chemical for a specified period (or "contact time") or by wet pasteurization (i.e., boiling for up to 30 minutes after cleaning). If a commercially prepared disinfectant is used, it should be used only as directed on the label, and the manufacturer's instructions should be followed exactly.

Sterilization is the complete destruction of all forms of microbial life, including bacterial spores. Either physical or chemical processes, such as steam under pressure, dry heat, ethylene oxide gas, or liquid chemicals, accomplish sterilization. The sterilization process is usually not performed by home or hospice care staff. Therefore, this chapter focuses primarily on disinfection.

LEVELS OF DISINFECTION

There are three levels of disinfection: low-level, intermediate-level, and high-level. When applied appropriately (i.e., at the recommended dilution and contact time), high-level disinfection destroys all microorganisms except bacterial spores. Intermediate-level disinfection destroys vegetative bacteria, mycobacterium tuberculosis, and most fungi; it neutralizes most viruses but does not kill bacterial spores. Low-level disinfection destroys most bacteria, fungi, and some viruses (e.g., human immunodeficiency virus [HIV], influenza viruses, adenovirus).

Products that can be used in home and hospice care for intermediate-level disinfection include (Rutala, 1996):

- sodium hypochlorite (5.25% household bleach), 1:50 dilution

- phenolic germicidal detergent solutions, diluted according to the product label
- iodophor germicidal solution (e.g., povidone-iodine), diluted according to the product label
- ethyl or isopropyl alcohol (70% to 90%)

OSHA's bloodborne pathogen regulations require that contaminated surfaces and items be decontaminated with an appropriate disinfectant. OSHA considers the following to be appropriate disinfectants:

- EPA-registered disinfectants with a tuberculocidal claim
- Solutions of 5.25% sodium hypochlorite (household bleach), diluted between 1:10 and 1:100 with water (OSHA, 1993)

Products that can be used to produce low-level disinfection include (Rutala, 1996):

- quaternary ammonium compounds, diluted according to the product label
- ethyl or isopropyl alcohol (70% to 90%)
- sodium hypochlorite (5.25% household bleach), 1:500 dilution
- phenolic germicidal detergent solutions (e.g., Lysol), diluted according to the product label
- iodophor germicidal solution (e.g., povidone-iodine), diluted according to the product label

Ethyl alcohol or isopropyl alcohol in concentrations of 60% to 90% volume per volume is appropriate for small surfaces (e.g., thermometer, central venous catheter injection cap) and stethoscopes; however, it should not be used for larger surfaces as alcohol evaporates quickly and makes extended surface contact time difficult to achieve (CDC, 2003).

GOVERNMENTAL OVERSIGHT

The Environmental Protection Agency (EPA) is the government agency responsible for overseeing the registration of sterilants, tuberculocidal disinfectants, disinfectants for HIV, disinfectants for HBV, and antimicrobial products. Germicides labeled as "hospital disinfectants" have passed the EPA's potency test for activity against three primary microorganisms (i.e., *Pseudomonas aeruginosa, Staphylococcus aureus,* and *Salmonella cholaerae-suis*) and are suitable for achieving low-level disinfection. Germicides labeled as "tuberculocidal hospital disinfectants" are suitable for intermediate-level disinfection, as the products have passed the EPA's germicidal potency test against mycobacterium (thus the label "tuberculocidal"). Mycobacteria have the highest intrinsic level of resistance among the vegetative bacteria, viruses, and fungi; therefore, if a germicidal product has "tuberculocidal" on the product label, the product is considered capable of inactivating a broad spectrum of pathogens that are much less resistant (CDC, 2003). Sodium hypochlorite (bleach) is inexpensive and effective against a broad spectrum of microorganisms. Despite evidence that sodium hypochlorite is an adequate germicidal against bloodborne pathogens, many chlorine bleach products available in retail grocery stores are not registered by the EPA for use as a surface disinfectant. The EPA tests products for safety and performance when the product is used according to the product label. Using non-EPA registered bleach as a surface disinfectant is considered by the EPA to be an "unregistered use"; users do so at their own risk. A list of products registered with the EPA as effective against HBV and Human HIV-1 (List D) can be located on the EPA's website at *http://www.epa.gov/oppad001/list_d_hepatitisbhiv.pdf*. List E includes the EPA's registered antimicrobial products registered as effective against *Mycobacterium spp,* Human HIV-1 virus, and HBV and can be found at *http://www.epa.gov/oppad001/list_e_mycobact_hiv_hepatitis.pdf.* These lists are updated regularly by the EPA and should be reviewed when making product purchase decisions.

OSHA's current policy is that EPA-registered disinfectants for HIV and HBV meet the requirement in the bloodborne pathogen standard and are "appropriate" disinfectants for cleaning contaminated surfaces, provided that such surfaces have not become contaminated with agent(s), volumes, or concentrations of agent(s) for which higher level disinfection is recommended (OSHA, 1999). This means that EPA-registered products from List D (i.e., products effective against HBV and HIV) would be an "appropriate disinfectant" under OSHA's bloodborne pathogen standard where HIV and HBV are the *only* pathogens of concern (e.g., in a research setting). In home and hospice care, it is generally not known what bloodborne pathogens may be present. Therefore, it would be prudent to use a registered product from List E (i.e., products effective against *Mycobacterium spp,* Human HIV-1 virus and HBV).

CLEANING AND DISINFECTING PATIENT CARE EQUIPMENT

Before the disinfection process begins, it is essential that the object be thoroughly cleaned and all organic matter removed. After cleaning, the object may be soaked, sprayed, or wiped down with chemical disinfecting solution, with the solution left on the object for the required period of contact time. When a piece of medical equipment, such as a commode, is picked up at a hospice patient's home by a delivery driver, the driver may decontaminate the equipment to make it safe for handling by spraying it down with a disinfectant and waiting the allotted time for it to dry before placing it in the delivery vehicle. When the equipment is returned to the facility, it will need to be properly cleaned and disinfected so that it is ready for another patient's use. The effectiveness of the disinfection process is determined by the following factors (Rutala, 1996):

- whether the object was cleaned before it was disinfected
- the object's organic load (i.e., the amount of soil and contamination)
- the type and level of microbial contamination
- the type, concentration, and contact time with the germicide
- the physical configuration of the object (i.e., flat surface versus a surface with crevices)
- the temperature and pH of the disinfectant

When disinfectants are used, home and hospice care staff members should take precautions to prevent or minimize exposure to either the chemical disinfectant solution or the microorganisms being removed from the equipment by using personal protective equipment such as gloves. A gown, mask, and goggles or face shield also may be needed if the cleaning method may result in the solution splashing. Utility gloves are recommended when equipment is being cleaned before the disinfecting procedure, because examination gloves can easily rip and cause exposure to the chemical solution as well as other potentially infectious material. When the equipment is handled after the exposure time period (i.e., contact time) to the disinfectant has been completed, gloves should be worn to prevent exposure to any remaining disinfectant solution.

Exhibit 9-1 How to Make Bleach Disinfecting Solutions (Intermediate-level)

To make a 1:10 bleach disinfecting solution:

Combine 1/2 cup bleach with 1 quart water

or

1/4 cup bleach with 2 1/4 cups water

To make a 1:5 bleach disinfecting solution:

Combine 1/2 cup bleach with 2 cups water

or

1/4 cup bleach with 1 cup water

How to Prepare a Bleach Disinfecting Solution

One of the chemicals most commonly used for disinfection is a homemade solution of household bleach and water. Bleach is inexpensive, easy to obtain, and is effective against HIV in a 1:10 solution of 5.25% sodium hypochlorite (household bleach). A 1:10 bleach solution is 1 part bleach to 9 parts water, and a 1:5 solution is 1 part bleach to 4 parts water (Rutala, 1996). The solution of bleach and water is easy to mix, nontoxic, and safe if handled properly, and it kills most infectious agents. It is important to note that some infectious agents are not killed by bleach. For example, *Cryptosporidium* species are killed only by ammonia or hydrogen peroxide. Exhibit 9-1 explains how to make two different bleach disinfecting solutions.

Bleach Disinfecting Solution Storage

A bleach and water solution loses its strength quickly, and can be weakened by organic material, evaporation, heat, and sunlight. Therefore, a 1:10 bleach solution should be mixed fresh each day to ensure that it is effective, and any leftover solution should be discarded down the sink or toilet at the end of the day. A 1:5 bleach solution may be stored for up to 30 days in an opaque (or brown glass container) at room temperature and out of sunlight. Bleach must never be mixed with anything but fresh tap water. Other chemicals may react with the bleach and release a toxic chlorine gas. The bleach and water solution should be stored in a cool place out of direct sunlight and out of the reach of children. Bleach is corrosive to metals, especially aluminum; it should not be used to decontaminate medical equipment with metallic parts.

Noncritical Item Disinfection Guidelines

As defined earlier, a noncritical item is one that will not come in contact with mucus membranes or nonintact skin. The most commonly used noncritical items in patient care in the home include stethoscopes, blood pressure cuffs, supply bags, scales, and pulse oximeters. Such items should be cleaned in between patient use and may undergo low-level disinfection. If a noncritical item is visibly contaminated with blood or other potentially infectious materials, the staff member should wear gloves and scrub the item with detergent and water, dry it with a disposable towel, and disinfect it with an intermediate-level disinfectant. Items that cannot be cleaned and disinfected without altering their physical integrity and function should not be reused. There is a risk of home or hospice care staff members transmitting infectious agents to patients if their hands become contaminated by touching a contaminated noncritical item. From this risk derives the importance of hand hygiene to prevent the spread of infection (CDC, 2002).

It is up to the staff member to use his or her judgment as to whether a noncritical item has become visibly soiled or contaminated. If it does become contaminated, it can be washed with a detergent or disinfectant-detergent, rinsed, and dried. Wiping blood pressure cuffs and aneroid gauges with 70% isopropyl alcohol or another appropriate disinfectant also may be effective in disinfecting the items. If a patient's skin is not intact, the staff member should wear gloves and place a disposable impermeable barrier between the patient's skin and the cuff to prevent soiling. Other options are to leave a blood pressure cuff in the patient's home to be picked up by the home or hospice care organization for cleaning and disinfecting when the patient is discharged or to provide the patient with a disposable blood pressure cuff.

Laboratory Supplies

When performing phlebotomy in the past, home and hospice care providers frequently removed the needle in order to reuse the blood tube holder and cleaned the blood tube holder in between patient use. OSHA's compliance directive CPL 2-2.69 at XIII.D.5 prohibits staff members from reusing blood tube holders and requires that the blood tube holder, with the needle attached, be immediately discarded into an accessible sharps container after the safety feature has been activated (OSHA, 2002). The reuse of blood tube holders places both the patient and the staff member at risk for exposure to bloodborne pathogens. A study conducted by the National Phlebotomy Association found that 50% to 80% of blood tube holders may be contaminated after just one use (Crawford, 2000).

Noncritical Equipment Provided to Patients

Noninvasive, reusable medical equipment, such as commode chairs, hospital beds, side rails, bedside equipment, walkers, canes, wheelchairs, and other equipment located in the home, should be cleansed and disinfected as soon as their use is discontinued or if they become soiled during use. Guidelines for selecting disinfectants can be found in Table 9-2. High-level disinfectants (e.g., Cidex) should not be used to disinfect noncritical instruments (e.g., ambulatory infusion pumps) and devices or any environmental surface, as this practice is not consistent with the manufacturer's instructions for use and these are toxic chemicals (CDC, 2003).

In the past, the Food and Drug Administration (FDA) identified that reusable (nondisposable) medical devices (e.g., ambulatory infusion pumps) rented or leased from third parties may not have been properly cleaned and disinfected before delivery to home care organizations. Also, when health care facilities exchanged equipment with other institutions, the equipment may not have been properly cleaned and disinfected either before or after patient use. Improper handling of devices between uses can contaminate facilities and expose individuals, including health care providers and couriers, to infectious, biohazardous material. Also, the presence of residual organic material on such equipment may compromise the effectiveness of the disinfection process. Therefore, the FDA recommends that home care organizations renting or leasing reusable medical devices from a third party, review all rental and leasing contracts, agreements, and other written documents to ensure that the parties responsible for cleaning, disinfecting, and/or sterilizing the equipment are clearly identified. If the home or hospice care organization is responsible for cleaning and disinfecting equipment for reuse, it should ensure that all appropriate personnel are aware of this responsibility and are properly trained and equipped to perform these tasks. If a third party is responsible for cleaning and disinfecting equipment for reuse, the home or hospice care organization should review the third party's operating procedures to determine that its facilities, equipment, processes, and personnel are adequate

to perform these operations. The home or hospice care organization should make sure that the third party is familiar with the manufacturer's instructions for cleaning, disinfecting, and/or sterilizing the devices. In addition, the organization must also ensure that its own personnel are properly trained and equipped to handle, package, and label contaminated equipment for shipment back to the supplier. In some cases, third-party suppliers may also reprocess or refurbish medical devices between uses. When the contract requires third-party suppliers to reprocess or refurbish medical devices, the home or hospice care organization should ensure that the supplier is familiar with the device manufacturers' specifications for the products (FDA, 1997).

Cleaning and Disinfecting Guidelines for Semicritical Items

Semicritical items come in contact with mucus membranes but do not enter tissue or the vascular system. Semicritical items should be subjected to either intermediate- or high-level disinfection prior to reuse on a different patient. Examples of semicritical items used in home care are given in Table 9-1. The only semicritical items used in home and hospice care that may be disinfected at an intermediate level are tubs used for soaking nonintact skin and thermometers. A tub used for soaking nonintact skin (e.g., foot ulcers) should be cleaned and subjected to intermediate-level disinfection by cleaning and then wiping down with a 1:50 or, if necessary, a 1:10 dilution of 5.25% household bleach (Rutala, 1996). The tub also may be cleaned and then sprayed with a tuberculocidal hospital disinfectant product, which should be left on the surface for the time required by the manufacturer (i.e., contact time) before being wiped off or rinsed.

Whenever possible, each patient should use his or her own thermometer. If a battery-operated digital thermometer from the nursing supply bag is utilized, a plastic protective sheath should be placed over the tip before it is inserted. After use, the plastic sheath should be discarded. And, the thermometer should be wiped with a 70% isopropyl alcohol or other appropriate disinfectant before being replaced in the carrying case. All other semicritical items should be subjected to high-level disinfection.

Disinfecting Guidelines for Critical Items

Critical items are those that enter the tissue or vascular system; these items require sterilization. Items that must be sterile are usually purchased as sterile. Home

Table 9-2 Methods of Sterilization and Disinfection

Object	Sterilization — Critical Items (will enter tissue or vascular system, or blood will flow through them) Procedure	Exposure Time (hr.)	Disinfection — High Level (semicritical items; will come in contact with mucus membrane or nonintact skin) Procedure (exposure time ≥20 min.)[b, c]	Disinfection — Intermediate Level (some semicritical items[a] and noncritical items) Procedure (exposure time ≤10 min.)	Disinfection — Low Level (noncritical items; will come in contact with intact skin) Procedure (exposure time ≤10 min.)
Smooth, hard surface[a]	A	MR	C	I	I
	B	MR	D	K	J
	C	MR	E	L	K
	D	6	F		L
	E	6	G[d]		M
	F	MR	H		
Rubber tubing and catheters[c]	A	MR	C		
	B	MR	D		
	C	MR	E		
	D	6	F		
	E	6	G[d]		
	F	MR			
Polyethylene tubing and catheters[c, e]	A	MR	C		
	B	MR	D		
	C	MR	E		
	D	6	F		
	E	6	G[d]		
	F	MR			
Lensed instruments	B	MR	C		
	C	MR	D		
	D	6	E	E	
	E	6	F	F	
	F	MR			
Thermometers (oral and rectal)[f]				I[f]	
Hinged instruments	A	MR	C		
	B	MR	D		
	C	MR	E		
	D	6	F		
	E	6			
	F				

A: Heat sterilization, including steam or hot air (see manufacturer's recommendations)
B: Ethylene oxide gas (see manufacturer's recommendations)
C: Glutaraldehyde-based formulations (2%) (caution should be exercised with all glutaraldehyde formulations when further in-use dilution is anticipated)
D: Demand-release chlorine dioxide (will corrode aluminum, copper, brass, series 400 stainless steel, and chrome with prolonged exposure)
E: Stabilized hydrogen peroxide 6% (will corrode copper, zinc, and brass)
F: Peracetic acid, concentration variable, but ≤1% is sporicidal
G: Wet pasteurization at 70°C for 30 min. after detergent cleaning
H: Sodium hypochlorite (1000 ppm available chlorine; will corrode metal instruments)
I: Ethyl or isopropyl alcohol (70%–90%)
J: Sodium hypochlorite (100 ppm available chlorine)
K: Phenolic germicidal detergent solution (follow product label for use-dilution)
L: Iodophor germicidal detergent solution (follow product label for use-dilution)
M: Quaternary ammonium germicidal detergent solution (follow product label for use-dilution)
MR: Manufacturer's recommendations

[a] See text for discussion of hydrotherapy.
[b] The longer the exposure to a disinfectant, the more likely it is that all microorganisms will be eliminated. Ten-minute exposure is not adequate to disinfect many objects, especially those that are difficult to clean, because they have narrow channels or other areas that can harbor organic material and bacteria. Twenty-minute exposure is the minimum time needed to reliably kill *M. tuberculosis* and nontuberculous Mycobacteria with glutaraldehyde.
[c] Tubing must be completely filled for disinfection; care must be taken to avoid entrapment of air bubbles during immersion.
[d] Pasteurization (washer disinfector) of respiratory therapy and anesthesia equipment is a recognized alternative to high-level disinfection. Some data challenge the efficacy of some pasteurization units.
[e] Thermostability should be investigated when appropriate.
[f] Do not mix rectal and oral thermometers at any stage of handling or processing.

Source: Reprinted with permission from W. A. Rutala, "Disinfection, Sterilization, and Waste Disposal" in *Prevention and Control of Nosocomial Infections* (pp. 540–541). © 1997, Williams & Wilkins.

and hospice care organizations generally do not perform sterilization procedures, but some medical equipment classified as critical items, such as urethral catheters used for intermittent catheterization, may be reused. The physician's orders, the patient's health status and home environment, and the patient's or caregiver's abilities will determine whether frequently used critical items, such as respiratory catheters or urethral catheters, can be disinfected between uses in the house or whether sterile products should be purchased and used on a one-time basis. The FDA, which regulates medical devices, covers only the first-time use of products and good manufacturing practices. The FDA does not determine whether a single-use device performs as intended after it has been cleaned and disinfected. Chapter 3 provides additional information about cleaning and disinfecting intermittent urethral catheters.

CLEANING AND DISINFECTING OTHER ITEMS IN THE HOME
Environmental Surfaces

Environmental surfaces carry a low risk of disease transmission and can be safely decontaminated using less rigorous methods than those used on equipment or used in patient care (CDC, 2003). Nonetheless, regular cleaning and removal of soil and dust is still required. Soap and water or a detergent/disinfectant, depending on the type of surface and the degree of contamination, should be used. Surfaces in the patient's home that are frequently touched by the patient or caregiver (e.g., door knobs, light switches, bathroom faucet handles) should be cleaned more frequently. Management of the home environment for a patient colonized or infected with a multidrug-resistant organism is addressed in Chapter 7.

Linens and Laundry

Although soiled linen may be a source of a large number of pathogenic microorganisms, according to the CDC the risk of actual disease transmission is negligible (CDC, 2003). Common sense should be used in the storage and processing of soiled linen. OSHA defines contaminated laundry as "laundry that has been soiled with blood or other potentially infectious material or may contain sharps (OSHA, 1991)." Home and hospice care staff members having contact with contaminated linen should wear protective gloves, hold the linen away from the body, and if necessary, wear an impervious gown if the linen is wet.

If the fabric can tolerate contact with chlorine bleach, it should be washed in a regular wash cycle in hot water with 1 cup of chlorine bleach per full load, along with regular detergent, and dried in an automatic dryer. A chlorine bleach substitute may be used, but the relative effectiveness of such a substitute in destroying microorganisms has not been determined (Belkin, 1998).

If a washing machine and dryer are not available in the patient's home, contaminated linens should be soaked in a receptacle or sink in cold, soapy water in a 1:10 bleach solution for 15 minutes. The linen should be washed and the fluids discarded down the toilet or drain; the staff member should wear gloves and other personal protective equipment as necessary during this washing. The linen should then be rewashed using the same procedure, but with hot soapy water. The clean linen should then be hung to dry outside in the sun. Once the linen is clean, it should be stored in the home in a manner that keeps it clean. In a residential setting such as home care, the CDC does not have any recommendations regarding a hot-water temperature setting and cycle duration. Hot water heated to at least 160°F ($\geq71^{\circ}$C) for a minimum of 25 minutes is needed to clean and sanitize laundry (CDC, 2003), although very hot water (≥120°F) can be a scalding hazard to children. Washing linens at lower temperatures (i.e., <160°F or $<70^{\circ}$C) with proper chemicals (such as bleach) and drying the linens with hot air can also be an effective way to clean and sanitize linens. Commercial dry cleaning of fabrics soiled with blood or other potentially infectious material does not eliminate the risk of pathogen transmission. Several studies have shown that dry cleaning alone is relatively ineffective in reducing the numbers of bacteria and viruses on contaminated linens, and that microbial populations are significantly reduced when dry-cleaned articles are heat pressed (CDC, 2003). Therefore, dry cleaning should be performed only when the fabric is not suitable for cleaning with water and detergent.

Dishes, Glasses, Cups, and Eating Utensils

No special precautions generally are needed for dishes, glasses, cups, or eating utensils. The best way to wash, rinse, and disinfect dishes and eating utensils is to use a dishwasher. If a dishwasher is not available, a multi-compartment sink or dishpan and a dish rack with a drain board should be used to wash the dishes with hot water and detergent.

STORAGE OF MEDICAL EQUIPMENT AND SUPPLIES IN THE HOME CARE OR HOSPICE ORGANIZATION'S FACILITY

Separate areas should be identified for the storage of clean equipment, dirty equipment, cleaning and disinfecting of equipment, equipment requiring repair or maintenance, obsolete inventory, and equipment that is ready for patient use. Physically separating clean and dirty equipment does not mean that the equipment must be kept in separate rooms or locations. As long as the dirty equipment is not physically comingled with the clean equipment, the equipment is considered properly separated. Equipment that is waiting to be cleaned and disinfected can be stored according to one or more of the following methods:

- placing a sticker on the equipment to indicate that it is dirty
- putting the equipment on a shelf that has a "to be cleaned" label on it
- putting the equipment in a red biohazard bag
- placing the equipment in an area that has colored tape on the floor or in confined quarters with a sign on the wall to designate it as an area for equipment to be cleaned
- storing the equipment in any other manner that is consistently followed and understood by the home care or hospice staff members (e.g., placing the item in a black plastic bag or storing the equipment in a certain room)

Once the equipment has been cleaned and disinfected, one or more of the following methods may be used to identify that it has been cleaned and is ready to be used by a patient:

- placing a tag on the equipment indicating that it has been cleaned
- putting the equipment on a shelf that has a "ready for patient use" label on it

- putting the equipment in a clear plastic bag
- placing the equipment in an area that has colored tape on the floor or in confined quarters with a sign on the wall to designate it as an area for equipment that is clean
- storing the equipment in any other manner that is consistently followed and understood by the home care or hospice staff members

Expiration dates on hand hygiene products, medical equipment and supplies, blood collection tubes, and culture medium vials stored in the home care or hospice organization's office should be checked on a regular basis (e.g., monthly) to ensure that the beyond dates have not been passed.

STORAGE OF MEDICAL EQUIPMENT AND SUPPLIES DURING TRANSPORT TO AND FROM THE PATIENT'S HOME

The cleanliness and sterility of items intended to be sterile should be maintained during storage and delivery by being kept in separate areas designated as clean or dirty/contaminated. During transport to or from the patient's home, clean equipment should be kept separate from dirty equipment so that the clean equipment does not become soiled or contaminated. Clean equipment can be separated from dirty equipment in the staff member's vehicle in one or more of the following ways:

- placing dirty equipment in a red or dark-colored plastic bag (rather than a clear bag, which generally designates that the equipment is clean) before placing it near clean equipment
- storing clean equipment and supplies in plastic bags or a trunk box
- storing clean and dirty equipment in any other manner that is understood and consistently followed by home care or hospice staff members

Once dirty equipment is returned to the home care or hospice organization's facility, it should be stored in a designated area and, if required, inspected between patient use (such as is required for infusion pumps). Once the reusable items are properly cleaned, they may be returned to the area designated for clean equipment or supplies.

Vehicles owned or leased by the home care or hospice organization or staff members' vehicles that are used to make home visits, should be cleaned and inspected on a regular basis at the frequency determined by the organization and any applicable law and regulation (e.g., state department of transportation). If an open-back vehicle, such as a pickup truck, is used to make deliveries, equipment and supplies should not be exposed to rain, snow, or other weather conditions that could impair the supplies' integrity or contaminate the equipment and supplies being delivered.

STORAGE OF MEDICAL EQUIPMENT AND SUPPLIES IN THE PATIENT'S HOME

Medical supplies taken into the patient's home should be stored away from pets and small children. The supplies should be placed in a sealable plastic bag, which should be kept closed at all times to prevent the contents from becoming contaminated—especially if the home is infested with pests. Sterile supplies should be stored in a manner that prevents them from becoming contaminated. For example, sterile gauze pads should not be stored under a kitchen or bathroom sink, where they may become wet.

If another health care organization (e.g., a home infusion provider or durable medical equipment provider) provides supplies to the patient, the home care and hospice staff member in the patient's home should verify the expiration date(s) before the products or supplies are used. If an expiration date has passed, the staff member should contact the provider immediately, and the expired products or supplies should be removed from the patient care area.

REFERENCES

Belkin, N. (1998). Aseptics and aesthetics of chlorine bleach: Can its use in laundry be safely abandoned? *American Journal of Infection Control, 16,* 149–151.

Centers for Disease Control and Prevention. (2003). Guidelines for environmental infection control in health-care facilities. *Morbidity and Mortality Weekly Report, (52)*RR10, 1–42.

Centers for Disease Control and Prevention. (2002). Guideline for hand hygiene in health-care settings: Recommendations of the Healthcare Infection Control Practices Advisory Committee and the HICPAC/SHEA/APIC/IDSA Hand Hygiene Task Force. *Morbidity and Mortality Weekly Report, 51*(RR16), 1–44.

Crawford, D. C. (2000). Case study. Phlebotomy: Reducing blood collection risks. *Advance for Administrators of the Laboratory, (9)*1, 70.

Danzig, L., Short, L., Collins, K., Mahoney, M., Sepe, S., Bland, L., & Jarvis, W. (1995). Bloodstream infections associated with a needleless intravenous infusion system in patients receiving home infusion therapy. *Journal of the American Medical Association, 273,* 1862–1864.

Do, A., Ray, B., Banerjee, S., Illian, A.F., Barnett, B., Pham, M., Hendricks, K., & Jarvis W. (1999). Bloodstream infection associated with needleless device use and the importance of infection control practices in home health care setting. *Journal of Infectious Diseases, 179,* 442–448.

Favero, M. S., & Bond, W.W. (2001). Chemical disinfection of medical and surgical materials. In S. S. Block (Ed.), *Disinfection, sterilization, and preservation,* 5th ed. (pp. 313–917). Philadelphia: Lippincott, Williams, & Wilkins.

Food and Drug Administration. Center for Devices and Radiological Health. (1997, April 17). *Public notice.* Washington, DC: Author. Retrieved 1/19/05 from *http://www.fda.gov/medwatch/safety/1997/device.htm.*

Friedman, M. (1996). Designing an infection control program to meet JCAHO standards. *Caring, 15,* 18–25.

Kellerman, S., Shay, D., Howard, J., Goes, C., Feusner, J., Rosenberg, J., Vugia, D., & Jarvis, W. (1996). Bloodstream infections in home infusion patients: The influence of race and needleless intravascular access devices. *Journal of Pediatrics, 129,* 711–717.

Occupational Safety and Health Administration. (2002). Reuse of blood tube holders. 1910.1030(d) (2) (vii) (A). *Standards Interpretations.* Retrieved 6/17/02 from *www.osha.gov/pls/oshaweb/owadisp.show_document?p_table=INTERPRETATIONS&p_id524040.*

Occupational Safety and Health Administration. (1999a). OSHA's policy regarding the use of EPA-registered disinfectants, 7/15/99. Retrieved 7/3/04 from *www.osha.gov/pls/oshaweb/owadisp.show_document?p_table5INTERPRETATIONS&p_id522767.*

Occupational Safety and Health Administration. (1999b). Glass capillary tubes: Joint safety advisory about potential risks. *Standards Interpretations.* 1910.1030 (d) (4) (ii) (A). Retrieved 6/30/04 from *www.osha.gov/pls/oshaweb/owadisp.show_document?p_table5INTERPRETATIONS&p_id522695.*

Occupational Safety and Health Administration. (1997). OSHA's Environmental Protection Agency approved quaternary ammonium disinfectant products. *OSHA Standards Interpretation and Compliance Letters.* Washington, DC: Author. Retrieved 1/19/05 from *http://www.osha-slc.gov/OshDoc/Interp_data/I19970515.html.*

Occupational Safety and Health Administration. (1993, February 1). Most frequently asked questions concerning bloodborne pathogen stantard. *OSHA Standards Interpretation and Compliance Letters.* Retrieved 1/23/05 from *http://www.osha.gov/pls/oshaweb/owadisp.show_document?p_table=INTERPRETATIONS&p_id21010.*

Occupational Safety and Health Administration. (1991). Occupational exposure to bloodborne pathogens: Final rule. 29 CFR 1910.1030. *Federal Register, 56,* 64003–64282.

Rutala, W. A. (1996). APIC guideline for selection and use of disinfectants. *American Journal of Infection Control, 24,* 313–342.

Spaulding, E. H. (1968). Chemical disinfection of medical and surgical materials. In C. A. Lawrence & S. S. Block (Eds.), *Disinfection, sterilization, and preservation* (pp. 517–531). Philadelphia: Lea & Febiger.

CHAPTER 10

Medical Waste Management

Each home care and hospice organization should have a medical waste management plan to ensure that its staff members—volunteers, patients, and family members—and the environment—both in the patient's home and the organization's office—are protected from medical waste that may be generated during the course of home care. One person in the home care and hospice organization should be designated to monitor, review, and administer the plan. The medical waste management plan should minimally meet the recommendations of the Environmental Protection Agency (EPA); the Occupational Safety and Health Administration's (OSHA) bloodborne pathogens regulations; and any applicable state, local, county, or municipal laws or regulations. Each state regulates the storage, transportation, and disposal of medical waste. Some states permit medical waste generated during the course of home care to be considered general waste and disposed of along with household waste. Other state, local, county, or municipal laws or regulations may be much stricter. They may consider waste generated during a patient care procedure to be medical waste and require that it be disposed of by a licensed biomedical waste hauler. Because of this variation, it is important that each home care and hospice organization have a copy of its state or local regulations addressing medical waste disposal. A directory of state agencies that regulate the management of infectious waste can be accessed at *www.safeneedledisposal.org/resswl.html.* The rule of thumb is to follow whatever laws or regulations (local, county, state, or federal) are the strictest.

NEEDLE STICK SAFETY AND PREVENTION ACT
Modifications to the Bloodborne Pathogen Standard

OSHA's bloodborne pathogen standard, which became effective in March 1992, requires that every employer perform a workplace exposure determination to identify hazards and implement proper controls. Although the requirement to implement safer medical devices is not new, the revised standard (OSHA, 2001) further clarifies what is meant by "engineering controls." These engineering controls include the use of safer medical devices, such as sharps with engineered sharps injury protection and needleless systems.

The term *sharps with engineered sharps injury protection* (SEISP) is defined as "a nonneedle sharp or a needle device used for withdrawing body fluids, accessing a vein or artery, or administering medications or other fluids, with a built-in safety feature or mechanism that effectively reduces the risk of an exposure incident" (OSHA, 2001a). The term *needleless systems* is defined as "a device that does not use needles for: the collection of bodily fluids or withdrawal of body fluids after initial venous or arterial access is established; the administration of medication or fluids; or any other procedure involving the potential for occupational exposure to bloodborne pathogens due to percutaneous injuries from contaminated sharps" (OSHA, 2001a). Refer to Chapter 4 for additional information regarding the use of needleless systems in infusion therapy.

Devices with Engineered Sharps Injury Protection Features

There are various ways that safety features have been incorporated into the most commonly used conventional needles and other sharp devices to protect healthcare workers from injury. Examples of engineering controls used in home care include needleless intravenous systems, needles that retract into a syringe after use, sliding sheath cover over a winged-steel "butterfly" needle, a hinged needle guard/shield attached to the needle hub used with Vacutainer needles for blood

drawing, and plastic (instead of glass) capillary tubes for infant heel sticks. Other products developed to promote safer work practices include devices used to stabilize a peripherally inserted central catheter that provide an alternative to suturing. These products can reduce the risk of percutaneous injuries to staff members; they can also improve patient care by reducing site trauma, inadvertent line removal, and the need to reinsert another catheter. A list of the features of devices with sharps injury protection is presented in Table 10-1. A list of the devices designed to prevent percutaneous injuries and

Table 10-1 Devices with Sharps Injury Prevention Features

Conventional device	Device with engineered sharps injury protection	Comment
IV delivery systems that use hypodermic needles to connect and access system components	Valved access ports and connectors. Prepierced septa for use with blunted cannulas. Recessed/protected needle connectors.	Needles generally cannot be used with valved ports. Needles can be used with prepierced septa systems and may be necessary in some situations. Assessment for compatibility with existing IV delivery systems in use in a facility, including IV pumps, is necessary before selecting a device. The number of parts can influence effective use of the system; fewer parts promote simplicity and safety.
Hypodermic needle with attached syringe	Syringe or needle with sliding sheath that covers needle after use.	Scope of needle/syringe use is not limited. No forcing function requires user to activate safety feature. Increases in waste volume should be considered.
	Hinged needle guard/shield that is attached to needle hub and is manually folded over needle after use; hinged guards also can be purchased separately.	Scope of needle/syringe use is not limited. Ability to permanently lock hinge in place over needle varies among devices with this feature. Compliance may be compromised if purchased as an add-on feature rather than being pre-attached at the time of manufacture. Hinge shield may promote compliance with safety feature activation; needle disposal is difficult if shield is not in place. Some interference with the procedure is possible if working in a confined area.
	Sliding shield needle guard that is attached to needle hub and is manually moved forward to cover needle after use.	Scope of needle/syringe use is not limited. No forcing function requires user to activate safety feature.
	Syringe with mechanical needle-retraction feature that isolates needle inside syringe; placing additional pressure on plunger upon completing injection activates feature.	Needle is completely isolated after use. Device can be used only for performing injections; fixed needle does not permit change of needle if needed; potential exists for creating aerosols if needle is retracted outside the body. Waste volume is reduced.
	Needleless jet injection devices.	Eliminates needle hazard. Scope of use is currently limited to giving injections, and only with certain drugs.

Table 10-1 Devices with Sharps Injury Prevention Features

Conventional device	Device with engineered sharps injury protection	comment
Intravenous (IV) insertion devices (catheters)	IV catheters (peripheral and midline) with sliding needle guard/shield. IV catheters with button or slide activated rigid needle encasement feature.	The stylet is permanently protected as it is withdrawn from the catheter. Some devices encase the entire stylet while others protect only the tip. Differences exist in the mode of safety feature activation (i.e., active versus passive). No device with engineered sharps protection feature is currently available for central line catheters. However, there are midline devices with safety features.
Blood collection tube/ phlebotomy needle assembly	Bluntable phlebotomy needle for use with reusable or single use tube holder.	Looks like a conventional phlebotomy needle. An internal cannula, advanced forward by pressing on the end of the blood tube, blunts the needle by extending beyond the tip. The safety feature can be activated while needle is still in the vein. No forcing function requires the user to activate the blunting feature.
	Hinged shield attached to needle for use with reusable or single-use tube holder. Single-use blood tube holder into which needle is *manually* retracted after use; hinged end at bottom of tube holder closes to encase needle. Single-use blood tube holder into which needle *mechanically* retracts after use; hinged cover at bottom of tube holder triggers retraction feature when closed. Single-use vacuum tube holder with attached sliding shield that protects needle after use.	Hinged shield may promote compliance with safety feature activation; needle disposal is difficult if shield is not in place. Completely protects both ends of needle, i.e., venipuncture needle and needle that punctures blood tube. No forcing function requires the user to activate the safety feature.
Winged steel (butterfly-type) needles for phlebotomy	Needle sheath that slides forward to cover the entire needle after use. Needle sheath into which the needle is withdrawn to cover the entire needle after use. Stainless steel needle tip guard that slides forward to cover the needle tip after use.	All devices require activation of the safety feature. No protection for boot end needle (tip that punctures the blood tube) is provided unless a single-use tube holder is used.
Finger/heel stick lancets	Single-use lancets with trigger that automatically protracts and retracts lancet. Reusable pen-like lancets with disposable end caps and lancets (available as separate components or as a combined unit).	With some devices, the lancet is not locked in place after use. The method of activation also varies. Pen-like devices should be assigned to individual patients to reduce the risk for cross-transmission of bloodborne pathogens.

Source: Adapted from *Workbook for Designing, Implementing, and Evaluating a Sharps Injury Prevention Program,* Centers for Disease Control and Prevention, 2004.

exposures to bloodborne pathogens was developed by the University of Virginia's International Health Care Worker Safety Center and can be accessed at *www. med.virginia.edu/epinet.* The problems associated with sharps injuries are often complex, and the factors related to their occurrence must be investigated to identify appropriate interventions. Table 10-2 contains problem-specific strategies for sharps injury protection.

DEFINITIONS

For the purposes of identification and safe handling, waste generated by home care staff members should be segregated into three distinct categories: *general waste, medical waste,* and *sharps.* The EPA uses the term *medical waste.* For home care and hospice purposes, and using the EPA's definition, medical waste would include any solid waste generated in the treatment or immuniza-

Table 10-2 Problem-Specific Strategies for Sharps Injury Prevention

Problem	Problem assessment	Possible prevention strategies
Recapping injuries	• Are recapping injuries associated with certain devices or procedures? • Are there certain locations where recapping injuries appear to be occurring? If so, what is different about these locations? • Is there a need to recap certain needles? • Are point-of-use needle disposal containers available so the home care staff members do not need to recap? • Is it likely that a device with a safety feature would prevent or deter recapping?	• Implement device(s) with sharps prevention features. • Install sharps disposal containers in more convenient locations. • Establish a policy/procedure for safe recapping when necessary for the procedure being performed. • Reinforce recommendations concerning recapping during annual bloodborne pathogen education.
Injuries during specimen transfer	• How are specimens being collected? • Is there an alternative means to perform specimen collection that would avoid the need for specimen transfer? • Is there a way to avoid the need for needles during specimen transfer? Would this create another hazard?	• Revise procedures for specimen collection. • Purchase new specimen collection devices with safety features. • Educate staff on safe means of collecting specimens.
Downstream injuries (i.e., injuries associated with improper disposal of sharp devices)	• Where are these injuries occurring? • Is there any pattern by occupation, location, or device? • Are sharps disposal containers available in all locations? • Are sharps disposal containers appropriate for all needs? • Are sharps disposal containers being used? If not, why not?	• Inform the organization as a whole (or branch, if problem is localized) of the problem and send written communication (e.g., memo, newsletter article). • Hold informal meetings with key staff members. • Encourage reporting of improperly disposed needles and other sharps, regardless of whether injuries occur.
Injuries during sharps disposal	• Where are these injuries occurring? • Is there any pattern by occupation, location, or device? • Does there appear to be a problem with the sharps disposal container being used? If so, is it the type of container? Or is it the location (e.g., height, proximity) of the container? • If a single type of device is involved, what is it about the device and/or the disposal container that contributes to the problem?	• Change the position of the sharps container. • Change to a different type of sharps container. • Reeducate staff about disposal hazards and provide instruction on safe practices.

Source: Adapted from *Workbook for Designing, Implementing, and Evaluating a Sharps Injury Prevention Program,* Centers for Disease Control and Prevention, 2004.

tion of human beings, including but not limited to soiled or blood-soaked bandages, needles, and lancets (EPA, 2004). OSHA uses the term *regulated waste* and defines it as liquid or semiliquid blood or other potentially infectious materials, contaminated items that would release blood or other potentially infectious materials in a liquid or semiliquid state if compressed, items that are caked with dried blood or other potentially infectious materials and are capable of releasing these materials during handling, contaminated sharps, and pathological and microbiological wastes containing blood or other potentially infectious materials (OSHA, 2001). For consistency, *medical waste* is used throughout the rest of this chapter to refer to waste that has been generated during the course of care and contaminated or visibly soiled with blood or other potentially infectious materials.

SEGREGATION OF WASTE

When waste generated in the home is segregated, it is important that it is stored in a proper container. If the state requires that medical waste generated in the home be disposed of as medical waste and not household waste, staff need to be aware of the difference between general waste and medical waste. Comingling medical waste and general waste increases the home care organization's costs for medical waste management. Staff should be careful to put only medical waste in a red bag or sharps container. Staff should also be aware of the difference between blood-saturated waste and blood-stained waste. Blood-stained waste is considered general waste and can be disposed of in the same manner as household waste, whereas blood-saturated dressings generated during a dressing change would be considered medical waste and should be placed in a red bag. Sterile wrappers and paper containers should be discarded as general waste.

General Waste

General waste is defined as materials that have not been contaminated or visibly soiled with blood or other potentially infectious materials. General waste includes products such as:

- paper towels used for drying hands
- dressing wrappers

- nonsoiled personal protective equipment (e.g., gowns, masks, or gloves) used by staff members
- old dressings that are not visibly soiled with blood or other potentially infectious materials
- diapers
- incontinence pads
- intravenous tubing (unless it has been used to administer blood or blood products in the home, in which case it would be considered medical waste)

General waste should be placed in a normal consumer trash bag, and the bag should be securely fastened. The bag may be discarded in the patient's regular waste receptacle.

Medical Waste

Medical waste may be generated by the patient, the patient's caregiver(s), or home care and hospice staff members. Items heavily contaminated with blood or other potentially infectious materials should be placed in a leak-proof, heavy-duty plastic bag. One plastic bag is adequate if the bag is sturdy and not overfilled. The contaminated items do not have to be double-bagged as long as they can be placed in the plastic bag without contaminating the outside of the bag or puncturing it. The bag should be appropriately labeled as biohazardous or color-coded in red, and it should be securely tied at the neck before removal from the patient's home.

Liquid waste such as urine, feces, povidone-iodine, irrigating solutions, suctioned fluids, excretions, and secretions may be poured carefully down the patient's toilet, which is connected to a sanitary sewer or septic tank. Body fluids in small amounts, such as the blood in a syringe withdrawn from a central venous catheter before a blood sample is obtained, may be discarded in a puncture-proof sharps container. State regulations may dictate the maximum volume of blood or body fluids that is permitted to be poured into the sanitary sewer.

Surgical masks used by a patient to prevent the spread of pulmonary tuberculosis as well as disposable respirators (i.e., N95 respiratory protective devices) certified by the National Institute for Occupational Safety and Health (NIOSH) used by a staff member as personal protective equipment may be disposed of as general waste.

All waste generated from home administration of chemotherapy is classified as *chemotherapy waste.* Chemotherapy waste disposal is a hazardous materials problem, not a potential transmitter of infectious disease. All items contaminated with antineoplastic agents, such as tubing, syringes, intravenous solution bags, and gloves, should be placed in a container specifically labeled "for chemotherapy waste only." Chemotherapy waste should be transported to the home care organization's facility in the trunk of a vehicle and segregated from other waste pending pickup from a licensed hazardous materials disposal company.

Sharps

The primary route of occupational exposure to blood-borne pathogens is accidental, percutaneous (through the skin) injury with nursing staff experiencing the highest number of needlestick injuries. The CDC estimates that each year 385,000 needlesticks and other sharps-related injuries are sustained by hospital-based health care personnel, an average of 1,000 sharps injuries per day. This data does not include exposures in home care (Panlilio, 2004). In order to determine the number of percutaneous injuries in home care staff, the CDC conducted a prospective study of home care organizations, with data from 11 agencies, over 33,000 visits, and 19,000 procedures (Bertrami, 2000). In this cohort, there were 0.6 percutaneous injuries per 1,000 procedures involving needles or lancets. Home care staff members handle sharps devices and equipment such as hypodermic needles, Huber needles, intravenous access devices, intravenous blood collection devices, and phlebotomy devices.

The factors most often related to sharps injuries include the following: inadequate design or inappropriate placement of the sharps disposal container, overfilling of the sharps disposal container, and inappropriate sharps disposal practices by the user during patient care.

If home care or hospice staff members clip patients' nails with nail clippers that are owned by the home care or hospice organization and the nail clippers are capable of penetrating the patient's skin, the clippers need to be stored in an impervious container, and the container needs to be appropriately labeled for storage and transport (OSHA, 1992).

Recapping a Needle

Used needles and other sharps should not be recapped, bent, removed from disposable syringes, or manipulated either by hands or by any technique that involves directing the point of the needle toward any part of the body unless the specific procedure requires that recapping be performed. Situations in which recapping may be required include the insertion of a needle into a vial of heparin or saline to prefill syringes used for flushing venous access devices and the prefilling of syringes from multidose vials when appropriate. When needle recapping is required for a specific procedure, or when no alternative is feasible, recapping must be performed by some method other than the traditional two-handed procedure—for instance, by means of a mechanical device or forceps. A properly performed one-hand scoop method (in which the hand holding the sharp is used to scoop up the cap from a flat surface) may be used; however, it must be performed in a safe manner and must be limited to situations in which recapping is necessary. If the home care or hospice organization claims that there is no alternative to recapping, the exposure control plan should include a written justification stating the basis for the determination that no alternative is feasible or specifying that a particular medical procedure requires that the needle be recapped. Needles that will not become contaminated by blood during use (e.g., needles used only to draw medication from vials) are not required to have engineering controls under this standard. Needles used for actual injections, however, must incorporate engineering controls (OSHA, 2001b).

Sharps Container

All used disposable sharp instruments, needles, syringes, and hypodermic units and other sharp items such as broken glass should be placed immediately in a puncture-resistant, leak-proof, impervious container for disposal. Even though sharps are now engineered with sharps injury protection features, the items must still be placed in a sharps container for disposal. The container should be labeled with a biohazard sign or color-coded, and it should remain upright. The container should be constructed with a secured lid that seals, so that the contents will not spill out if it is knocked over and injuries will not result from handling the container. The container should be readily accessible and located as close as possible to the patient care or work area. Puncture-resistant sharps containers should be brought into the work area any time syringes and needles are used for a procedure.

Vacuum container needles should not be removed from the blood tube and must not be reused. Once the needle safety device is activated, the entire set (needle, safety device, and blood tube) should be placed in the sharps container for disposal (OSHA, 2002). Broken glass that may be contaminated should not be picked up directly by hand; rather, a forceps, tongs, or a brush and dustpan should be used. NIOSH has developed safety performance criteria for selecting and using sharps disposal containers; these are presented in Table 10-3 (CDC, 1998).

Sharps Storage in the Patient's Home

When a staff member brings a sharps container into a patient's home for use during a home visit, he or she should be cautious about where the sharps container is placed. The staff member should consider, for example, whether there are small children or drug abusers in the home. Under either of those circumstances, the staff member should keep the portable sharps container in his or her possession at all times. The portable sharps container should also be positioned close to where the staff member sets up for a procedure in which sharps will be used. The sharps container should be placed within arm's reach. Once the container has been used, the lid should be closed to prevent spillage or protrusion of the contents during storage and transport. Appendix 10-A contains a brochure that can be provided to patients and families

to educate them in the proper methods for disposing of sharps and other medical waste; Appendix 10-B contains information regarding disposal methods and additional information geared toward the staff member. Appendix 10-C contains a brochure intended for diabetics on the proper disposal of lancets in the home.

Sharps containers can be stored in the patient's home between staff member visits. Sharps containers should be stored in the closed position and away from pets and small children. Care should be taken not to fill the sharps container above the indicated safe fill line placed on the container by the manufacturer. Once the sharps container fill capacity has been reached, the lid should be closed tightly and the container should be returned to the home care or hospice organization for disposal. The container can be disposed of as household waste if this is permitted by state regulations.

Sharps Storage in the Staff Member's Possession

Sharps containers should be stored in the staff member's possession or carried in and out of the patient's home as long as there is no immediate hazard to the home care or hospice staff member carrying the container; common sense should prevail. Factors to consider in determining the proper storage of a sharps container include the size of the container and whether the container can be completely sealed. As long as the sharps container is closed and the external surface is not visibly contaminated, it may be hand carried, placed in a separate bag, placed inside the staff mem-

---

Table 10-3 Criteria for Selection and Use of Sharps Containers

Criterion	Recommendation
Functionality	The sharps container should be durable, leak resistant, and puncture resistant under all normal environmental conditions during use.
Accessibility	The sharps container must be accessible to home care staff members who use, maintain, or dispose of sharps devices. There must be sufficient numbers of containers of sufficient volume conveniently placed with safe access to the disposal opening.
Visibility	The sharps container fill status and warning labels must be visible to the home care staff members who use it.
Accommodation	Proper selection and use of sharps disposal containers are important.
	Prevention strategies through training, personal protective equipment, and engineering controls such as needleless intravenous systems and safe needle-bearing products should be considered part of a needlestick prevention plan.

Source: Reprinted from *Selecting, Evaluating, and Using Sharps Disposal Containers,* Centers for Disease Control and Prevention, National Institute for Occupational Safety and Health, January 1998.

ber's supply bag, or placed in a side pocket or attachment to the supply bag.

Decontaminating Sharps Before Transport and Disposal

Some states that permit medical waste generated in the home to be disposed of as household waste strongly recommend that sharps first be decontaminated. If the home care or hospice organization's state requires decontamination before disposal, the staff member can decontaminate the contents of a 1-gallon-size sharps container by adding 1/2 teaspoon bleach and 1 and 1/2 tablespoons water to the container, closing the container tightly, and gently shaking the contents to disinfect them. Medical waste that has been decontaminated does not have to be labeled or color-coded (OSHA, 1991).

Sharps Disposal

Some states permit waste generated in the home to be disposed of in the public solid waste system as household waste. Disposing of sharps as household waste poses a potential risk of injury and infection to the public. In addition, used needles may place others at risk for exposure to bloodborne pathogens. There currently are no federal regulations for the safe disposal of sharps. In August of 2002, the Coalition for Safe Community Needle Disposal was formed to support federal policies governing the safe disposal of sharps by individuals; establish state and local laws that provide safe community disposal programs for sharps; encourage community-based disposal solutions that are available, affordable and discreet; and provide effective public education about safe needle disposal for all "at-home" users of sharps. The Coalition for Safe Community Needle Disposal is a collaboration of businesses, community groups, and nonprofit and government organizations that includes the American Association of Diabetes Educators, American Diabetes Association, American Medical Association, American Pharmacists Association, National Association of Chain Drug Stores, National Association of County and City Health Officials, National Association of Home Care and Hospice, National Recycling Coalition, National Solid Wastes Management Association, and U.S. Conference of Mayors. Additional information on the Coalition for Safe Community Needle Disposal's efforts can be accessed at *www.safeneedledisposal.org.*

WASTE STORAGE DURING TRANSPORT TO THE HOME CARE OR HOSPICE ORGANIZATION

Some home care organizations, especially home infusion organizations, properly pick up sharps containers that have been filled by the patient or caregiver during the course of care. When the sharps container is taken out of the patient's home, it should be completely sealed. In the vehicle, the container should be placed in a location that would not cause injury to the driver or passengers if the driver needed to stop quickly and the sharps container were to overturn and spill its contents.

During transport, the sharps container should be placed upright in the trunk of a vehicle, the back seat of a vehicle if the vehicle does not have a trunk, a cargo box in an open-bed pickup truck, or a closed container in an open cargo van. The waste should be not exposed to rain, snow, or other weather conditions that might impair the container's integrity.

SEPARATING WASTE FROM CLEAN EQUIPMENT AND SUPPLIES

During transport from the patient's home to the home care or hospice organization, medical waste must be kept separate from clean equipment so that the clean equipment does not become soiled or contaminated. Medical waste can be separated from clean equipment in the staff member's vehicle by storing it in a red plastic bag. Sharps containers should also in some manner be stored separate from clean equipment and supplies (i.e., in a box or other container). Clean equipment and supplies can be stored in clear plastic bags or trunk boxes. Medical waste and clean equipment can also be separated in any other manner selected by the home care organization that is consistently understood and followed by home care or hospice staff members.

MEDICAL WASTE STORAGE IN THE HOME CARE OR HOSPICE ORGANIZATION

If medical waste and sharps cannot be disposed of at the patient's home, the biohazard bags and sharps should be either brought back to the home care or hospice organization for storage or brought to another facility with which the home care or hospice organization has made arrangements. If the medical waste is returned to the home care or hospice organization, it should be stored in a designated area until it is picked up for final disposal. The medical waste and sharps containers should be placed in a secondary box or containment device provided by the biomedical waste hauler, or in another appropriate container labeled with the international biohazard symbol or color-coded. The secondary container should be of the appropriate size and material required by the state's regulations and should be stored in a well-ventilated, low-traffic area within the facility or in a storage area with limited access. Medical waste should be stored in the home care or hospice organization for as short a time as possible—or at the most for the maximum time permitted by the state's regulations. If the secondary container is full, the contracted medical waste hauler should be contacted for a pickup. Some hospital-based home care or hospice organizations store medical waste in their offices, and another hospital department comes to the organization to pick it up. Regardless of who is the party responsible for pickup, the medical waste should be picked up on a routine basis to prevent overfilling of the container. Medical waste should not be compacted by home care or hospice staff members.

MEDICAL WASTE TRANSPORT

In the practice of home care and hospice, the home care and hospice organization is considered the medical waste generator and is responsible for the medical waste until it is destroyed. Therefore, a commercial, licensed medical waste hauler should be used to transport waste for treatment and final disposal unless the organization has other capabilities (e.g., incineration) for the final disposal. For example, a hospital-based home care or hospice organization may store its medical waste in its office and have it picked up at regular intervals by a hospital staff member, to be incinerated along with the hospital's medical waste. Whatever method is used, all final disposal methods should be in compliance with federal, state, and local regulations.

Department of Transportation

The Department of Transportation's (DOT) requirements for transporting infectious substances, including regulated medical waste, were revised in 2002. They provide a complete exception for medical waste generated from households collected by local sanitation workers along with trash, garbage, and other nonmedi-

cal household waste, and transported in accordance with applicable state or local requirements. The exception also applies to regulated medical waste generated through the home treatment of medical conditions by professional health care providers when these health care providers remove the regulated medical waste and transport it elsewhere for disposal (DOT, 2002).

United States Postal Service

Most regulated medical waste and sharps waste may be shipped via the United States Postal Service (USPS). The USPS requires that anyone who mails these items to use USPS-authorized mailing packages. These packages have been tested to meet the DOT's hazardous materials packaging standards to prevent leaking and damage, and most importantly to protect postal workers from injury or exposure to bloodborne pathogens. The mailable medical waste and sharps waste must also meet labeling, marking, and documentation requirements. Examples of labeling, marking, and documentation requirements include a USPS authorization number, a container identification number, the name of the manufacturer or distributor, a display of the universal biohazard symbol, and the name "Regulated Medical Waste—Sharps, UN 3291 or Regulated Medical Waste, UN 3291" noted on the package. Each sharps mailing container must include a resealable envelope affixed to the outside of the package that contains a completed USPS manifest identifying the mailer and the destination facility and including an emergency phone number in case the package is damaged in the mail. The USPS manifest must include any additional information required by the state from which the package is mailed (USPS, 2005).

OSHA LABELING REQUIREMENTS

OSHA requires that a biohazard warning label be affixed to containers of medical waste. Containers should be fluorescent orange or orange-red with letters or symbols in a contrasting color. A biohazard warning label is shown in Figure 10-1. The biohazard label can be either part of the container or affixed by a method that will prevent loss or removal, such as taping. If the container or bag is red, a biohazard label or sticker is not required.

If a refrigerator is used in the home care organization to store blood specimens until they are picked up by a

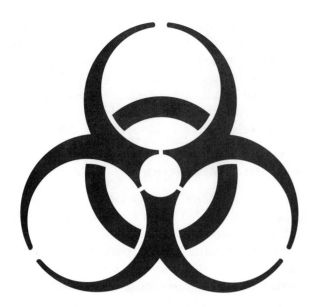

Figure 10-1 Biohazard Symbol

Source: Reprinted from *Occupational Exposure to Bloodborne Pathogens: Final Rule,* 29 CFR 1910.1030, Federal Register, Occupational Safety and Health Administration, 1991.

laboratory courier, the refrigerator must have a biohazard label on the front. The refrigerator that is used for storing laboratory specimens should not be used to store medications or staff members' food.

After blood specimens are obtained in the patient's home, they should be placed in an impervious container for storage or transport. If a non-red container, such as a Rigid food storage container, is used to store blood specimens during transport, it should have a biohazard label affixed to the top. Some home care organizations teach their patients to dispose of their sharps in other impervious household containers. If it is the home care organization's policy to pick up non-red sharps containers for disposal, the container must be placed inside a red bag or labeled with a biohazard label for transport and storage. Bags of cross-matched blood, blood components, or other blood products that are labeled as to their contents and that have been released for transfusion are not required to be labeled as biohazardous (OSHA, 1991).

BLOOD SPILLS IN THE HOME

Environmental surfaces in the home may become contaminated by a blood spill, such as may occur if a blood collection tube is broken. OSHA does not require that

each staff member be issued a blood spill kit containing prepackaged items such as a blood-solidifying product, a brush, and a dust pan to clean the blood spill. However, this is an option that home and hospice care organizations can consider. Staff members do need to have personal protective equipment (e.g., gloves and possibly a gown and goggles) available to protect himself or herself against exposure to the blood while cleaning the blood spill. He or she also needs supplies (e.g., disposable paper towels, a red plastic bag) to wipe up and dispose of the blood and contaminated items. Disposable towels and/or wipes should be used to wipe up the spill. Once the gross blood is removed, the surface should be cleaned and disinfected. If the blood is not wiped up first, the diluted bleach solution or other appropriate disinfectant will not be effective, because disinfectants do not work in the presence of blood. A hard, nonporous surface can be disinfected with a 1:10 dilution of 5.25% household bleach or another intermediate-level disinfectant or product from the EPA's List D, or preferably List E. The product should be used according to the manufacturer's instructions for dilution and contact time. Refer to Chapter 8 for additional information regarding EPA-registered products. The paper towels used to contain and clean the blood spill and to disinfect the spill area should be bagged to prevent leakage and exposure. A heavy-duty plastic bag should be used for this purpose, and it should either be color-coded or have a biohazard label.

Blood Spills on Carpeted Surfaces

OSHA does not have any evidence to determine if decontamination of plush carpets is possible. However, it is OSHA's opinion that carpeted surfaces cannot be decontaminated. Therefore, a home care provider should make a reasonable effort to clean and sanitize carpeting and plush surfaces with carpet detergent or cleaning products (OSHA, June 1994). Wearing gloves, the staff member should first wipe up the blood spill with disposable towels and then clean the carpet. The carpet should then be disinfected with a solution that does *not* contain 5.25% household bleach, because bleach will remove the color from the carpet fibers as well as chemically damage the tensile strength of the fibers and backing. Any other EPA-approved germicide may be used. The disinfectant should be applied according to the instructions on the label and should be allowed to remain on the carpet to air dry.

REFERENCES

Beltrami, E., McArthur, M., Mc Geer, A., Armstrong-Evans, M., Lyons, D., Chamberland, M., & Cardo, D. (2000). The nature and frequency of blood contacts among home healthcare workers. *Infection Control and Hospital Epidemiology, 21*(12), 765–770.

Centers for Disease Control and Prevention. (2003). Guidelines for environmental infection control in health-care facilities. *Morbidity and Mortality Weekly Recommendations and Reports, 52*(RR10).

Centers for Disease Control and Prevention, National Institute for Occupational Safety and Health. (1998, January). Selecting, evaluating, and using sharps disposal containers. Atlanta: Retrieved 1/23/05 from *http://www.cdc.gov/niosh/sharps1.html.*

Department of Transportation. (2002). Hazardous materials: Revision to standards for infectious substances. Final rule. Research and Special Programs Administration, 49 CFR Parts 171, 172, 173, 177, and 178. *Federal Register, 67*(157). Retrieved 1/23/05 from *http://hazmat.dot./gov/regs/rules/final/678R/67fr/53118.htm*

Environmental Protection Agency. (2004). *Medical Waste.* Retrieved April 27, 2004, from *www.epa.gov/epaoswer/other/medical.*

Occupational Safety and Health Administration. (2002). Re-use of blood tube holders. 1910.1030(d) (2) (vii) (A). *Standards Interpretations.* Retrieved 6/17/02 from *www.osha.gov/pls/oshaweb/owadisp.show_document?p_table=INTERPRETATIONS&p_id524040.*

Occupational Safety and Health Administration. (2001). Occupational exposure to bloodborne pathogens; Needlestick and other sharps injuries. Final Rule. 29 CFR 1910.30 (b). Retrieved 1/23/05 from *http://www.osha.gov/pls/oshaweb/owadisp.show_document?p_table=STANDARDS&p_id510051.*

Occupational Safety and Health Administration. (2001a). Enforcement procedures for the occupational exposure to bloodborne pathogens. CPL 2-2.69. November 27, 2001. Retrieved 1/23/05 from *www.osha.gov/pls/oshaweb/owadisp.show_document?p_table=DIRECTIVES&p_id52570.*

Occupational Safety and Health Administration. (1999). OSHA's policy regarding the use of EPA-registered disinfectants. July 15, 1999. *Standards Interpretations.* Retrieved 1/23/05 from *www.osha.gov/pls/oshaweb/owadisp.show_document?p_table=INTERPRETATIONS&p_id522767.*

Occupational Safety and Health Administration. (1994, June 10). Decontamination of a plush carpet surface after a spill. *OSHA Standards Interpretation and Compliance Letters.* Retrieved 7/3/04 from *http://www.osha.gov/pls/oshaweb/owadisp.show_document?p_table=INTERPRETATIONS&p_id521511.*

Occupational Safety and Health Administration. (1991). Occupational exposure to bloodborne pathogens. Final rule. 29 CFR 1910.1030. *Federal Register, 56,* 64003–64282.

Occupational Safety and Health Administration. (1992, April 4). Infectious materials and nail and tissue clippers as sharps. *OSHA Standards Interpretation and Compliance Letters.* Retrieved 1/23/05 from *http://www.osha-slc.gov/OshDoc/Interp_data/I19920404.html.*

Panlilio, A. L., Orelien, J. G., Srivastava, P. U., Jagger, J., Cohn, R. D., Cardo D. M.; NaSH Surveillance Group; EPINet Data Sharing Network (July 2004). Estimate of the annual number of percutaneous injuries among hospital-based healthcare workers in the United States, 1997–1998. *Infection Control and Hospital Epidemiology. 25*(7):556–62.

United States Postal Service. (2005, January 6). Domestic Mail Manual CO23 Hazardous Materials. Issue 58. Retrieved 1/23/05 from *http://www.usps.com.*

Needle Disposal

Traveling with Needles

Don't forget, safe needle disposal is important no matter where you are—at home, at work, or on the road. Never place used needles in the trash in hotel rooms, on airplanes, or in public restrooms, where they could injure the cleaning staff or other people.

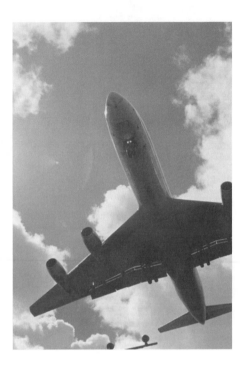

Sharps and Air Travel

Before you fly, check the Transportation Security Administration (TSA) Web site (www.tsa.gov) for up-to-date rules on what to do with your needles when you travel. To make your trip through airport security easier, make sure your medicines are labeled with the type of medicine and the manufacturer's name or a drug store label, and bring a letter from your doctor.

Be prepared—ask about options for safe needle disposal when you make travel reservations, board an airplane, or check into a hotel or cruise ship. If you aren't sure that needle containers will be available where you're going, be sure to buy a needle container that you can take with you to hold your used needles until you can throw them away the right way.

United States
Environmental Protection Agency
5305W
Washington, DC 20460

EPA530-F-04-004
October 2004
www.epa.gov/osw

Recycled/Recyclable—Printed with Vegetable Oil-Based Inks on 100%
Postconsumer, Process Chlorine-Free Recycled Paper

Protect Yourself, Protect Others

Safe Options for Home Needle Disposal

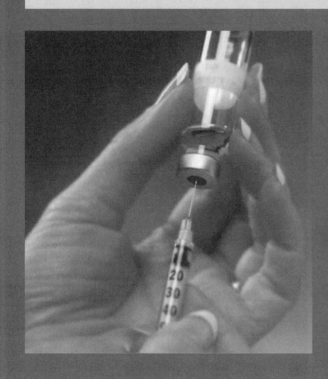

A 44-year-old trash collector was stuck in the leg with a needle from someone's trash. A year later, he started having stomach pains. His doctor told him that he had caught Hepatitis C, probably from being stuck by the needle. Doctors have not been able to help him, and he is now in chronic liver failure. He will likely die from this disease.

It's not just trash workers who are at risk of needle sticks—it's also your neighbors, children, janitors, housekeepers, and pets. That's why used needles should not be thrown in the garbage.

Why are used needles dangerous?

Used needles and lancets are dangerous because they can:

◆ Injure people

◆ Spread germs

◆ Spread diseases such as HIV/AIDS, hepatitis, tetanus, and syphillis

All needles should be treated as if they carry a disease. That means that if someone gets stuck with a needle, they have to get expensive medical tests and worry about whether they have caught a harmful or deadly disease. Be sure you get rid of your used needles the safe way to avoid exposing other people to harm.

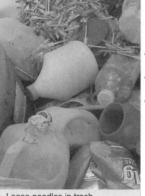
Loose needles in trash

DON'T

◆ Throw loose needles in the garbage

◆ Flush used needles down the toilet

◆ Put needles in recycling containers

DO

Use one of the recommended disposal methods in this brochure

Remember, not all of the options listed in this brochure are available in all areas. Check carefully to see what options are available near you—it could save a life!

Appendix 10-A   145

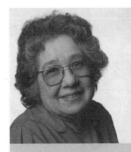

Recommended Needle Disp

Community Services

Drop-off Collection Sites	"Household Hazardous Waste" Centers	Residential "Special Waste" Pickup Service
Some communities offer collection sites that accept used needles—often for free. These collection sites may be at local hospitals, doctors' offices, health clinics, pharmacies, health departments, community organizations, police and fire departments, and medical waste facilities. Don't just leave your needles at one of these places —make sure the site accepts them, and be sure to put needles in the right place.	Many communities have a disposal site already set up that accepts "household hazardous waste" items like used oil, batteries, and paint. In some places, these centers also accept used needles. If your area has a hazardous household waste center, be sure it accepts used needles before you go, and put needles in the right place when you drop them off.	Some communities offer a "special waste" pickup serv that collects your full conta of used needles from your house. Some services requ you to call for a pickup, wh others collect used needles a regular schedule.

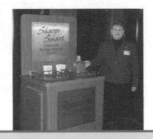
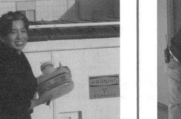

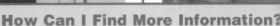

How Can I Find More Information?

- ◆ Call your trash or public health department, listed in the city or county government (blue) pages your phone book, to find out about programs available in your area.

- ◆ Check the Centers for Disease Control (CDC) Web site at <www.cdc.gov/needledisposal> for a lis of needle disposal rules in your state, along with needle disposal programs near you.

- ◆ Ask your health care provider or local pharmacist if they can dispose of your used needles, or if they know of safe disposal programs near you.

- ◆ Contact the Coalition for Safe Community Needle Disposal at (800) 643-1643 or visit the Web sit at <www.safeneedledisposal.org> to find out about safe disposal programs near you.

- ◆ Visit the Earth 911 Web site at <www.earth911.org>. You can go to the "Household Hazardous Was section of the site and search for a needle disposal program near you by entering your ZIP code.

- ◆ To learn more about rules regarding medical waste disposal, consult EPA's Medical Waste Web site <www.epa.gov/epaoswer/other/medical>.

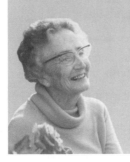

al Options for Self-Injectors

National Services

...ringe Exchange Programs	Mail-back Service	Home Needle Destruction Devices
...se programs let you trade ...r used needles for new ...s. The group that runs the ...vice will dispose of your ...d needles safely.	You can buy this service, which comes with a needle container and mail-back packaging. You fill the needle container with your used needles and mail it back in the package that is provided by the company. You have to pay for this service, and the price usually depends on the size of the container you pick.	Several manufacturers offer products for sale that allow you to destroy needles at home by burning, melting or cutting off the needle—making it safe to throw in the garbage. Prices vary depending on the product.

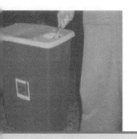 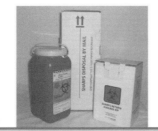 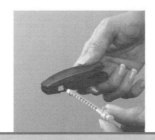

How Can I Find More Information?

| ...tact the North American ...inge Exchange Program at ...3) 272-4857 or visit the ... site at <www.nasen.org>. | For a list of mail-back service companies, contact the Coalition for Safe Community Needle Disposal at (800) 643-1643 or visit the Web site at <www.safeneedledisposal.org>. When contacting a mail-back service company, be sure to ask them if the service is approved by the U.S. Postal Service. | Contact the Coalition for Safe Community Needle Disposal at (800) 643-1643 or visit the Web site at <www.safeneedledisposal.org> for a list of companies that make home needle destruction devices. |

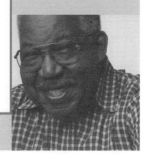

APPENDIX 10-B

Staff Education

NURSES and HEALTH EDUCATORS

What Do I Tell My Patients?

SafeNeedleDisposal.Org

**Coalition for Safe
Community Needle Disposal**

1 800 643 1643

The Environmental Protection Agency (EPA) recently revised its recommendations on safe disposal of used needles. EPA now discourages patients from placing containers of used needles (syringes) in the household trash. This practice creates needle stick hazards for workers in the waste and other industries. The new EPA information (http://www.epa.gov/epaoswer/other/medical/sharps.htm) specifically states that patients should "ask your local health care provider or pharmacist if they offer disposal, or if they know of safe programs in the area." Healthcare providers are well positioned to educate patients on safe needle disposal. Some health care facilities, especially those with services dedicated to patients with diabetes, also offer disposal to their patients.

KNOW YOUR PATIENTS – ASK THE RIGHT QUESTIONS

"How long will you be injecting this medication, short-term or long-term?"

Short-Term. Some patients inject for a short period of time (infertility, allergy and interferon treatments) and often the best solution for this group is a onetime sharps mail back program.

Long-Term. Other patients may be injecting daily over an indefinite period of time for diseases such as diabetes, arthritis or HIV. In this case, cost may be a factor in proper disposal. While needle destruction devices may be high in the initial cost, over time they could prove to be the most cost effective. A needle clipper is usually inexpensive and can collect hundreds of needles, however, the patient will also need to purchase a sharps container (mail back – possibly) to properly dispose of the needles when it is full.

"How do you plan to dispose of your used needles?"

Public Health Concern. If your patient is injecting for a highly infectious disease such as HIV, Hepatitis B, or Hepatitis C insist that your patient use one of the many safe disposal options. Again any of the programs will work, but help the patient to understand how imperative it is to the community that they use or purchase a program that provides safe disposal for their used needles.

"What factors are most important to you in safe needle disposal?"

Understand Your Patient. Is disposal cost a concern? Is anonymity a concern? Is convenience a concern? Mail backs and destruction devices provide both anonymity and convenience, while community drop-off programs and household hazardous waste programs are inexpensive (often free) but don't always offer the convenience or anonymity some patients desire. Research your community – find out if the household hazardous waste program (collection site for used paint and oil) will accept used needles. Does your local hospital or community health clinic accept used needles? Call the local medical waste processor in your community and find out if it will accept used needles from individuals; if so, at what cost and what type of container is acceptable. Knowing this information can help you help your patient transition into safe disposal.

"Do you need more information?"

Safe Disposal Resource. The Coalition for Safe Community Needle Disposal is a collaboration of businesses, community groups, non-profit organizations and local, state and federal government entities that promotes public awareness and solutions for the safe disposal of needles, syringes and other sharps in the community. For more information on safe needle disposal contact the Coalition for Safe Community Needle Disposal at 800-643-1643 or www.safeneedledisposal.org. The Coalition website offers disposal solutions for individuals by zip code.

YOU CAN MAKE A DIFFERENCE – HOW DO I HELP MY PATIENTS?

- *Work Together.* Changing behavior isn't easy. It will take the efforts of everyone involved to ultimately change the way people dispose of their used needles at home. Work with other health care providers (doctors, nurses, educators, pharmacists, hospital administrators) and public health officials and waste officials to determine what disposal solutions may work best for your community.

- *Promote Local Needle Disposal Programs.* If you are aware of programs in your community for safe needle disposal, share information about those programs with your patients.

- *Research Disposal Program Availability.* If you are not aware of programs in your community contact your local solid waste department (city or county government pages in your phonebook) to determine if there are drop-off programs such as household hazardous waste programs that accept used needles at these facilities. In addition, the CDC has a special website that identifies at-home needle disposal regulations for each state. This is a good place to get started if you are trying to determine what is available in your community (http://www.cdc.gov/needledisposal).

- *Be a Community Leader.* Work with other health care providers (doctors, nurses, educators, public health officials) and develop a community-based program for your community. Don't re-invent the wheel; contact the Coalition for Safe Community Needle Disposal at 800-643-1643 for help or ideas on getting a program started in your community.

- *Know Your Patients.* Understand that many patients who use syringes to treat medical conditions already face significant economic challenges due to these conditions. Work with appropriate groups and individuals in the community and/or state to make safe disposal programs free when possible.

- *Recommend Products.* If there are no programs available, encourage patients to purchase one of the disposal options currently available on the market. In addition, the Coalition (www.safeneedledisposal.org) features disposal solutions on its website. This lists some current products available on the market and will link patients directly to the vendor of the product.

  a. Mail back programs are abundant and vary in cost depending on the size ($20-$50). Listed are some products currently on the market:

      Becton, Dickinson and Company – 877-927-8363 or www.bd.com
      Sharps Compliance, Inc. – 800-772-5657 www.sharpsinc.com

  b. At-home needle destruction devices. Many of the products on the market sever, burn or melt the needle and the patient can throw the syringe or plunger in the garbage. The cost of these items vary ($8 - $180). Listed are some products currently on the market:

      BD – Needle Clipper (clips the needle into a small container) www.bd.com

Agencies and businesses working on this issue include: American Association of Diabetes Educators, American Diabetes Association, American Medical Association, American Pharmacists Association, National Alliance of State and Territorial AIDS Directors, National Association of Chain Drug Stores, National Association of County and City Health Officials, National Association for Home Care and Hospice, National Recycling Coalition, National Solid Wastes Management Association, U.S. Conference of Mayors, Waste Management, Sharps Compliance, and Becton, Dickinson and Co.

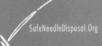 SafeNeedleDisposal.Org

WWW.SAFENEELEDISPOSAL.ORG   1 800 643 1643

Lancet Disposal

Handle With Care

How To Throw Out Used Insulin Syringes and Lancets At Home

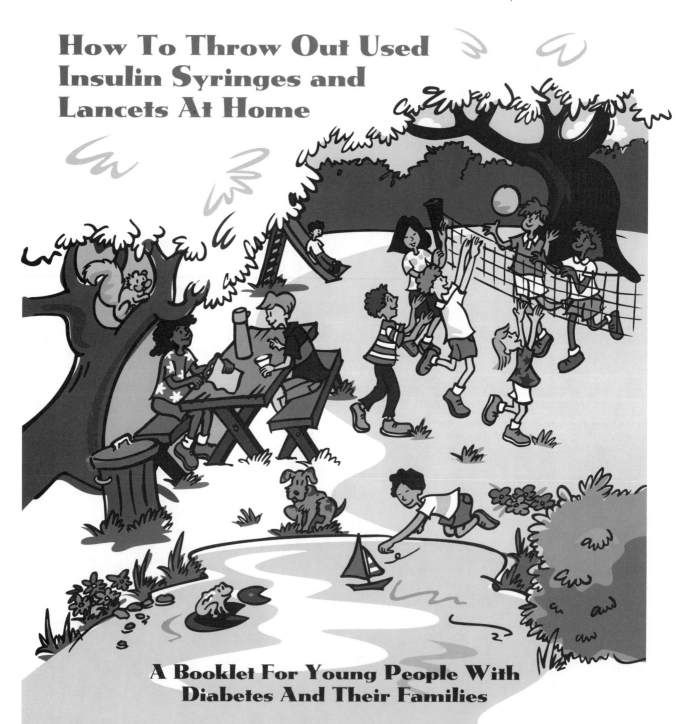

A Booklet For Young People With Diabetes And Their Families

A Note To Adults

This booklet is for young people with insulin-dependent diabetes and for you.

People living in the United States use more than **one billion** (1,000,000,000) syringes, needles, and lancets **each year** to take care of their diabetes. This booklet shows you the safe way to handle <u>and</u> throw out used insulin syringes and lancets at home.

It's simple. The easy directions on the following pages show you how to protect your family and waste handlers from injury—and help **keep the environment clean and safe!**

While you are reading this booklet, keep in mind that your state, county, or town may have special rules about how to dispose of syringes and lancets. They may also have a special collection center for these items. You should ask your doctor, diabetes educator, or community representative how to find out about any rules or collection programs in your area.

**United States
Environmental Protection
Agency**

November 2003
EPA530-F-98-025C
www.epa.gov/osw

New Information About Disposing of Medical Sharps

The Coalition for Safe Community Needle Disposal, comprised of medical, government and waste association and private sector companies, is working with the Environmental Protection Agency to evaluate and promote alternative disposal methods for used needles and other medical sharps.

Improper management of discarded needles and other sharps can pose a health risk to the public and waste workers. For example, discarded needles may expose waste workers to potential needle stick injuries and potential infection when containers break open inside garbage trucks or needles are mistakenly sent to recycling facilities. Janitors and housekeepers also risk injury if loose sharps poke through plastic garbage bags. Used needles can transmit serious diseases, such as HIV and hepatitis.

The Coalition has identified several types of safe disposal programs for self-injectors. Instead of placing sharps in the trash, self-injectors are encouraged to use any of these alternative disposal methods:

- **Drop Box or Supervised Collection Sites**
Sharps users can take their own sharps containers filled with used needles to appropriate collections sites: doctors' offices, hospitals, pharmacies, health departments, or fire stations. Services are free or have a nominal fee. Check with your pharmacist or other health care provider for availability in your area.

- **Mail-back Programs**
Sharps users place their used sharps in special containers and return the container by mail to a collection site for proper disposal. This service usually requires a fee. Fees vary, depending on the size of the container. Check with your health care provider, pharmacist, yellow pages, or search the Internet using keywords "sharps mail back."

- **Syringe Exchange Programs (SEP)**
Sharps users can safely exchange used needles for new needles. Contact the North American Syringe Exchange Network at 253-272-4857 or online at <www.nasen.org>.

- **At-home Needle Destruction Devices**
Several manufacturers offer products that allow you to destroy used needles at home. These devices sever, burn, or melt the needle, rendering it safe for disposal. Check with your pharmacist or search the internet using keywords "sharps disposal devices." The prices of these devices vary according to product type and manufacturer.

For More Information:
- Call your local solid waste department or public health department to determine the correct disposal method for your area.

- Ask your health care provider or local pharmacist if they offer disposal, or if they know of safe disposal programs in the area.

- Contact the Coalition for Safe Community Needle Disposal at 1-800-643-1643. Ask about the availability of safe disposal programs in your area or for information on setting up a community disposal program. Visit *www.epa.gov/epaoswer/other/medical*. This website also offers a list of all state health and solid waste/sanitation department contacts.

Did You Know?

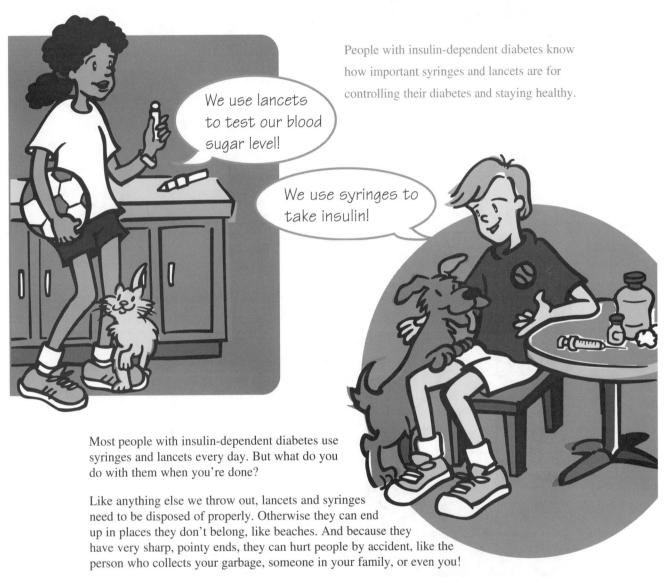

People with insulin-dependent diabetes know how important syringes and lancets are for controlling their diabetes and staying healthy.

We use lancets to test our blood sugar level!

We use syringes to take insulin!

Most people with insulin-dependent diabetes use syringes and lancets every day. But what do you do with them when you're done?

Like anything else we throw out, lancets and syringes need to be disposed of properly. Otherwise they can end up in places they don't belong, like beaches. And because they have very sharp, pointy ends, they can hurt people by accident, like the person who collects your garbage, someone in your family, or even you!

But there's a simple way you can help protect people <u>and</u> the environment. It's quick and easy!

Just follow these **TWO** steps ☞

1

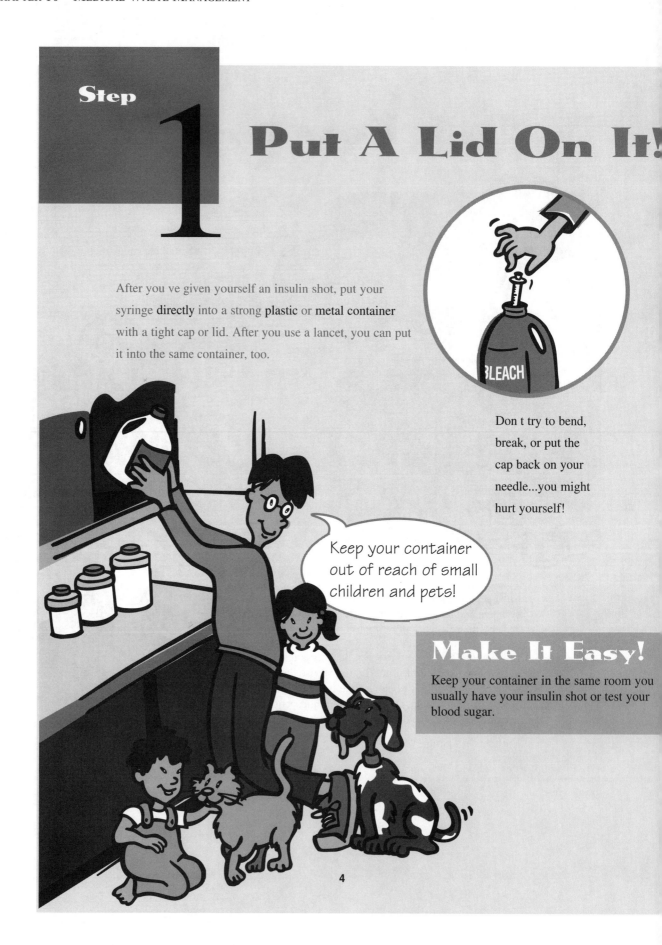

Step

1

Put A Lid On It!

After you ve given yourself an insulin shot, put your syringe **directly** into a strong **plastic** or **metal container** with a tight cap or lid. After you use a lancet, you can put it into the same container, too.

BLEACH

Don t try to bend, break, or put the cap back on your needle...you might hurt yourself!

Keep your container out of reach of small children and pets!

Make It Easy!

Keep your container in the same room you usually have your insulin shot or test your blood sugar.

4

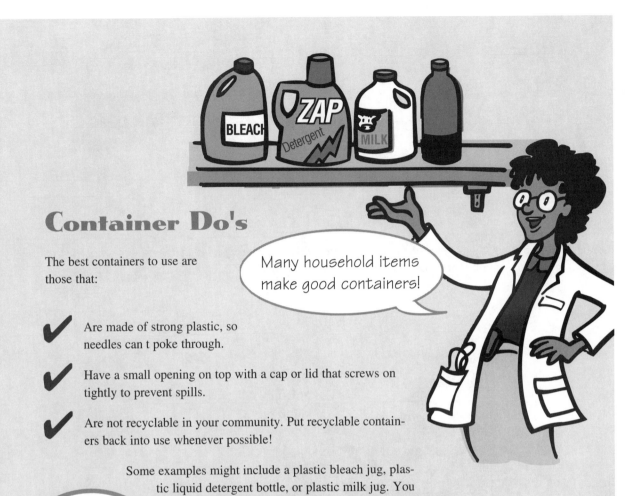

Container Do's

The best containers to use are those that:

Many household items make good containers!

✔ Are made of strong plastic, so needles can t poke through.

✔ Have a small opening on top with a cap or lid that screws on tightly to prevent spills.

✔ Are not recyclable in your community. Put recyclable containers back into use whenever possible!

Some examples might include a plastic bleach jug, plastic liquid detergent bottle, or plastic milk jug. You can use a coffee can, too. But when it gets full, close the lid tightly and seal it with strong tape.

Container Don'ts

✘ Don t use glass containers (they can break), or light-weight plastic containers.

✘ Don t use any container that will be returned to a store.

✘ If you use a recyclable container to dispose of syringes and lancets, be sure it doesn t end up in the recycling bin by mistake. These items are not recyclable, and could affect the safe and effective recycling of other items in the bin.

Step 2

Pitch In!

When the container is full, tightly secure the lid and reinforce it with heavy-duty tape before throwing it in the trash. Be sure not to put it in the recycling bin.

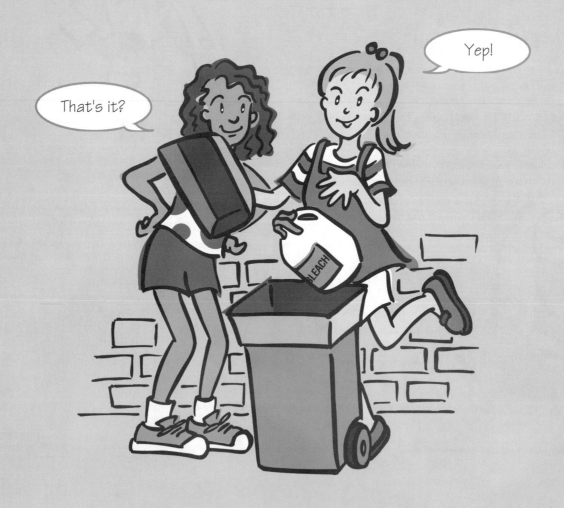

Word Scramble

1. Put your syringes and lancets into a strong_ _ _ _ _ _ _ or
(CLIPAST)

_ _ _ _ _ container and tighten the _ _ _.
(LATME)   (DLI)

2. When it gets full, reinforce the lid with_ _ _ _and throw
(PETA)

your_ _ _ _ _ _ _ _ _ into the _ _ _ _ _ !
(RENTANOIC)   (SHART)

CUT OUT THE BOTTOM OF THIS PAGE AND KEEP IT NEAR YOUR CONTAINER AS A REMINDER.

Remember

Step 1:
Put A Lid On It!

After you use a syringe or a lancet, put it
directly into a strong **plastic** or **metal**
container with a tight cap or **lid**.

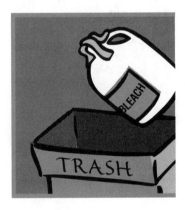

Step 2:
Pitch In!

When the **container** is full and tightly sealed
with heavy-duty tape, throw it out in the
trash. Don't put this container in your
recycling bin.

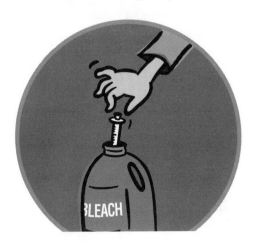

7

Congratulations!

Now you know how to handle and throw out used insulin syringes and lancets safely.

Pass It On!

Do you know others with insulin-dependent diabetes? Tell them what you've learned about handling and safe disposal of used syringes and lancets. By spreading the word, you can help others keep the environment clean and safe!

For additional copies of this booklet, please call the RCRA Hotline
Monday through Friday, 9 a.m. to 6 p.m., Eastern time.
The national toll-free number is 800 424-9346; for the hearing impaired it is TDD 800 553-7672.
In Washington, DC, the number is 703 412-9810; TDD 703 412-3323.

This booklet may be photocopied.

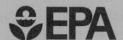

United States
Environmental Protection
Agency

EPA530-K-99-008
September 1999
www.epa.gov

 Printed on paper that contains at least 30 percent postconsumer fiber.

CHAPTER 11

Surveillance of Home Care-Acquired Infections*

Wherever health care is delivered—whether in the hospital, home, long-term care facility, or a hospice facility—there is some risk that the patient may acquire an infection related to the care rendered. It is incumbent upon the home care and hospice organization and its professional staff members to recognize this risk and to use appropriate infection control and prevention strategies to reduce the risk and prevent infection. Even with the best infection control efforts, however, the risk of infection can never be completely eliminated because it depends on the host's ability to resist infection (intrinsic factors) as well as on the many circumstances that surround the delivery of care (extrinsic factors). Home care and hospice professionals have the responsibility to measure the occurrence of home care–acquired infection in their patient population, estimate risk more accurately, and determine whether infection control procedures are effective. Risk assessment is accomplished through surveillance activities.

INFECTION SURVEILLANCE

Surveillance is defined as "the ongoing, systematic collection, analysis, and interpretation of health data essential to the planning, implementation, and evaluation of public health practice, closely integrated with timely dissemination of these data to those who need to know" (CDC, 1988). Surveillance is based on epidemiological principles and methods and can be applied to many types of health data (e.g., cancer incidence, mortality statistics, and risk factors for a specific disease). Infectious disease epidemiology, among the oldest applications of the science, related initially to the study of epi-

demics to determine their causes and develop interventions to control them. A classic case is represented by the Broad Street cholera epidemic, which occurred in 1849 in London, in which many thousands of people became ill and died. The source of the infection was determined through the now-famous epidemiological study conducted by John Snow, which associated drinking water from the public well with the occurrence of cholera (Snow, 1965). More recently, infectious disease epidemiology has succeeded in determining the cause and risk factors for new diseases such as West Nile virus (CDC, 2000) and Sudden Acute Respiratory Syndrome (SARS) (CDC, 2003a).

Hospital epidemiology is a developing field that began in the United States in the early 1970s with newly established infection control programs (see Chapter 1). Infection control practitioners (ICPs)—usually nurses or microbiologists—and hospital epidemiologists—usually physicians with training in infectious diseases or microbiology—developed surveillance programs specifically to study nosocomial infections. The study of nosocomial infection allowed ICPs and hospital epidemiologists to determine the expected frequency of infection (endemic rates), identify risk factors (e.g., indwelling Foley catheters), and measure the effectiveness of interventions and strategies to reduce infection (e.g., maintaining a closed urinary drainage system). These efforts are greatly enhanced through the support of the Centers for Disease Control and Prevention (CDC) and the National Nosocomial Infection Surveillance (NNIS) System study. The NNIS program has developed standard definitions of nosocomial infection and has standardized methods for data management (Emori *et al.*, 1991; Garner *et al.*,

---

*Home care-acquired infection refers to infections related to home and hospice care.

1988). Many U.S. hospitals participate in NNIS and submit their data regularly for analysis and comparison. In early 2000, there were approximately 315 hospitals submitting data to one or more of the NNIS programs. As a result, there are published rates of site-specific infection that provide a basis for comparison with other hospitals (CDC, 2004; CDC, 2003b).

ICPs and others involved in health care quality are now challenged to develop surveillance methods for studying health care–associated infections in settings outside the hospital. Standardized surveillance systems are needed in home care, ambulatory care, long-term care, subacute care facilities, and other settings in which patients are at risk for the development of an infection related to the care they are receiving. Standardized methods (e.g., definitions, data collection, and data analysis) are needed so that the occurrence of infection from nonhospital settings can be measured, compared, and reduced. Although surveillance definitions and methods used in hospitals provide an excellent model for the study of infections in other settings, in most cases both the definitions and the surveillance methods must be modified to accommodate the differences. For example, the NNIS definitions rely upon culture results for many sites of infection. This reliance on culture results may not be suitable in home care and hospice due to physicians' less frequent use of cultures to diagnose and treat infection in that setting. Although hospitalized patients may represent the most severely ill in the health care system, there is increasing acuity among patients in other settings, especially home care, which puts them at risk for infection. This chapter focuses on the development of surveillance methods for the study of home care–acquired infections. Information about current efforts to organize surveillance programs in home care as well as some early results are also provided.

WHY STUDY HOME CARE-ACQUIRED INFECTIONS?

Ongoing surveillance and the study of endemic and epidemic nosocomial infections provide scientifically valid information for identifying risk factors and reducing risk, which contributes to the focus on evidence-based practice. *Endemic infection* is the usual or expected rate of infection in a specific population within a defined time period. For example, a certain proportion of patients with indwelling Foley catheters de-

velop a urinary tract infection (UTI); the frequency is never zero percent even with the best infection control efforts. Occasionally, staff members notice that several patients have similar health care-associated infections within a limited timeframe (e.g., several patients that had surgery at the same facility may have surgical site infections within a two-week period). If they are not otherwise related, this might be referred to as a cluster of infections that may or may not be investigated. However, when the frequency of infection is much higher than expected, an outbreak is said to have occurred. For example, an outbreak of bloodstream infections related to the use of needleless systems was recognized and confirmed when the rate of infection was demonstrated to be greater than expected for the population and setting (Danzig *et al.,* 1995; Do *et al.,* 1999).

Published "normal" or "expected" endemic rates of infection can be used to compare a hospital's nosocomial infection rate with that of other hospitals. The NNIS publishes the results of the infection data submitted to the CDC (CDC, 2003b; CDC, 2004). These reports provide data that other hospitals can use to compare and evaluate their own rates of infection. However, even when the same definitions and methods for surveillance are employed, caution must be used when infection rates are compared directly (CDC, 1991). There may be a number of differences from one organization to another in the patient populations and associated risk factors, as well as in the manner of care delivery that must be considered when results are compared. Many of these factors are discussed in Chapter 3. A home care organization providing services to Medicare patients may have more older women with long-term indwelling Foley catheters and therefore a higher endemic rate of UTIs than an organization caring for pediatric patients with less frequent long-term urinary catheter use. A more valid comparison for a home care organization providing Medicare services would be another Medicare-certified agency with a similar patient population.

Reports of outbreaks have also allowed ICPs to identify potential causes of infection and eliminate them. Publication of these outbreaks, the results of the investigational methods, and the risk reduction strategies provide important references for others in the field that may experience a similar situation. A limited number of outbreaks in home care, all involving home infusion therapy, have been reported in the literature (Danzig *et al.,* 1995; Kellerman *et al.,* 1996; Do *et al.,* 1999).

Several authors have studied the incidence of health-care-associated infections in hospice patients (Pereira, 1998; Vitetta, 2000). While the occurrence of infection in terminally ill patients may not impact their outcome, it may have a negative impact on their comfort and quality of life. Thus, professionals providing hospice care should track the incidence of infection in their patients in order to identify exposures (e.g., use of indwelling urinary catheters) that might increase the risk of infection, which may be accompanied by pain and discomfort. As hospice providers are prioritizing to plan surveillance activities, they should consider those infections that most affect the patients' comfort and quality of life.

Given the many competing demands for resources, the progress in developing standardized methods and definitions for the surveillance of home care–acquired infections has been slow—but it's been steady. Two interested groups have published definitions for home care–acquired infections: the Association for Professionals in Infection Control and Epidemiology (APIC) (Embry & Chinnes, 2000) and the Missouri Alliance for Home Care (MAHC, 2004). The MAHC has sustained its support for the Infection Surveillance Project (ISP) since it began organizing in 1993. The ISP began its project by developing definitions for two sites of infection, catheter-associated urinary tract infections and central venous catheter infections (Schantz, 2001), and in 2004 it added a definition for surgical site infections (MAHC, 2004). The ISP provides training and guidance for infection surveillance. It also produces quarterly reports that allow participating home care organizations to compare the results of their surveillance activities to those of other organizations in the program. Results of catheter-associated UTIs and central venous catheter infection surveillance since 1999 can be viewed at the ISP website: *http://www.infectioncontrolathome.org.*

To date, no national organization or federal agency has come forward to standardize the definitions and methods or to organize the reporting of home care–acquired infection—the steps that would lead to publication and comparison of results. In addition to the ISP's surveillance results, however, others have published their results in the literature, as summarized in Table 11-1. Most authors have reported results of studies related to central venous catheter-associated infections; others have reported results for catheter-associated UTIs.

A home care organization can compare these results to their own experience, but any comparison of data must be done with caution and consideration. The rates of infection presented on Table 11-1 *cannot be used for direct comparison* without considering the definitions used by the authors, the methods of identifying cases, and the populations under study. In several of the studies, a specific population, such as patients with HIV (Skiest, 1998), were the target population, whereas others included patients with a variety of diagnoses who were receiving home care (Tokars, 1999). Some of the studies cited were performed using retrospective review (Tokars, 1999), whereas others were done in a concurrent manner (Gorksi, 2004). Probably the most

Table 11-1 Selected Published Results of Home Care-Acquired Infection Rates

Author/date of publication	Catheter-associated UTIs (rate per 1000 catheter days)	Central venous catheter-related infections* (rate per 1000 catheter days)
Missouri Home Care Alliance (ISP) (2004)	3.9	0.817 (BSI and site)
Gorski (2004)		0.77 (BSI)
Moureau (2002)		0.19 (BSI)
		0.26 (site)
Long (2002)	4.4	
Leuhm (1999)	2.79	0.54
Woomer (1999)	3.4	
Tokars (1999)		0.99 (BSI)
Skiest (1998)		1.4 (BSI)
		2.8 (site)
Rosenheimer (1998)	4.5	1.1 (BSI)

*Includes bloodstream infections (BSI) and catheter site infections (site), using various definitions of each; studies include various types of central IV catheters in a variety of populations.

important consideration when using data for comparison is the author's definition of infection.

The definitions for hospital-acquired infections have been standardized by the CDC through the NNIS study (Garner *et al.*, 1988). Because NNIS has published their definitions, hospitals that use the same definitions and methods for the appropriate populations can compare their data to the NNIS rates. However, NNIS definitions do not work as well in home or hospice care due to their reliance on laboratory data and cultures. Therefore, if a home care or hospice organization wants to compare its rate of infection with any of the data cited in Table 11-1 or other published data, it must consider all the factors mentioned previously, including most importantly the definition of infection used by the author(s). As outlined below, these definitions vary considerably. In an analysis of the definitions used for catheter-associated urinary tract infection (CAUTI) and those used for infections related to central venous catheters (bloodstream infections and exit-site infections) cited on Table 11-1, the authors organize risk variables into three main categories: (1) physical signs and symptoms, (2) laboratory findings, and (3) physician interventions. These are then incorporated in varied approaches. Please note that although APIC has not published any aggregate results of home care–acquired infection using their definitions, the variables found within their draft definitions are included in this discussion (Embry, 2000).

As an example of varying definitions, the APIC draft definition for symptomatic urinary tract infection in catheterized or noncatheterized patients includes the presence of three of four of the listed signs and symptoms accompanied by abnormal findings in a urinalysis (e.g., pyuria and positive nitrite and/or leukocyte esterase) or a positive urine culture ($>10^5$ cfu/ml of bacteria and no more than two organisms). The MAHC definition, on the other hand, requires the observance of changes in the character of the urine (e.g., color, odor, sediment) plus two or more signs and symptoms of infection, such as an increased serum white blood cell (WBC) count or physical signs and symptoms such as pain or a positive urine culture. However, a physician's order for antibiotics alone also meets the MAHC definition. These and another published definition are compared on Table 11-2.

The variables considered for surveillance of central venous catheter (CVC)–associated infections are even more diverse. The APIC, Rosenheimer, and Gorski all define the finding of a positive blood culture with a known pathogen and no other site of infection as a laboratory-confirmed bloodstream infection (APIC, 2000) or CVC-related sepsis (Rosenheimer, 1998; Gorski, 2004). If no cultures have been obtained, APIC provides a definition for clinical sepsis that includes the presence of fever, hypotension, and oliguria and no other site of infection and a physician's order for antibiotic therapy. Gorksi and the MAHC both refer to "catheter-related infections", but do

Table 11-2 Definitions of Symptomatic Urinary Tract Infection

Source	Signs and symptoms	Laboratory results	Physician orders
APIC (2000)	Three of four signs/symptoms: 1. Fever (>100.4°F) or chills 2. Flank pain, suprapubic pain, tenderness, frequency, or urgency 3. Worsening of mental status/functional status 4. Changes in urine character **and**	Urinalysis showing pyuria and nitrites or leukocytes	Not included
MAHC (2003)	Change in urine character: • hematuria • increased sediment • foul odor; • plus two or more signs and symptoms: – Fever >100.4°F – New flank or suprapubic pain – Elevated serum WBC – Worsening or change in mental status or a positive urine culture	Urine culture considered with other signs and symptoms **or**	Physician order for antibiotics
Rosenheimer (1998)	One sign or symptom **and**	Urine culture with >10⁵ CFUs **or**	Physician order for antibiotics

not differentiate between bloodstream infections and IV exit-site infections. It appears that both combine these incidences into one rate. However, Gorski refers to "systemic" infection when providing results of her 7-year study (Gorski, 2004). A summary of various definitions for CVC–associated infections is included in Table 11-3.

Publications from the peer-reviewed literature provide a range of results in the surveillance of home care-

Table 11-3 Definitions of Central Venous Catheter-Associated Infections

Author/source	Definition
Embry/APIC (2000)	Primary bloodstream infection (includes laboratory-confirmed bloodstream infection and clinical sepsis) 1. Recognized pathogen isolated from blood culture and pathogen is not related to infection at another site 2. One of the following signs and symptoms: fever, chills, or hypotension and one of the following: • Common skin contaminate isolated from two blood cultures drawn on separate occasions and organism is not related to infection at another site • Common skin contaminant isolation from blood culture from patient with intravascular access device and physician institutes appropriate antimicrobial therapy Clinical sepsis Must meet one of the following clinical signs or symptoms with no other recognized cause: fever (>100.4°F), hypotension (systolic pressure <90 mm), or oliguria (<20 cm³/hour), and all of the following: 1. Blood culture not done or no organisms detected 2. No apparent infection at another site 3. Physician institutes antimicrobial therapy for sepsis
Missouri Home Care Alliance (2004)	Define central venous catheter (CVC) site related infection occurrence of a patient with a central venous catheter as: 1. Two or more of the following signs/symptons are present: • Erythema associated with central line • Pain associated with central line • Purulent drainage from the exit site • Elevated serum WBC* • Fever 100.4°F or greater* **or** 2. A physician prescribes a course of antibiotic treatment for a suspected or confirmed CVC infection **or** 3. A physician orders the CVC to be pulled due to suspected or confirmed infection
Rosenheimer (1998)	Bloodstream infection in a patient receiving intravenous therapy; a recognized pathogen has to be isolated from a blood culture and the pathogen cannot be related to an infection at another site.
Gorksi (2004)	Must have a Central Venous Access Device (CVAD) present and the finding (by blood culture) of bacteriemia **or** CVAD present and two of the following: • Temperature >2°F or 1°C over the patient's baseline or chills • Significant local pain and redness associated with central catheter or exit site • Hypotension (<90 mm HG systolic) • Physician suspects central line infection is present and initiates therapy (changes/removes line or starts antibiotics) • WBC count >10,000 **or** Pus, cellutitus, or significant pain present at exit site of central catheter
Tokars (1999)	Bloodstream infection is diagnosed if all of the following features are present: 1. One or more positive blood cultures 2. Antimicrobial therapy or catheter removal 3. No infection at another site that could have caused the bacteremia
Skiest (1998)	Define catheter-related bacteremia: Isolation of the same organism from blood culture and either from a catheter tip by the Maki roll plate technique or in association with purulence, erythema, and growth of the same organism at the skin exit site. Probable catheter-related bacteremia: Bacteremia with an organism known to be a cause of catheter-related infections (two positive blood cultures are required for a diagnosis of bacteremia secondary to coagulase-negative staphylococci) in the absence of another source of bacteria.
Moureau (2002)	Catheter infection is defined an infectious event involving an intravenous catheter documented through laboratory findings (e.g., positive blood culture and catheter cultures). Can be either a local site infection or a systemic primary bloodstream infection.

*Need to rule out other possible causes of infection

acquired infections. One can observe in Table 11-1 that the reported range for catheter-associated UTI is 2.79 to 4.5 infections per 1000 catheter days. The range and comparison of infection rates related to CVCs is a bit more complicated, due to the wider variety of risk variables, definitions, and methods. The reported range of CVC-related bloodstream infections incorporated in Table 11-1 is 0.19 to 1.4 per 1000 catheter days. A catheter insertion site infection also varies widely, with a reported range of 0.26 to 2.8 per 1000 catheter days. As mentioned above, the definition and methods for the ISP from the MHCA combine both BSI and site infection, resulting in a combined rate in summary reports from 1999 through 2003 of 0.36 to 0.97 infections per 1000 catheter days (MHCA, 2004). Home care professionals involved in infection control and the provision of home infusion therapy should continue to monitor the literature for additional studies as well as reports of further efforts toward standardization of definitions and methods.

The remainder of this chapter focuses on the application of epidemiologic principles and methods for surveillance in home and hospice care. This information can be used in the development of surveillance programs; it can also be used to examine and evaluate current and future reports in the literature.

ASSESSMENT OF THE POPULATION

There are specific steps that should be followed in the development of a surveillance system in a home care or hospice organization (Lee *et al.*, 1998; Exhibit 11-1). First, the patient population must be assessed to identify characteristics that may affect health status as well as intrinsic and extrinsic factors that may affect risk

---

Exhibit 11-1 Steps in Developing a Surveillance Program

1. Assess the patient population.
2. Select the outcome or process for surveillance.
3. Develop or select definitions.
4. Develop data collection methods.
5. Calculate infection rates and analyze data.
6. Apply risk stratification methods.
7. Use data and information for risk reduction and quality improvement.

---

for developing an infection. Intrinsic risk factors are related to the host and his or her immune status. For example, patients with chronic diseases, such as insulin-dependent diabetes or chronic obstructive pulmonary disease, are at increased risk for infection. Extrinsic factors are related to the care being provided and the environment in which it is provided. Home infusion therapy presents specific risks because it involves an invasive procedure and an indwelling medical device.

In light of limited resources, surveillance efforts should focus on patients and services that represent the greatest risk for home care–acquired infection. For example, surveillance for bloodstream infections in children receiving home infusion therapy and CVC care and maintenance should be a priority because of the risks related to the age of the patients and to the therapy provided. When the decision must be made about where to focus surveillance efforts, priority should be given to those infections that (1) are the direct result of home care services and interventions and (2) can be reduced through specific procedures under the control of the home and hospice care staff. Infections that are not directly related to home care or hospice services (e.g., UTIs in uncatheterized older female hospice patients) may not be a priority for measurement. Identification of infection for surveillance purposes (to reduce overall risk) must be differentiated from identification of an infection so that the patient's physician can provide appropriate treatment. Both are important, but they have different purposes.

Although home care and hospice professionals know the general characteristics of their patient population and the types of services being provided, a more explicit assessment should be done when planning for surveillance. Exhibit 11-2 provides a list of population characteristics and types of services that may be considered when designing a surveillance program for a home care or hospice organization. If possible, actual data and statistics from the past 1 to 2 years that describe the home or hospice care organization's population (e.g., Medicare patients or pediatric patients) and the types of care the patients have received (e.g., wound care or home infusion therapy) should be used to profile the population. This assessment helps ensure that the limited resources available for surveillance activities are used in the most effective manner.

Exhibit 11-2 Assessment of the Population

Patients served	Services provided
Age	Homemaker/companion
• Newborn	services
• Pediatric	Home health aide
• Adult	services
• Geriatric	Skilled nursing services
Gender	Behavioral health care
Race	Respiratory therapy
National origin	Home infusion therapy
Language spoken in the	Home hemodialysis
home	Ambulatory peritoneal
Level of education	dialysis
Socioeconomic status	Medical equipment and
Living conditions and	supplies
sanitation	Neonatal/infant/
Demographics	pediatric care
• Urban	Hospice care
• Suburban	Physical therapy
• Rural	Occupational therapy
Frequency of disease	Speech-language
Common diagnoses	pathology
Chronic illnesses	Medical social services
	Perinatal/postpartum care
	Nutritional assessment
	and consultation

SELECTION OF OUTCOMES OR PROCESSES FOR MEASUREMENT

Selection of the specific outcomes for measurement is the next important step in planning a home or hospice care surveillance program. Surveillance activities in home care should not include identification and measurement of community-acquired infections. Community-acquired infections may include upper and lower respiratory infections (e.g., colds, influenza, and pneumonia), gastrointestinal infections (e.g., nausea, vomiting, diarrhea, and viral gastroenteritis), and other common illnesses that may occur as a result of exposure in the community through visitors and family members. Although home care and hospice staff members can advise patients and their families on how to avoid the risk of community-acquired infection (e.g., by offering an influenza vaccine and recommending immunization of family members),

they do not have control over patients or family members. In fact, community-acquired infections may frequently come from a family member living in the patient's home; this risk is difficult to avoid.

In some home and hospice care organizations, surveillance activities measure all home care–acquired infections in all home care patients. For several reasons, this approach of performing total surveillance is not recommended. First, it may not be necessary for the purpose of quality improvement to detect all infections. Some infections may not be preventable because of intrinsic risk factors. Second, unless significant resources are provided to support surveillance activities and ensure the accuracy and reliability of data, the data may be inaccurate and misleading. Finally, as has been demonstrated in nosocomial surveillance, conducting surveillance of all infections and calculating a single infection rate is ill advised. An overall rate is not specific or focused enough to draw conclusions or make reasonable plans for risk reduction. A reportedly low rate may be unreliable and may not reflect actual incidence and risk in certain high-risk patients. In addition, external agencies and organizations, such as accrediting bodies or purchasers, may request this rate and rely on its accuracy. Requests for such data should be denied, with an explanation of why they are not reasonable or valid (Bryant, 1997).

Home and hospice care organizations should measure home care–acquired infections; that is, those infections that occur as a result of the home care provided. The term *home care–acquired infection* is preferred over other recently suggested terms, such as *nosohusial infection* or *homocomial infection* (Friedman, 1996). Rather than attempt to measure all health care–acquired infections, home care and hospice organizations should assign priority to a given measurement by considering factors related to risk and preventability. These factors may include the following (Lee et al., 1998):

* frequency of infection
* negative impact, such as increases in morbidity, mortality, and/or cost
* potential for prevention by home care or hospice staff
* specific needs and risks in the patient population served

- requirements of external customers (e.g., reporting requirements of managed care organizations)
- requirements of accrediting bodies
- the organization's mission and strategic goals
- relationship of the infection outcome with the process of care
- resources available for surveillance

Infections are generally categorized by body site. A list of the types of home or hospice care-acquired infections that can be considered for surveillance is provided in Exhibit 11-3. Not all infections in this list must or should be monitored. Each home care or hospice organization must decide which infections to measure based on the factors discussed above, the assessment of the home care or hospice population served, and the knowledge gained from the surveillance planning process.

Data demonstrate that a large proportion of nosocomial infections are related to medical devices. These devices (e.g., urinary catheters, CVCs, and tracheotomies) interrupt (urinary catheter) or breech (CVC) normal anatomical barriers to infection and provide a portal of entry for microorganisms that is not normally present. They may also provide a protective environment for bacteria to grow and cause infection (Goldmann & Pier, 1993). Patients with indwelling devices have a greater extrinsic risk for infection than those without devices. Device-related infections should receive priority when sites are selected for surveillance because home care and hospice staff members are responsible for care and maintenance of the device. Home care organizations providing home infusion therapy should minimally select central line-associated bloodstream infections as part of their surveillance activities.

Exhibit 11-3 Sites of Home Care-Acquired Infection

IV-related infections
- central line-associated bloodstream infection
- contaminated infusate–related bloodstream infection
- exit-site infection
- pocket or tunnel infection

Urinary tract
Respiratory tract
Skin and soft tissue (e.g., pressure ulcers)
Gastrointestinal system
Surgical site
Eye, ear, nose, throat, mouth

Although many home care organizations monitor wound infections in their surveillance activities, surgical site infections are not usually home care–acquired infections. Surgical site infections begin (are seeded) in surgery. Once the surgical wound is closed, there is little risk for external contamination of the wound if there is primary closure and no drains are left in place. Generally, the wound seals in about 12 hours. For a surgical-site infection to become a home care–acquired infection, the wound would either have to be open or have some type of drain or catheter in place that is cared for in the home. If the wound has a drain (e.g., a Jackson-Pratt drain after head and neck or breast surgery or a chest tube), the drainage system is usually closed. A home care–acquired surgical site infection might occur if a closed drainage system is entered carelessly and thereby contaminated. Routine surveillance of true home care–acquired surgical site infections may not be of great value, because the frequency is normally very low.

A home care organization may decide to identify surgical site infections in postoperative patients for other purposes. Because most surgical site infections have an incubation period of 7 to 10 days (or longer), they are usually not evident before hospital discharge. Although most surgical site infections become evident while the patient is receiving home care services, the infection should be considered nosocomial if the infection occurs within 30 days of surgery. A home care organization might consider identifying, recording, and reporting surgical site infections to the referring hospital's infection control department or to the ambulatory surgery center to assist in its surveillance efforts. If the home care or hospice organization is JCAHO-accredited, this reporting is required (JCAHO, 2004). The information can be helpful because many surgical procedures are now performed on an ambulatory basis and because the length of postoperative stay for those who are admitted to the hospital has decreased significantly in the past several years. This makes surgical site infection surveillance difficult for hospital ICPs. Home care staff members can greatly improve the surveillance of nosocomial surgical site infections by reporting them to the infection control program of the hospital where the surgery was performed or to the ICP in the ambulatory surgery center. Other infections recognized during the course of home or hospice care and suspected to be of nosocomial origin can also be reported to the hospital infection control program.

Wound infection surveillance for home care–acquired infections may more logically focus on infected pressure ulcers and soft tissue infections that are the result of skin breakdown. Although there are many intrinsic host factors that affect the risk for pressure ulcers and general skin integrity, there are a variety of interventions that may reduce the risk. These are logical targets for surveillance and improvement efforts, especially in hospice patients.

DEVELOPING DEFINITIONS FOR HOME CARE-ACQUIRED INFECTIONS

Although home care and hospice staff members can recognize infections, definitions provide specific criteria for measuring home care–acquired infections in a consistent manner. Otherwise, one staff member may interpret various clinical signs and symptoms as an infection more frequently than another staff member. Consistency among staff members in identifying and measuring infections for surveillance is referred to as *interrater reliability*. Ideally, the same conclusion about the presence of an infection should be reached no matter who is performing surveillance. Application of specific criteria within a definition facilitates this consistency. In addition, standard definitions are necessary if rates of infection are to be compared with those reported by other home and hospice care organizations.

The NNIS has published a full set of definitions for nosocomial infections (Garner et al., 1988). Although these definitions are widely used in hospital surveillance programs, they are not easily adapted to home care. Legitimately, the NNIS definitions rely heavily on diagnostic tests (e.g., cultures, laboratory tests, and radiological imaging) to identify and define infection. Obtaining specimens for cultures and laboratory tests is not common practice in home care or hospice. Frequently, a physician makes the diagnosis of an infection based on signs and symptoms, the patient's history and current health status, and extrinsic risk factors. Diagnosis is made for the purpose of treatment, not surveillance. The physician will more often presume that the patient is infected and treat the infection empirically than underdiagnose and increase the potential for additional complications. Some home care and hospice organizations use a physician's diagnosis of infection or prescription for antibiotic therapy as the sole criterion for the definition of a home care–acquired infection. This may result in

a higher than actual infection rate due to the lack of specific definitions for infection. A set of definitions has been developed for infections acquired in long-term care that are less reliant on laboratory data than the NNIS definitions are. These may be helpful in developing definitions for home care–acquired infections (McGeer *et al.*, 1991).

The definitions of infection for the purposes of surveillance should be based on several considerations. First, clinical data, including the typical signs and symptoms that would occur in a normal host with the infection in question, should be incorporated into the definition. Signs and symptoms vary according to the site of infection and age of the patient. For example, symptoms of a UTI include frequency of urination, burning, pain, and fever. Signs may include cloudy urine. A skin or wound infection may result in symptoms of redness, pain, and tenderness at the site. Purulent drainage may also be observed as a sign of infection. Definitions of infection should take into account the fact that signs and symptoms may vary in different age groups. Neonates, infants, and children exhibit different signs and symptoms of infection than adults. For example, neonates may not develop a fever if they have a bloodstream infection, and their body temperature may be below normal. These differences must be incorporated into the definitions of infection if different age groups are served by the home care organization.

Second, some type of laboratory data should be included in the definition of a home care–acquired infection as objective evidence of infection. This is more difficult because the diagnosis of infection for the purpose of treatment in home care and hospice patients is more often empirical (based on the physician's assessment of the signs and symptoms reported) and less often based on laboratory tests. The diagnosis of a UTI, for instance, is frequently based on signs and symptoms, and antibiotics are ordered without a culture. For surveillance purposes, however, it is preferable to have some confirmatory laboratory data whenever possible. Table 11-4 provides some criteria for consideration in the development of definitions for home care–acquired infections by site.

The surveillance of infections related to home infusion therapy (see Chapter 4) is important, but it may be the most challenging in terms of the development of definitions. To accurately determine the incidence of infections related to intravenous (IV) therapy and identify specific risks, definitions for various types of IV-related

Table 11-4 Criteria for Definition of Infection by Site

Site of infection	Clinical data	Laboratory data
Catheter-associated UTI	Change in characteristics of urine Fever Pain	Elevated serum white blood cell (WBC) count Evidence of UTI on urinalysis Evidence of WBCs on urine dipstick test Positive urine culture ($>10^5$ colony-forming units of a single organism per milliliter of urine)
Postoperative pneumonia	Change in character of sputum Decreased breath sounds Increase in rales and rhonchi Fever Shortness of breath Pain	Elevated serum WBC count Evidence of respiratory infection on sputum Gram stain Positive sputum culture Positive chest radiograph
Central line-associated bloodstream infection	Fever with chills and rigors Redness, tenderness, pain at insertion site Purulent drainage at site	Elevated serum WBC count Positive blood culture Positive catheter culture (after catheter removal)
Skin and soft tissue (includes infected pressure ulcer)	Pain, swelling, tenderness at site Inflammation and warmth Purulent drainage Fever	WBCs and organisms on Gram stain Positive culture Elevated serum WBC count
Endometritis in postpartum patients	Uterine tenderness and abdominal pain Purulent vaginal drainage (lochia) Foul-smelling lochia Fever	Positive Gram stain of lochia Positive culture of lochia Elevated serum WBC count

infections must be developed. Both clinical signs and symptoms (e.g., fever and redness at the exit site) and laboratory data (e.g., positive blood cultures) should be incorporated in the definitions. Bloodstream infection should also be distinguished by its source. Bloodstream infection may be secondary to an infection at another site (e.g., secondary to pneumonia), or it may be secondary to contaminated IV fluid. Bloodstream infection may also arise from a colonized CVC, or it may be related to an exit-site infection. To assess the risk accurately, the specific source must be distinguished in the definition of bloodstream infection. In addition to clinical signs and symptoms, the definition of central line-associated bloodstream infection should include positive blood culture results with cultures drawn from two separate sites. One culture specimen should be drawn through the IV catheter, and the second should be ob-

tained through a percutaneous blood draw. If both cultures grow the same organism (genus and species) with the same antibiotic sensitivity pattern, the infection can be considered a central line-associated bloodstream infection (CDC, 2002b).

Local IV-related infections must also be specifically defined according to the type of IV access device. Signs and symptoms of infection (e.g., redness, tenderness, and purulent drainage) may be incorporated into a definition of exit-site infection related to percutaneous catheters (such as a peripherally inserted central catheter). A tunnel infection may occur in surgically implanted catheters (such as a Hickman catheter). A tunnel infection is one that is below the skin and exit site; it affects the subcutaneous tract that was created to "tunnel" the catheter below the skin and into a major vein. Subcutaneously implanted access devices or ports have surgically created pockets that may become infected. They, too, should be considered in the development of definitions for IV-related infection (CDC, 2002b).

The definitions of home care–acquired infection must also consider the incubation period for the infection. The incubation period is the time from the initial exposure to the pathogen to the time the infection is evident. Most bacterial infections have an incubation period of 48 to 72 hours, but the period may be shorter or longer. The incubation period varies for viral infections; for chicken pox it is 10 to 21 days, and for influenza it is 24 to 48 hours. The incubation period must be considered to avoid counting nosocomial infections (or infections that originated at other sites of care) as home care acquired. Therefore, if a patient discharged from a hospital with an indwelling Foley catheter exhibits signs and symptoms of a UTI within 48 hours of admission to home care, the infection should not be counted as home care acquired because it is probably nosocomial. Specific circumstances should be considered, however. Some home care–acquired infections can occur within the first 72 hours of home care. For example, if a patient receiving home parenteral nutrition develops a fever with shaking chills and rigors the first or second day at home and immediately after a new bag of IV fluid has been hung, this should be counted as a home care–acquired bloodstream infection.

There are two specific conditions that should *not* be included as home care–acquired infections: colonization and inflammation. As explained in Chapter 2, colonization describes the presence of bacteria without multiplication and damage to the host tissue. A positive culture may detect colonization, but the application of the definition of infection should avoid inclusion of a case of colonization as a home care–acquired infection. For example, a patient may be colonized with MRSA (methicillin-resistant *Staphylococcus Aureus*) but not infected. Inflammation may occur without infection, as in the case of phlebitis from a peripheral venous catheter. Again, a consistent definition of infection should be applied to avoid the identification of an inflammation as an infection.

DATA COLLECTION METHODS

Once the site definitions of infection are selected or developed, the home care organization must determine what additional information about each infected patient should be collected and analyzed. The general tendency is to collect more information than is useful, such as the name and dose of the antibiotic ordered to treat an in-

fection. This approach should be avoided because data collection can be time consuming, adding to the expense of performing surveillance. To determine what specific information should be recorded, the home care or hospice organization must consider the value and future use of the specific information in elucidating more about home care–acquired infection. If the data will not be useful in describing the occurrence of home care–acquired infections and identifying risk factors, it should probably not be collected. Useful data, however, may include the specific organism cultured from the site of infection; such data may lead to the recognition of an outbreak or a specific reservoir of infection.

The data collected and recorded should include patient demographic data, data to describe the infection, and some risk data. Demographic data may include age, gender, and diagnosis. Other variables about the patient may be helpful but should be limited to only what is considered useful in defining risk. For example, when information is collected about bloodstream infection in children receiving home infusion therapy, in addition to the patient's identification number the demographic data could include the child's age, gender, primary diagnosis, and primary caregiver. If the home care organization provides care in an urban setting to a diverse ethnic population, the primary language spoken in the home may be an important demographic variable. In an elderly patient population, information about living arrangements (e.g., lives alone, lives with daughter, lives with disabled elderly spouse) may be important.

A description of the infection should include the site of infection, the date of infection onset (the day signs and symptoms were first observed), and the results of cultures, if available. It is usually not useful to collect data on the antibiotic sensitivity report for routine surveillance. If the organism demonstrates multidrug resistance (e.g., methicillin-resistant *Staphylococcus aureus* or VRE), that information should be noted in the infection surveillance report (see Chapter 8).

The risk data collected depend on the site of infection. Some examples of risk elements are provided in Table 11-5. For example, information about IV catheter–related infections should include the type of catheter (e.g., Broviac or Hickman) and the number of lumens, because these may be important risk factors. Information must be recorded in a practical, useful manner. Thus it must be categorized or coded so that it can be either entered into a database or easily counted and summarized in a table. Descriptive information written in sentences or

Table 11-5 Risk Factors for Home Care–Acquired Infection by Site

Site of infection	Risk factors
Catheter-associated UTI	Date of insertion Urethral versus suprapubic catheter
Central line-associated bloodstream infection	Type of catheter (Hickman, Broviac, peripherally inserted central, midline) Central or peripheral Percutaneous or implanted Number of lumens Date of insertion Type of infusion therapy (total parenteral nutrition, antibiotics)
Postoperative pneumonia	Date and type of surgery
Gastrointestinal infection in patients receiving enteral nutrition	Type of enteral therapy (prepared in home or preprepared) If prepared in home, how and by whom
Peritonitis in continuous ambulatory peritoneal dialysis (CAPD) patients	Type of catheter Date of placement

phrases does not lend itself to easy analysis. Dependence on a written narrative to provide information about home care–acquired infection should be avoided. Thus an infection report form should be designed with check boxes and minimal "fill in the blank" fields. An example of an infection control report form is provided in Exhibit 11-4.

Period of Surveillance

A specified period for which data are collected and analyzed should be determined before data collection is initiated. Hospitals use surveillance periods of 1 month. Most home care and hospice organizations aggregate surveillance data on a monthly basis and report on a quarterly basis. Based on anecdotal experience and limited data (White, 1992), however, it appears that home care–acquired infections do not occur as frequently as hospital-acquired infections do. Home care surveillance periods should be longer than 30 days when there is not a sufficient sample size for data analysis, drawing conclusions, and planning risk-reduction activities. Eventually, annual rates of infection by site can be calculated, but the trending of rates over short periods, such as monthly or quarterly, is much more meaningful and sensitive, provided that there is a sufficiently large sample.

Defining Denominators

Infections should never be reported as a number of events (e.g., 12 UTIs in May and 16 UTIs in June). Infections should be reported, analyzed, and trended as rate-based data by infection site. To develop rate-

based data, it is necessary to have a numerator (number of infections) and a denominator. The denominator is the number of patients at risk for that infection (e.g., postoperative patients at risk for postoperative pneumonia during the surveillance period) or the number of days patients are at risk (e.g., total number of catheter days for all patients with indwelling urinary catheters during the surveillance period). Days at risk provides the more accurate estimate of risk when the rate of device-related infections is calculated. The alternative measure, the number of patients with a device (no matter how long they had the device), does not adequately or accurately represent the risk because risk for infection increases with exposure time. The longer a device is in place, the greater the risk for infection.

A specific denominator must be developed or selected for each site of home care–acquired infection. Suggested denominators for various sites of infection are found in Table 11-6. It is important to define the denominator before surveillance begins because this determines which patients will be monitored for the infection. Methods for identifying patients with the infection of interest are discussed next.

Retrospective Versus Concurrent Data Collection

Infections should always be identified concurrently (as they occur) rather than retrospectively (after the fact). Retrospective surveillance is usually based on chart review. Retrospective clinical record review should not be performed as the routine method of

Exhibit 11-4 Infection Screening Report

Date of Report: _____   Completed by: _____

Patient Name: _____   Identification Number: _____ SOC date: _____

Primary Diagnosis: _____   Physician Name: _____

Instructions: The staff member observing the signs and symptoms should complete sections one and two and submit the report to infection control practitioner. _____

Section One: Patient Signs and Symptoms (Check all that apply)

Signs and Symptoms and Date Observed: _____
- ☐ Fever ≥100.5° F (oral)
- ☐ Chills and rigors
- ☐ Elevated serum WBC   Date: _____   Results: _____ or ☐ Copy of lab results attached
- ☐ New antibiotic order   Date: _____   Order: _____
- ☐ New culture order—Site and date: _____
- ☐ Positive culture results or ☐ Copy of lab results attached
  Date culture obtained: _____ Site of culture: _____
  Organism(s) isolated: _____
  Drug resistant organisms: ☐ Yes ☐ No   Describe _____

Section Two: Potential Infection Site(s)

Possible catheter-associated UTI
- ☐ Change in character of urine (Check all that apply: ☐ increased sediment, ☐ cloudiness, ☐ foul odor, ☐ hematuria)
- ☐ New flank pain or suprapubic pain
- ☐ Change or worsening mental status
- ☐ WBC's in dipstick urine test

Possible bloodstream infection
- ☐ IV central line-associated bloodstream infection
- ☐ IV infusate-related bloodstream infection
- ☐ Secondary to other infection site
  Primary site (e.g., pneumonia, peritonitis): _____

Possible IV catheter-related infection (Check One: ☐ exit site ☐ tunnel ☐ pocket)
- ☐ Insertion/exit site, tunnel or pocket (Check all that apply: ☐ redness, ☐ pain, ☐ swelling)
- ☐ MD ordered catheter to be removed
- ☐ Pain, tenderness at pocket site
- ☐ Pain, tenderness along tunnel
- ☐ Purulent drainage—Describe: _____
  Date of catheter insertion: _____

Possible skin or soft infection
Specific site: _____
Check all that apply: ☐ redness ☐ pain or tenderness ☐ swelling
- ☐ Purulent drainage—Describe: _____
- ☐ Evidence of cellulitis—Describe: _____

Possible wound infection (Check One: ☐ wound ☐ drain site ☐ decubitus)
- ☐ Redness, tenderness
- ☐ Swelling
- ☐ Purulent drainage—Describe: _____
- ☐ Post-operative wound Date and type of surgery: _____

Continues

Exhibit 11-4 continued

Possible Pneumonia
☐ Change in sputum (Check all that apply: ☐ color, ☐ purulence, ☐ thickness)
☐ Increase in rales and rhonchi
☐ Decrease in breath sounds
☐ Pain in chest/thorax
☐ Change or worsening mental status
☐ Shortness of breath

Possible Postpartum Endometritis
☐ Uterine tenderness
☐ Abdominal pain
☐ Foul-smelling lochia

Possible Peritonitis
☐ Abdominal pain
☐ Rebound tenderness

Possible Gastrointestinal
☐ Sudden onset of nausea and vomiting
☐ Diarrhea

Source: Copyright © 1999, Emily Rhinehart and Mary Friedman.

Elements from Exhibit 11-4 can be combined with elements of Exhibit 11-5 to develop a single form for screening and recording home care-acquired infections.

Table 11-6 Denominators for Infection by Site

Infection site (numerator)	Denominator	Type of rate
Catheter-associated UTI	Total number of catheter days for all patients with indwelling Foley catheters	Incidence density
Postoperative pneumonia	Number of patients admitted during surveillance period for postoperative care	Cumulative incidence
Central line-associated bloodstream infection	Total number of catheter days for all patients with venous access devices (or by device if there is a sufficient sample)	Incidence density
Skin and soft tissue infection in patients with diabetes	Number of patients with insulin-dependent diabetes mellitus admitted or cared for during surveillance period	Cumulative incidence
Gastrointestinal infection in patients receiving enteral nutrition	Number of patients receiving enteral nutrition or total number of days for which all patients received enteral nutrition	Incidence density
Endometritis in postpartum patients	Number of postpartum patients admitted during surveillance period	Cumulative incidence
Peritonitis in patients receiving continuous ambulatory peritoneal dialysis (CAPD)	Total number of days during surveillance period	Incidence density

case finding mainly because it may be inaccurate. This method relies solely on what is written in the patient record and may not include important signs and symptoms; also, it is labor intensive. In addition, if the home care or hospice staff member who cared for the patient is asked to clarify information in the clinical record, his or her recall may be incomplete or inaccurate. Finally, if a retrospective approach is taken, current problems and outbreaks of infection may be missed.

It may also be preferable to collect denominator data concurrently, depending on the type of data required. For example, if the denominator is the number of patients admitted for CVC care and the data is captured from a clinical documentation or billing system, the counting at the end of the month will likely be accurate and feasible. If the denominator is the total number of days for which all patients had indwelling urinary catheters, however, a daily count (concurrent) may be necessary. The choice of concurrent versus retrospective capture of denominator data may depend on what data are available electronically in a clinical record or billing system and what data must be compiled manually.

Identifying Home Care-Acquired Infections

Once the specific definitions for home care–acquired infections are developed and denominators are selected, case finding to identify patients with the infection of interest can begin. The home or hospice care organization must decide who will be responsible for identifying the cases and reporting or recording them for the purpose of surveillance and data analysis. In some organizations, all professional home or hospice care staff are responsible for identifying and recording infections. This may result in poor interrater reliability, however, if too many individuals are applying the definitions and counting infections. To improve the reliability of surveillance data, the home care or hospice organization may decide to conduct surveillance in two phases: (1) screening all patients at risk for the specified infection and (2) applying the specific definition. In this approach, all professional staff members are required to report any patient with signs and symptoms of an infection. This may include patients with a fever, local signs and symptoms of infection, and/or a new prescription for an antibiotic. Reports should not be verbal; a screening form should be completed (a sample form is provided in Exhibit 11-5)

and forwarded to the individual who has been designated as the infection control practitioner (ICP) responsible for surveillance.

The designated ICP should review the screening form to determine whether the infection meets the criteria for home care-acquired infection as specified in the organization's definitions. The ICP should make this determination based on additional information obtained by reviewing the clinical record, speaking with the professional who filled out the infection control screening form, speaking with the patient's physician if necessary, reviewing laboratory data if available, and/or actually visiting the patient to assess for infection. Once the ICP has determined that the patient meets the definition of infection, he or she records information about the patient, the infection, and risk factors for aggregation and further analysis. The infection reporting form (Exhibit 11-4) and the sample screening form (Exhibit 11-5) can be combined into a single surveillance form if preferred, but the two-phase approach, which improves data reliability, should be kept in mind.

The ICP should be a registered nurse who has had some training or additional education in infection control, including surveillance methods. In this role, the nurse is not only responsible for surveillance but also may be responsible for developing and maintaining current infection control policies and procedures, providing staff education related to infection control, and serving as the primary resource for infection control questions (see Chapter 13).

AGGREGATION AND ANALYSIS OF INFECTION DATA

At the end of the surveillance period, all the numerator and denominator data should be aggregated. Analysis can then be performed. If surveillance data are aggregated and reported quarterly, the ICP should review them at the end of each month to ensure the completeness and accuracy of the infection reports. Denominator data should also be obtained monthly or at the end of the quarter if they have not already been collected. Data collection for a particular surveillance period usually cannot be completed until 7 to 10 days after the end of the period. This delay allows for recognition and reporting of all infections evidenced within the time period and for other systems to complete the tally of denominator data. Once a complete set of numerator data

Exhibit 11-5 Confirmed Home Care-Acquired Infection Report

Patient Name: _____   Identification Number: _____

Age: _____ Gender: M F Primary Diagnosis: _____

Lives alone ☐   Lives with spouse or family ☐

Primary language spoken: ☐ English ☐ Other: _____

Confirmed Site of Infection:	***Culture Results (if available):***

☐ Cathether-associated UTI
☐ Bloodstream infection:
  ☐ IV catheter-related bloodstream infection
  ☐ IV infusate-related bloodstream infection
  ☐ Secondary to other infection
☐ Central-line associated bloodstream infection
  ☐ Exit site infection
  ☐ IV tunnel infection
  ☐ IV pocket infection
☐ Skin or soft tissue infection
  ☐ Pressure ulcer
  ☐ Other
☐ Surgical site infection
☐ Wound drain or G-tube site infection
  ☐ Pneumonia
  ☐ Postpartum endometritis
  ☐ Peritonitis
☐ Gastrointestinal infection
	☐ Attach a copy of culture results
	   OR complete as follows:
	Date obtained: _____
	Site of culture:
	☐ Urine
	☐ Blood
	☐ Wound drainage of lochia
	☐ Sputum
	☐ Other
	Organism(s) isolated:_____
	_____
	Multidrug-resistant ☐ Yes ☐ No
	If yes, describe: _____

UTI

Indwelling foley   Date of original insertion: _____   Date of last insertion: _____

Indwelling suprapubic catheter   Date of original insertion: _____   Date of last insertion: _____

IV-Related infection

☐ Central Venous Access Device   Date of insertion: _____
  ☐ Nontunneled CVC—Number of lumens: _____
  ☐ Hickman/Broviac—Number of lumens: _____
  ☐ Implanted port—Number of lumens: _____
    ☐ Single lumen
    ☐ Double lumen
    ☐ Triple lumen
  ☐ PICC—Number of lumens: _____
  ☐ Other _____
☐ Peripheral Venous Access Device
  Type: _____ Date of insertion: _____
  ☐ Short line
  ☐ Midline

Pneumonia

☐ Post-operative
☐ Immobility (non-stop-op) including stroke. Cause of immobility: _____
☐ Ventilator dependent
☐ Tracheostomy tube
☐ Enteral feeding
☐ Respiratory therapy (e.g., oxygen, nebulizer)
  Type: _____

Exhibit 11-5 continued

Surgical site infection
G-tube site infection
Type and date of surgical procedure or G-tube insertion: _____

Gastrointestinal infection
☐ Enteral feeding
   Feedings prepared by: _____
   Feedings provided by: _____

Peritonitis
☐ CAPD
☐ Other _____

Previous hospital or long-term care admission (date of discharge): _____

Other risk factors:
_____
_____

To be completed by infection control practitioner
_____

Screening Results
(Check One): ☐ Home care-acquired infection ☐ Nosocomial infection ☐ Community-acquired infection

Infection reported to, as applicable:
☐ Physician (Name and date): _____
☐ Hospital/ICP facility (Name and date): _____
☐ Pharmacist (Name and date): _____
☐ Department of Health (Name and date): _____

Reviewed by: (Name and date) _____

Recorded for surveillance period of: ☐ 1st Quarter, ☐ 2nd Quarter, ☐ 3rd Quarter, ☐ 4th Quarter   Year _____
Additional Comments: _____
_____

Source: Copyright © 1999, Emily Rhinehart and Mary Friedman.

---

and denominator data is available, however, the ICP should not delay in preparing the infection report.

An additional form or tool that can be used at this time to analyze the organization's infection surveillance data is a line listing. This form contains summary information for all infections identified at a specific site. A line listing can be compiled manually or generated as part of a computerized surveillance program. A line listing frequently is helpful in that all key information about the infections can be viewed on one page, facilitating recognition of a specific risk factor or the frequency of a specific organism. A sample line listing is provided in Exhibit 11-6.

At a minimum, the individual preparing the infection report should provide a summary of the infections that have occurred, calculate rates, and provide some analysis of the current incidence of home care–acquired infection. As discussed previously, some infection rates use the number of patients at risk as the denominator, and some use days at risk (i.e., device days). These two types of rates are referred to as cumulative incidence and incidence density, respectively. The formulas for calculating each are given in Exhibit 11-7.

The individuals in the home care or hospice organization who review infection surveillance data usually prefer to have data provided in simple charts, graphs,

Exhibit 11-6 Line Listing for IV Catheter–Related Bloodstream Infections

Patient ID	Age and gender	Dx	Date of catheter insertion	Date of onset	Type of catheter	Number of lumens	Type of IV therapy	Culture results
19837204	64 yo/M	Bowel obst	12/12/97	3/19/04	Broviac	1	TPN	N/A
19827684	45 yo/F	Endocarditis	1/14/98	2/2/04	PICC	1	Atb therapy	S. epidermidis
19875385	18 mo/F	Short gut	2/3/98	3/18/04	Hickman	3	TPN, meds	E. faecalis
19885490	70 yo/M	Ca bowel	1/29/98	2/28/04	Portacath	1	Chemo and meds	S. aureus
19865075	35 yo/M	AIDS	11/23/97	1/14/04	Hickman	3	Meds and Atb	C. albicans
19860974	56 yo/F	Ca—breast	2/5/98	3/22/04	PICC	1	Chemo	N/A
19892755	22 yo/M	Osteo	3/12/98	3/29/04	Peripheral	1	Atb	N/A
19843847	3 yo/F	Leukemia	1/14/98	3/15/04	Hickman	2	Chemo, Atb	E. cloacea

Exhibit 11-7 Formulas for Calculation of Infection Rates

Cumulative incidence

$$\frac{N\ (\text{Number of infections})}{D\ (\text{Number of patients at risk})} \times 100 = \text{Rate}$$

N = Number of patients with postoperative pneumonia
D = Number of postoperative patients

$$\frac{4}{164} \times 100 = 2.4\% \text{ infection rate}$$

Incidence density

$$\frac{N\ (\text{Number of infections})}{D\ (\text{Number of days at risk})} \times 1000 = \text{Rate per 1000 days}$$

N = Number of central line-associated bloodstream infections
D = Number of IV central line-associated device days

$$\frac{4}{1820} \times 1000 = \frac{2.2 \text{ central line-associated bloodstream infections}}{\text{per 1000 catheter days}}$$

and tables rather than in lengthy written or verbal reports. These tables and graphs should be used to summarize data by site. Table 11-7 presents a summary of CAUTI data displayed by quarter for 2003 and 2004. In this home care organization, the risk reduction ef-

fort was focused on reducing the number of patients with Foley catheters to reduce the days of exposure. Table 11-7 shows that in the first two quarters of 2004 the home care organization was able to accomplish both goals. This apparently led to the reduction in the

Table 11-7 Catheter-Associated UTI Data by Quarter

Quarter	Number of patients with Foley catheters	Total catheter days*	Mean (range)†	Number of infections	Incidence density‡
1st Q 03	108	6912	64 (3–90)	26	3.76
2nd Q 03	112	8064	72 (2–90)	32	3.96
3rd Q 03	102	4896	68 (4–90)	34	6.94
4th Q 03	115	6900	78 (2–90)	28	4.05
1st Q 04	98	6468	66 (2–88)	22	3.40
2nd Q 04	88	4928	56 (2–78)	18	3.65

* Obtained by adding all the catheter days from all patients with catheters.
† Mean calculated by adding all catheter days and dividing by number of patients.
  Range is the fewest number of catheter days in one patient to the greatest number of catheter days in one patient.
‡ Number of UTIs/Total number of catheter days × 1000 = Incidence density

Table 11-8 Summary of Bloodstream Infections

Quarter	Number of patients receiving IV therapy	Number of bloodstream infections	Pediatric/ adult patients (%)	Peripheral/ central catheters (%)	Number (%) of infected patients on total parenteral nutrition	Number (%) of infected patients receiving antibiotics	Number (%) of infected patients receiving chemotherapy
1st Q 03	230	6	66/34	36/64	2 (33%)	1 (16%)	3 (50%)
2nd Q 03	184	2	72/28	22/88	0 (0%)	0 (0%)	2 (100%)
3rd Q 03	192	4	56/44	44/56	1 (25%)	0 (0%)	3 (17%)
4th Q 03	225	8	82/18	21/89	3 (38%)	1 (12%)	4 (50%)
1st Q 04	212	3	76/24	38/62	1 (33%)	0 (0%)	2 (66%)
2nd Q 04	198	1	68/32	28/82	0 (0%)	0 (0%)	1 (100%)

number of CAUTIs as well as the risk per 1000 catheter days.

Other descriptive data about patients with home care-acquired infections, including data about the frequency of infection related to specific risk factors, can be placed in a table or graph. Table 11-8 summarizes information about central line-associated bloodstream infections, including information about catheter placement (peripheral or central) and type of therapy. The frequency of home care-acquired infections caused by specific organisms can also be illustrated. Figure 11-1 is a pie chart depicting the proportion of various organisms causing IV-related bloodstream infections. The

bar graph in Figure 11-2 illustrates the proportion of home care-acquired infections by site for six consecutive quarters.

Incidence data should be tracked and trended. This requirement lends itself to the representation of data on a line or run chart. Figures 11-3 and 11-4 depict time on the horizontal axis and the rate of infection on the vertical axis. This allows for ready identification of increases and decreases in the rate of infection over time.

No single table, graph, or chart may be sufficient to allow for identification of all important variables or causes of home care-acquired infections. The ICP may want to experiment with displaying the data in various

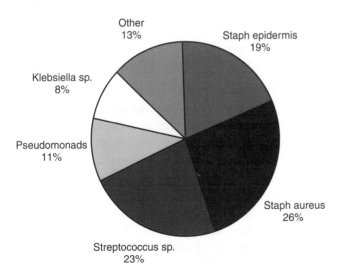

Figure 11-1 Organisms Causing Central Line-Associated Bloodstream Infections, 2004

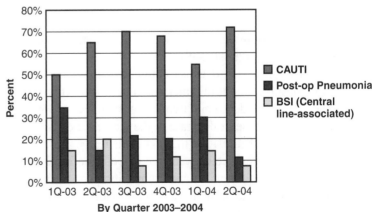

Figure 11-2 Proportions Summary of Home Care-Acquired Infection by Site, 2003–2004

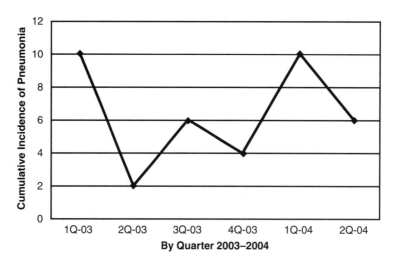

Figure 11-3 Post operative Pneumonia (Cumulative Incidence)

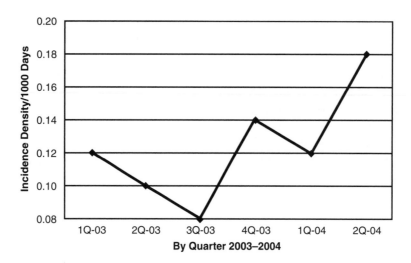

Figure 11-4 Central Line-Associated Bloodstream Infection (Incidence Density)

ways, and the individuals who examine the data can determine which is most useful.

Once a full year of data is accumulated, there may be more questions about the interpretation of the data beyond simple incidence and trends over time. For example, is the increase or decrease in the incidence density of CAUTIs in Table 11-7 in 2004 statistically significant? Is the difference between the risk of bloodstream infection related to total parenteral nutrition versus that related to chemotherapy in Table 11-8 statistically significant? Although these questions are important, it is more important to look for trends than for statistical significance. In the CAUTI example (Table 11-7), the or-

ganization has demonstrated a decrease in the risk associated with the use of Foley catheters, the length of time they are in place, and the number of infections. This demonstrates significant quality improvement and risk reduction regardless of whether it meets statistical significance. The proportion of central line-associated bloodstream infections in patients receiving chemotherapy appears to be at least two times greater than in those receiving total parenteral nutrition. This may be related more to the diagnoses among the patients and their intrinsic risk than to the infusion therapy.

Once the ICP and the organization become competent in surveillance skills, further application of biostatistical methods may be sought (Lee & Baker-Montgomery, 2000). Initially, however, the ICP and the organization should stick to the basics.

USE OF DATA FOR IMPROVEMENT OF PATIENT CARE

As discussed throughout this chapter, the purpose of infection surveillance is to reduce risk. Once confidence in the data is established and there is at least 1 year of data, the home care or hospice organization should select a specific area for risk reduction. Notes and minutes from surveillance planning meetings may be useful, especially with reference to criteria for selection of the outcome of interest. The selection can be made in collaboration with the quality improvement activities of the organization. Although the ICP can participate in the risk reduction project, other knowledgeable clinical staff members should lead and participate as well. The ICP can provide continued support through data collection and analysis.

Risk-reduction projects should use surveillance data to identify some risk factors and provide baseline measurement. In addition, resources from the literature will be necessary to fully explore identified risks and their potential reduction. Most projects focus on clinical policies and procedures that can be changed and improved to reduce risk. For example, the procedure for CVC dressing changes might be revised to specify the use of a different skin antiseptic (e.g., chlorhexidine). Various strategies for improving urinary continence might be implemented to reduce urinary catheter days and CAUTIs. Whatever the project, the plans should be well researched and then implemented. Remeasurement and comparison should not begin until the new protocol is fully in place.

Ongoing Measurement

To determine whether the revised or redesigned approach to care has resulted in a reduction in risk and infection, the rate of infection should be remeasured on an ongoing basis. It is essential that the same definitions and surveillance methods be used in the postintervention period as were used previous to it. Any change can affect the data, leading to potentially inaccurate measurement of improvement (or lack of improvement). Focusing a revised procedure on a particular infection site may actually result in an increase in the number of infections identified. This may be due to increased interest and sensitivity in detecting the infection. It also may occur that there is an actual decrease in infection during the initial months in which the new procedure is in place and a subsequent gradual increase over time. Surveillance for a targeted infection should continue long enough to ensure that the organization is able to "maintain the gain," i.e., to sustain a reduction in the infection rate over time.

VALIDATING SURVEILLANCE DATA

Accuracy of surveillance data has been a concern in nosocomial infection surveillance, and it is a concern in home care and hospice as well. Ideally, infection rates should be as close to the actual occurrence as possible. Efforts to improve accuracy may increase the cost of surveillance, however. Because home care and hospice resources are so precious, the home care or hospice organization must determine how much can be invested in surveillance to get acceptably accurate data, knowing that most systems are not 100 percent accurate. The two main factors that influence the accuracy of infection rates are the case finding methods and the definitions of infection. The methods used to screen patients for home care–acquired infection should be sensitive, acknowledging that once the definition is applied it will be determined that some of the patients identified do not have a home care–acquired infection. Infection rates are more likely to be underestimated if the identification and screening methods are insufficient. They may be overestimated if the definition is too broad.

To perform some quality control and validation of infection data, the ICP may employ several strategies, depending on how much time is allotted for surveillance and how much electronic data is available. For example, to determine whether all patients with symptoms of a CAUTI are being reported on screening reports, the ICP may obtain a list of all patients with indwelling Foley catheters during a specific time period (e.g., 1 month) in the past. Through clinical record review, the ICP can determine whether there were additional patients with signs and symptoms of a CAUTI who were not identified or reported. A broader review to identify patients who should be reported via screening would involve obtaining a list of all patients with new antibiotic orders within a selected month and comparing that list with the screening forms submitted for the same time period. Alternatively, the clinical records from 1 month of all patients with CVCs can be reviewed. Patients with evidence of bloodstream infection can be compared with those patients who are included on the line listing for that month. There might also be some coded information within an electronic clinical record system that could be used to validate surveillance data.

To validate the application of the definitions of home care–acquired infection, the ICP may ask a colleague to review the records of patients whom he or she has determined meet the definition and see whether there is agreement. This colleague may be the ICP from another location in a multisite organization or the ICP from the corporate office in a national organization. In a hospital-based home care organization, the hospital ICP may perform the record review.

USE OF SOFTWARE FOR SURVEILLANCE

There are many software programs available specifically for the management and analysis of nosocomial infection data. Currently, there are no software programs for home care surveillance. If a home care or hospice organization is large and sees many thousands of patients each year, computerization of surveillance data may be beneficial and necessary. Initially, however, the ICP who is developing skills in home care surveillance should rely on a sharp pencil, paper, and a hand-held calculator. Common computer applications, such as Microsoft Office (which includes Access and Excel), can be used to produce graphs, charts, and tables. Once the basics of surveillance are mastered, the ICP may wish to enter the surveillance data routinely into a database for analysis. Many database programs, including Access, are suitable for this task.

GETTING STARTED

Surveillance of any type requires the development of definitions and methods. Skills in applying those definitions and methods must also be developed. Skills development requires some education and training followed by practice. A home care or hospice organization initiating a serious surveillance program should anticipate a reasonable time period for developing definitions and methods. This can be 3 to 6 months, depending on the degree of reliance on outside sources, such as APIC and the MAHC, compared with development of internal definitions. Data collection methods require development time as well. The ICP and others participating in surveillance projects need time and resources. Once the surveillance begins, a pilot period of 1 to 3 months should be planned for training of staff and skill development. The data from the pilot period should not be used in reporting because they will probably not be reliable initially. The reliability of data will improve as the ICP skills improve. Development of knowledge and skills related to infection surveillance often benefits other quality measurement and improvement projects. All the activities involved in infection surveillance should be performed in the context of the overall quality improvement program.

REFERENCES

Bryant, J. (1997). Organized systems of care. *American Journal of Infection Control, 25,* 363–364.

Centers for Disease Control and Prevention. (2003a). Outbreak of Severe Acute Respiratory Syndrome—worldwide, 2003. *Morbidity and Mortality Weekly Report, 52*(11), 226–228.

Centers for Disease Control and Prevention. (2003b). National nosocomial infections surveillance system report; data summary from January 1992 to June 1993. *American Journal of Infection Control, 31*(8), 481–498.

Centers for Disease Control and Prevention. (2004). National Nosocomial Infection Surveillance (NNIS) System Report, data summary from January 1992 through June 2004, issued October 2004, *American Journal of Infection Control, 32,* 470–485.

Centers for Disease Control and Prevention. (2002b). Guidelines for the prevention of intravascular catheter–related infections. *Morbidity and Mortality Weekly Report, 52*(RR10), 1–29.

Centers for Disease Control and Prevention. (2000). Guidelines for surveillance, prevention and control of West Nile Virus infection—United States. *Morbidity and Mortality Weekly Report, 49*(02), 25–28.

Centers for Disease Control and Prevention. (1991). National nosocomial infections surveillance system. Nosocomial infection rates for interhospital comparison: Limitations and possible solutions. *Infection Control and Hospital Epidemiology, 12*(10), 609–621.

Centers for Disease Control and Prevention. (1988). Guidelines for evaluating surveillance systems. *Morbidity and Mortality Weekly Report, 37*(S5), 1–18.

Danzig, L., Short, L., Collins, K., Mahoney, M., Sepe, S., Bland, L., & Jarvis, W. (1995). Bloodstream infections associated with a needleless intravenous infusion system in patients receiving home infusion therapy. *Journal of the American Medical Association, 23,* 1862–1864.

Do, A. N., Banerjee, R., Barnett, B., & Jarvis, W. (1999). Bloodstream infection associated with needleless device use and the importance of infection control practices in the home health care setting. *Journal of Infectious Diseases, 179,* 442–448.

Embry, F., & Chinnes, L. (2000). Draft definitions for surveillance of infections in home health care. *American Journal of Infection Control, 28,* 449–453.

Emori, I., Culver, D., & Horan, T. (1991). National Nosocomial Infections Surveillance System (NNIS): Description of surveillance methods. *American Journal of Infection Control, 19,* 259–267.

Friedman, M. (1996). Designing an infection control program to meet JCAHO standards. *Caring, 15,* 18–25.

Garner, J., Jarvis, W., Emori, T., Horan, T., & Hughes, J. (1988). CDC definitions for nosocomial infection. *American Journal of Infection Control, 16,* 28–40.

Gaynes, R., Edwards, J., Jarvis, W., Culver, D., Tolson, J., & Martone, W. (1996). Nosocomial infections among neonates in high-risk nurseries in the United States. National Nosocomial Surveillance System. *Pediatrics, 98,* 357–361.

Goldmann, D., & Pier, J. (1993). Pathogenesis of infections related to intravascular catheterization. *Clinical Microbiology Review, 6,* 176–192.

Gorski, L. (2004) Central venous access device outcomes in a homecare agency: A 7-year study. *Journal of Infusion Nursing, 27*(2), 104–111.

Joint Commission on Accreditation of Healthcare Organizations. (2004). *CAMHC Update,* September 2004. (IC-7). Oakbrook Terrace, IL.

Kellerman, S., Shay, D., Howard, J., Goes, C., Feusner, J., Rosenberg, J., Vugia, D., & Jarvis, W. (1996). Bloodstream infections in home infusion patients: The influence of race and needleless intravascular access devices. *Journal of Pediatrics, 129,* 711–717.

Kunin, C., & McCormack, R. (1966). Prevention of catheter-induced urinary tract infections by sterile closed drainage. *New England Journal of Medicine, 274,* 1155–1162.

Lee, T., & Baker-Montgomery, O. (2000). Surveillance. In J. Pfeiffer (Ed.), APIC text of infection control and epidemiology (pp. 13-1 to 13-15). Washington, DC: APIC.

Lee, T., Baker, O., Lee, J., Scheckler, W., Steele, L., & Laxton, C. (1998). Recommended practices for surveillance. *American Journal of Infection Control, 26,* 277–288.

Leuhm, D., & Fauerbach, L. (1999). Task force studies infection rates, surgical management, and Foley catheter infections. *Caring, 18*(11), 30–34.

Long, C., Anderson, C., Greenberg, E., & Woomer, N. (2002). Defining and monitoring indwelling catheter–related urinary tract infections. *Home Healthcare Nurse, 20*(4), 255–262.

Lorenzen, A., & Itkin, D. (1992). Surveillance of infection in home care. *American Journal of Infection Control, 20,* 326–329.

Martone, W., Gaynes, R., Horan, T., Danzig, L., Emori, T., Monnet, D., Stroud, L., Wright, G., Culver, D., & Banerjee, S. (1995). National Nosocomial Infections Surveillance (NNIS) semiannual report, May 1995. *American Journal of Infection Control, 23,* 377–385.

McGeer, A., Campbell, B., Emori, T., Hierholzer, W., Jackson, M., Nicolle, L., Peppler, C., Rivera, A., Schollenberger, D., & Simor, A. (1991). Definitions of infection for surveillance in long-term care facilities. *American Journal of Infection Control, 19,* 1–7.

Missouri Home Care Alliance, Infection Surveillance Project. (2004). *www.infectioncontrolathome.org/bc_group_rate.htm.*

Moureau, N., Poole, S., Murdock, M., Gray, S., & Semba, C. (2002). Central venous catheters in home infusion care: Outcomes analysis in 50,470 patients. *Journal of Vascular and Interventional Radiology, 13*(10), 1009–1016.

Pereira, J., Watanabe, S., & Wolch, G. (1998). A retrospective review of the frequency of infections and patterns of antibiotic utilization on a palliative care unit. *Journal of Pain and Symptom Management, 16*(6), 374–381.

Rosenheimer, L., Embry, F., Sanford, J., & Silver, S. (1998). Infection surveillance in home care: Device-related incidence rates. *American Journal of Infection Control, 26*(3), 359–363.

Schantz, M. (2001). Infection control comes home. *Home Health Care Management and Practice, 13*(2), 126–133.

Skiest, D., Grant, P., & Keiser, P. (1998). Nontunneled central venous catheters in patients with AIDS are associated with lower infection rate. *Journal of Acquired Immune Deficiency Syndrome, 17*(3), 220–226.

Snow, J. (1965). *Snow on cholera.* Cambridge: Harvard University Press.

Tokars, J., Cookson, S., McArthur, M., Boyer, C., McGeer, A., & Jarvis, W. (1999). Prospective evaluation of risk factors for bloodstram infection in patients receiving home infusion therapy. *Annals of Internal Medicine, 131*(5), 340–351.

Vitetta, L., Kenner, D., & Sali, A. (2000). Bacterial infections in terminally ill hospice patients. *Journal of Pain Symptom Management, 20*(5), 326–334.

White, M., & Ragland, K. (1993). Surveillance of intravenous catheter–related infections among home care clients. *American Journal of Infection Control, 21,* 231–235.

White, M. (1992). Infection and infection risks in home care. *Infection Control and Hospital Epidemiology, 13,* 535–539.

Woomer, N., Long, C., Anderson, C., & Greenberg, E. (1999). Benchmarking in home health care: A collaborative approach. *Caring, 18*(11), 22–28.

CHAPTER 12

Outbreak Investigations

WHAT IS AN OUTBREAK?

The term *outbreak* is commonly used when the expected frequency of infection (endemic rate) is greatly exceeded. Public health professionals use the term *epidemic*. For the purposes of home and hospice care infection control, however, the term *outbreak* refers to an incidence of home care–acquired infection that is greater than expected or the occurrence of an unusual infection, even if it is only a few cases. The term is used to alert the home or hospice care organization's leaders that something out of the ordinary may be occurring and should be investigated. There is no specific arbitrary or statistical threshold that signals the occurrence of infectious disease, nosocomial infection, or home care–acquired infection in "epidemic proportions." Detection is more a matter of judgment based on experience and, if available, data. When Severe Acute Respiratory Syndrome (SARS) first appeared in Asia, it could have been assumed to be influenza. However, public health officials recognized that the pneumonia and the clinical course appeared to be different than that of influenza and that there was higher mortality among all age groups (CDC, 2003a). The cause of the pneumonia was eventually determined to be a new coronavirus (SARS-CoV). Eventually, many cases were seen in Toronto, including occupationally-acquired illness in health care workers (CDC, 2003b). This broadspread epidemic involved a new virus with a different epidemiology than has been seen with other respiratory viruses, had a significant mortality rate, and eventually involved a number of health care providers who were observing normal infection control procedures.

WHY OUTBREAKS SHOULD BE INVESTIGATED AND REPORTED

The SARS epidemic began as a community-based outbreak, and then hospital-based transmission became evident. In home care organizations, outbreaks occur as well. Not all outbreaks are recognized or reported, but several have been reported in the infection control and medical literature. Outbreak investigation and reporting are important for several reasons. The occurrence should be investigated so that a source can be identified and eliminated and so that other patients can avoid infection. The results of the outbreak investigation and the control measures implemented should be reported to the organization's leadership. Beyond the specific organization and its patients, it is important that outbreak investigations and findings be reported in the literature as a reference for other health care providers in case they recognize a similar occurrence in their practice setting.

IDENTIFYING THE CAUSE OF AN OUTBREAK

New sources, organisms, and causes of outbreaks are reported every year, but these are usually hospital-based occurrences. At the time of this writing, only three home care–based outbreaks have been reported in the infection control literature (Danzig et al., 1995; Kellerman et al., 1996; Do, 1999). These reports describe the investigation of an outbreak that was recognized by home care staff when the occurrence of bloodstream infections was much greater than expected. The outbreak investigations that were performed applied epidemiological methods to collect variables about the patients involved and to determine the probable cause(s) of the outbreak. In these outbreaks, the investigations revealed that the increase in bloodstream infections was associated with the use of needleless intravenous (IV) delivery systems.

Outbreaks may be associated with a single organism, a single source, or a single cause of infection. A single organism may be a multidrug-resistant microorganism, such as methicillin-resistant *Staphylococcus aureus* (MRSA) or a vancomycin-resistant enterococcus that is recognized to colonize or infect a number of patients (Rhinehart *et al.*, 1987; Rhinehart *et al.*, 1990). A single environmental source, such as a contaminated sink in an intensive care unit (Dandalides, Rutala, & Sarubbi, 1984) or a contaminated antiseptic solution (Sobel *et al.*, 1982), may be identified as the reservoir of infection. A single source may also arise from an inanimate object used from one patient to another, such as an electronic thermometer (Livornese, Dias, & Samel, 1992). A person may also be a single source of infection if he or she is colonized or infected with an organism such as *S. aureus*. In the home care–based outbreaks mentioned above, the bloodstream infections were not caused by a single or unusual organism but rather were related to the improper use and management of needleless IV administration sets. These outbreaks had a common cause rather than a single source or common reservoir.

In home and hospice care, when an increase in respiratory infections is recognized, the increase may be associated with an outbreak in the community rather than directly related to home or hospice care services. This is the case most common in the winter months, when influenza and other respiratory illnesses occur at increased rates. These outbreaks should not be considered home care–acquired infections. Home and hospice care staff, however, should educate patients and families about the risk of community-acquired infections and recommend strategies to reduce the risk. In most cases, these would involve staying out of crowded public areas, such as malls and sites of public events, and minimizing the number of visitors in the home. If there is an outbreak of community-acquired infection, the family should request that visitors not come into the home if they are symptomatic. Any family or household member that cannot be excluded from the home should practice cough etiquette, as prescribed by the CDC (CDC, 2004).

STEPS IN AN OUTBREAK INVESTIGATION

It is sometimes difficult to determine when an outbreak investigation should be undertaken. As mentioned earlier, there is no particular threshold or trigger to be used. In general, if a home care or hospice organization suspects or has the impression that something is out of the ordinary—either more infections than normally seen or one or two cases of an unusual infection—an investigation should be initiated. It is better to be prudent and gather the facts in an organized fashion and determine that there is no problem than to wait and determine later that there is a significant problem that involves many more patients than had been initially recognized.

Many infections in patients who are already ill, such as pneumonia in hospice patients, may not be preventable. By definition, infections related to an outbreak are preventable because they arise from a single source or cause. An outbreak investigation is undertaken to identify the source of the outbreak and to eliminate it. That is why it is so important to conduct an outbreak investigation using the specific steps described below. If information is not gathered in an organized fashion and carefully examined, erroneous assumptions about the cause of the outbreak may be made, and the steps taken to end the outbreak will not be effective. This may lead to much wasted time and further incidence of infection. It is preferable to approach the investigation in a planned, scientific manner rather than to guess at the cause.

There are specific steps that have been prescribed for carrying out an outbreak investigation (Table 12-1; Checko, 2000). On the first suspicion that an outbreak is occurring, the infection control practitioner (ICP) must verify the diagnosis or identify the organism involved. For example, a home care staff member may observe that several patients receiving home infusion therapy have purulent exit-site infections. Although the staff member has seen exit-site infections before, he or she suspects that there have been more infections in the past 2 weeks than usual. When this is reported to the ICP, he or she must verify the diagnosis. The ICP would want to interview the staff member reporting the infections to determine their specific nature and the time frame in which they have occurred. If any cultures were performed, the results should be obtained immediately. If some patients had cultures and others did not, a physician's order for cultures should be obtained for those who did not.

Table 12-1 Outbreak Investigation

Steps to take	What to do
1. Verify the diagnosis and identify the organism.	When the potential or suspicion is reported, obtain objective, scientific data (cultures, blood tests, physician's diagnosis) to substantiate that all the potential cases have a common diagnosis, organism, or source.
2. Confirm that an outbreak exists.	Review the known cases and compare their occurrence with the expected occurrence, or determine whether a single case or small cluster of cases is so unusual that an outbreak investigation is warranted.
3. Formulate a case definition and search for additional cases.	Formulate a case definition based on the diagnosis or organism, and look for additional cases among the patient population.
4. Characterize cases for common elements or exposures such as time, place, or person.	Review all the cases to look for a temporal relationship and a common exposure or risk.
5. Formulate a hypothesis.	Based on information gained in step 4, formulate a possible cause of the outbreak.
6. Test the hypothesis.	Go back to each case and analyze it based on the hypothetical cause to determine whether the theory is potentially correct in all or most cases.
7. Develop control measures and implement them.	Once the potential cause is determined, develop and implement strategies to eliminate the cause.
8. Evaluate the control measures.	Continue to watch for new cases to determine whether the control measures were effective.
9. Write a report.	Summarize the outbreak investigation findings and interventions.

It may take a few days to confirm that these exit-site infections are occurring and that the same organism is involved in all of them. The ICP may find that there are more exit-site infections than usual but that they are caused by different bacteria. To determine whether the causative organism is the same in each case, the ICP would review the culture results. The genus and species of the organisms may be the same (e.g., *Staphylococcus aureus*), or the cultures may show that some of the infections are caused by *S. aureus* and others by *S. epidermidis* or some other organism. If the same genus and species are found, further review of the culture results is necessary. Although many bacteria have a common pattern in their sensitivity and resistance to specific antibiotics that are tested in the microbiology laboratory (as discussed in chapter 8), the bacteria causing the outbreak infections may have a different pattern, which can differentiate the "outbreak strain." When a culture is performed, a sensitivity test for a specifically selected set of antibiotics is also done; this is referred to as "sensitivity testing." Gram positive organisms, such as staphylococci and enterococci, are tested against a different panel of antibiotics than Gram negative organisms, such as *Pseudomonas* and *Klebsiella* species. The results of the sensitivity testing are referred to as an "antibiogram." Organisms of the same genus and species

frequently have different antibiograms. This provides a means of differentiating one bacterial strain from another. For example, some strains of *S. aureus* are sensitive to gentamicin and others are resistant, just as some are sensitive to methicillin and MRSA is not. Although gentamicin is not used to treat staphylococcal infections, the resistance or sensitivity in the antibiogram can differentiate one staphylococcal strain from another.

The ICP in home care can review the antibiograms to see if there are differences or similarities in them. Some assistance in the review and analysis can be sought from the microbiologist at the laboratory that performed the cultures. The antibiogram can be helpful in recognizing the common pattern of sensitivity and resistance (the so-called "garden variety") and discriminating it from a pattern that may be more unusual. If the antibiogram of the bacteria from the patient is different from that usually seen but the same as the one from all or most of the outbreak cases, that evidence is helpful in confirming an outbreak and identifying its cause. If the organisms cultured from the patients are different, this does not necessarily mean that there is not an outbreak. It may mean that there is an increase of infection caused by different organisms.

The next step is to search for additional cases that were not identified in the initial report. Now the ICP can develop a case definition to identify new cases. This is sometimes difficult because at this point in the investigation not much is known. The definition may be based on a combination of factors, such as the site of infection, the organisms or other laboratory data, or other clinical factors, such as the type of care (e.g., home infusion therapy) that the patients are receiving or have undergone. The case definition may initially be broad and then changed as more information is collected (Beck-Segue, Jarvis, & Martone, 1997). The ICP must formulate a case definition, however, to continue the investigation and to focus on the patients most likely to be included as cases. As part of the investigation of an exit-site infection outbreak, the ICP might formulate the following case definition: "patients receiving central venous catheter care and maintenance who have had signs and symptoms of an exit-site infection within the past 30 days." Although this definition narrows the field to those patients receiving home infusion therapy, it is not so narrow as to focus only on a specific type of catheter, IV therapy, or organism. If the definition is too narrow at this early phase of the investigation, cases may be missed.

Once the case definition has been formulated, the ICP can identify additional cases. These patients can be identified through a record review or by interviewing staff members and asking them to recall potential cases. A review of all culture reports could also be used to identify cases. Further culturing of patients who have signs and symptoms of exit-site infections may be necessary. This can be accomplished by calling the patients' physicians, explaining that a potential outbreak is occurring, and requesting an order for a culture.

Collection of data and information about the patients who are potential cases in the outbreak should be accomplished using a data collection form specifically developed for the outbreak investigation. This will assist the ICP in ensuring that the same information is collected for each patient in an organized fashion; it should also minimize the need to go back to information sources to gather further data or ask more questions. A sample data collection tool for the investigation of an exit-site infection is provided in Exhibit 12-1.

Once the cases that meet the case definition are identified, more data on each case must be collected.

Exhibit 12-1 Data Collection Tool for Outbreak Investigation

Patient's name_____   Record # _____ Date of admission _____

Date of onset of signs and symptoms of exit-site infection _____

Type of catheter _____   Date placed _____

Setting where CVC placed _____   Physician who placed CVC _____

Type of dressing _____   Frequency of dressing change _____

Who performs dressing changes?   Home care nurse (name) _____
                                                        Family member or other? (name) _____

Have cultures been obtained?   Yes _____   No _____

Culture results:

Date of culture _____

Organism(s) cultured _____

Provide antibiogram for each organism.

The information can be put into a line listing, as described in Chapter 11 (see Exhibit 11–6). From these data the ICP looks for particular factors related to time, place, and person that the cases have in common. One would expect, for instance, that all the cases in an outbreak would occur in a narrow time frame. Six cases of *Staphylococcus aureus* exit-site infection over 2 months may not constitute an outbreak (depending on the total number of patients at risk), but six cases over 2 weeks would be more suspicious. A simple graph, referred to as an "epidemic curve," can be drawn to illustrate how many cases have occurred and their relationship in time (see Figure 12-1). In home care, the place component may be related to a referral hospital where the patients were admitted or had their central venous catheters (CVCs) placed. Place may also refer to a common pharmacy that prepared the IV fluids if there was an increased occurrence of bloodstream infection related to contaminated infusate. Person refers to a common person who may have been involved in the care of the patients. In home care, a single staff member may be involved in the care of home infusion therapy patients with exit-site infections caused by *S. aureus*.

Once there is enough information to characterize the infections and the ICP has drawn some conclusions about what the patients have in common, he or she can develop a hypothesis about the cause. The hypothesis should be tested by applying it to the cases that have been gathered, to determine whether it fits. If it does fit the majority of cases, control measures based on the assumed cause should be developed to stop the outbreak. If it does not fit the majority of cases, it may be necessary to gather further information about the cases; there

may be important data or risk factors missing. Occasionally, observation of patient care activities may provide additional information or clues as to the cause of an outbreak. For example, if CVC exit-site infections are occurring, the ICP may go on home visits and observe dressing changes and other aspects of home infusion therapy care by several home care staff members or the patient or family members. Interviews with home care staff about how they provide care or education to patients and family members about performing CVC care and maintenance may be helpful in identifying risks and potential sources of an outbreak.

Sometimes these first steps of an outbreak investigation can occur rapidly; in other cases, they may occur over a few days or even a few weeks. For example, an outbreak involving contaminated IV fluids may be recognized quickly if several patients exhibit signs and symptoms in the course of a day or two. Once the second or third case is reported, the ICP should suspect right away that an outbreak related to IV fluids is occurring. Culture results may not be available, but the fact that the fluids are from the same pharmacy would be evident, and the pharmacy would be notified immediately. The pharmacy may provide home infusion therapy services to other home care organizations and have reports of similar episodes from those organizations. In this case, the investigation would quickly focus on the pharmacy. On the other hand, it can take a few days or weeks to identify a problem with exit-site infections. Once the ICP recognized that more infections than usual are occurring, he or she would focus on this problem and initiate an investigation.

CONTROL OF AN OUTBREAK

The nature of control measures obviously depends on the assumed cause of the outbreak. If equipment is suspected, the equipment should be removed from use and inspected. Cultures of the equipment could be helpful in indentifying it as a source. In the contaminated fluid example from the previous paragraph, all IV fluid from the infected patients should be collected and returned to the pharmacy. The suspected IV fluid and tubing, as well as any other admixtures in the home, should be secured (clamped off at the distal end). The pharmacy staff should have a record of who mixed the IV fluid and the batch or lot numbers from the manufacturer of the main fluid as well as any solution in the admixture. All the suspected fluid should be sent to a microbiology

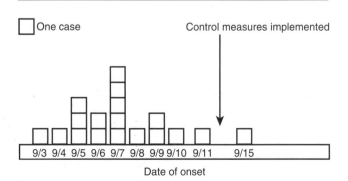

Figure 12-1 Epidemic Curve—Exit-Site Infections

laboratory, where specific techniques for culturing the fluid would be applied.

If a person is suspected as the potential cause or source of an outbreak, the individual should be interviewed and possibly should undergo a physical examination to obtain specimens for culture. This would occur most often in an outbreak of *Staphylococcus aureus* or other organisms that can be transmitted by a human carrier. A *carrier* is an individual who is colonized by an organism but may not have signs or symptoms of active infection; the carrier state is therefore unrecognized until the organism causes infection in someone else. An individual who is an index case (i.e., source of the infectious agents) may have signs and symptoms of infection, such as a draining wound or pustule.

Once control measures are in place, the home care organization and the ICP must evaluate their effectiveness by continuing surveillance and staying alert for new cases. If new cases occur, it must be determined whether they are the result of the already-identified source and whether the exposure occurred before or after the control measures were put in place. If it was before, the new cases are added to the data. If it was after or if they are not related to the identified source, some factor may have been overlooked and all the cases, along with the new cases, must be reexamined and new or additional control measures must be developed and implemented. Eventually, the control measures will be effective, the outbreak will cease, and new cases will no longer occur.

Although a formal investigation is performed in many hospital outbreaks, frequently the specific cause of the outbreak is not identified or proven, but the outbreak terminates nevertheless. It may remain unknown whether the termination is due to the specific control measures that were implemented. There are several possible reasons for this common scenario. First, many experts believe that if the cause of the outbreak was not a single source but rather a combination of factors that increased the risk of transmission, even though a specific cause is not identified, the outbreak ends as a result of the Hawthorne effect. The *Hawthorne effect* refers to the phenomenon in which people who know that they are being observed in a critical manner tend to perform more carefully. Home care staff members may wash their hands more frequently when their supervisor or a Joint Commission on Accreditation of Healthcare Organizations surveyor is with them in the home,

for instance. During an outbreak, health care professionals become aware of the outbreak and consciously and unconsciously improve their infection control efforts (e.g., hand hygiene and compliance with Standard Precautions). Thereby the chain of transmission is broken and the outbreak stops, but no specific source or cause is ever identified.

DOCUMENTATION OF AN OUTBREAK INVESTIGATION

A record of the steps taken in the outbreak investigation should be maintained. Some documentation may occur in internal reports or memos. Most of the documentation will be recorded by the infection control practitioner as the investigation unfolds. All handwritten notes or messages should be retained for future reference. The ICP will have ongoing verbal communication about the outbreak with the home or hospice care organization's leaders. When decisions are made, more information is obtained, and specific steps are taken, some type of interim documentation (notes, memos, or brief interim reports) should be created to ensure accuracy if recall is needed. Eventually, a full report of the outbreak investigation should be written. This report will be used to communicate specifics of the event with the group or committee in the home care organization that oversees infection control. It will also serve as a reference document if questions arise in the future. Although the document ideally should be protected from discovery if a lawsuit or claim is brought by a patient, it can also serve to demonstrate that a prudent and organized effort was undertaken to investigate the outbreak and to control it.

EXTERNAL ASSISTANCE

If a serious outbreak occurs—that is, an outbreak involving either an unusual infectious disease or organism or a large number of patients—the home care or hospice organization should consider obtaining assistance from outside experts. In most states, the state health department can provide epidemiologists to assist in the investigation. The CDC has a specific division, the Epidemiologic Intelligence Service (EIS), that also can be called upon. Although some EIS officers are based in Atlanta, others are based within state health departments to assist in investigations. Neither the state health department nor the CDC's/EIS's charges for its services. In many cases, telephone consultation is of sufficient assistance to the home care ICP and leaders in the investigation and analysis. In other cases, the public health consultants must come on site to review clinical records and other information. Home and hospice care organizations must also be aware of any state requirements about reporting an outbreak of home care–acquired infections, even if the organization does not need assistance from the state.

In a hospital-based home care organization, the hospital ICP and epidemiologist should be called upon to help determine whether an outbreak is occurring and to consult on and guide the investigation. Use of hospital-based ICPs and epidemiologists by freestanding home care organizations may depend on the relationship with a specific hospital and other resources that are available.

COMMUNICATION TO STAFF AND PATIENTS

Communication during an outbreak investigation can be tricky. On the one hand, a home care or hospice organization does not want to announce that there is a potential problem and cause undue concern among patients and families or draw the attention of the media. On the other hand, if there are rumors in the community that need to be corrected, some type of communication to staff members as well as to patients and families may be necessary and prudent. Home care or hospice staff should be reminded of the constant obligation to maintain confidentiality of all patient care information. They also should be reminded that discussion of any potential outbreak situation outside specified parameters must be avoided. They should not discuss the situation in general or ever discuss specific patients with other patients and families. They should not discuss the situation in public places. Any discussion should be conducted within the offices of the home care or hospice organization. If telephone discussions are necessary, they should be conducted in a manner that ensures the privacy of all parties. Any information or facts that are shared outside the organization must come only from the organization's leadership. If a staff member is questioned by a patient or family member, he or she should direct the questions and concerns to a specifically designated person within the organization, such as the ICP or a member of senior management. These individuals should provide information as necessary and agreed upon by the organization's leaders.

As home care and hospice expands its services to more acutely ill patients and provides more skilled, high-technology services, it can be expected that more outbreaks will occur. Although there are currently only three outbreak reports of home care-acquired infection in the literature, it is probably safe to assume that others have occurred and were either unrecognized or unreported. It is imperative that more home and hospice care organizations take the time to investigate outbreaks and report their findings and experiences at professional meetings and in the literature. This will benefit all providers and their patients.

REFERENCES

Beck-Segue, C., Jarvis, W., & Martone, W. (1997). Outbreak investigations. *Infection Control and Hospital Epidemiology, 18,* 138–145.

Centers for Disease Control and Prevention. (2004). Draft guideline for isolation: Preventing transmission of infectious agents in healthcare settings. Retrieved 6/15/04 from *http://www.cdc.gov/ncidod/hip/isoguide.htm.*

Centers for Disease Control and Prevention. (2003a). Outbreak of Severe Acute Respiratory Syndrome—Worldwide. *Morbidity and Mortality Weekly Report, 52*(11); 226–228.

Centers for Disease Control and Prevention. (2003b). Cluster of Severe Acute Respiratory Syndrome cases among protected health-care workers—Toronto, Canada. *Morbidity and Mortality Weekly Report, 52*(19); 433–436.

Checko, P. (2000). Outbreak investigation. In J. Pfeiffer (Ed.), APIC text of infection control and epidemiology (pp. 15-1–15-9) Washington, DC: APIC.

Dandalides, P., Rutala, W., & Sarubbi, F. (1984). Postoperative infections following cardiac surgery: Association with an environmental reservoir in a cardiothoracic intensive care unit. *Infection Control, 5,* 378–384.

Danzig, L., Short, L., Collins, K., Mahoney, M., Sepe, S., Bland, L., & Jarvis, W. (1995). Bloodstream infections associated with a needleless intravenous infusion system in patients receiving home infusion therapy. *Journal of the American Medical Association, 273,* 1862–1864.

Do, A. N., Banerjee, R., Barnett B., & Jarvis W. (1999). Bloodstream infection associated with needleless device use and the importance of infection control practices in home health care setting. *Journal of Infectious Diseases, 179,* 442–448.

Kellerman, S., Shay. D., Howard, J., Goes, C., Feusner, J., Rosenberg, J., Vugia, D., & Jarvis, W. (1996). Bloodstream infections in home infusion patients: The influence of race and needleless intravascular access devices. *Journal of Pediatrics, 129,* 711–717.

Livornese, L., Dias, S., & Samel, C. (1992). Hospital-acquired infection with vancomycin-resistant *Enterococcus faecium* transmitted by electronic thermometers. *Annals of Internal Medicine, 117,* 112–116.

Rhinehart, E., Shlaes, D., Serkey, J., & Keys, T. (1987). Nosocomial clonal dissemination of methicillin-resistant *Staphylococcus aureus:* Elucidiation by plasmid analysis. *Archives of Internal Medicine, 147,* 521–524.

Rhinehart, E., Smith, N., Wennersten, C., Gorss, E., Freeman, J., Eliopoulos, G., Moellering, R., & Goldmann, D. (1990). Rapid dissemination of beta-lactamase–producing, aminoglycoside-resistant *Enterococcus faecalis* among patients and staff on an infant–toddler surgical ward. *New England Journal of Medicine, 323,* 1814–1818.

Sobel, J., Hashman, N., Reinherz, G., & Merzbach, D. (1982). Nosocomial *Pseudomonas cepacia* infection associated with chlorhexidine contamination. *American Journal of Medicine, 73,* 183–186.

CHAPTER **13**

Planning for Occupational Health

The health and well-being of the employees in a home care or hospice organization represent an important priority. Although little is known about the actual risk and incidence of occupationally acquired infectious diseases among home care and hospice staff members, there are many reports of the occurrence of these illnesses in health care providers in other settings, especially in acute care. With care continuing to shift from the hospital to home, long-term, and subacute care, and various ambulatory settings, health care staff members outside acute care may be at increased risk for occupational exposure to and illness from infectious diseases. Surveillance data for human immunodeficiency virus (HIV) and hepatitis B virus (HBV) have been maintained for many years. Although there are no reports of occupational HIV infection in home care or hospice providers to date, data reprinted in early 2003 indicate that 57 health care workers have acquired HIV through occupational exposures such as needlesticks (Do, 2002a). Immunization with HBV vaccine has significantly reduced the risk for contracting HBV since its introduction in 1982. Health care staff in all settings (Panlilio, 2004), however, continue to experience needlestick injuries and other exposures to bloodborne pathogens, even though the Occupational Safety and Health Agency (OSHA) implemented a rule requiring the use of safe needle devices (OSHA, 2001).

From a practical standpoint, employee absence due to illness or injury, whether occupational or nonoccupational, presents significant challenges to the scheduling and provision of patient care. In addition, occupationally acquired-illnesses and injuries add to workers' compensation costs. Therefore, home care and hospice

organizations must take a proactive approach to identifying occupational health needs and in planning, supporting, and managing an occupational health program.

Considering that occupational health and safety programs involve many infection control issues (e.g., immunizations, follow-up of exposures, and workers' compensation claims), many home care and hospice organizations have incorporated these programs into a single management function. The occupational health program in home care or hospice should include structural elements such as policies and procedures, responsibility and authority, and organization oversight; processes for implementation, management, day-to-day application of the policies and procedures, and oversight of outsourced services; education and training of staff at all levels; and specific methods for annual assessment of the program's effectiveness.

As with other areas in the infection control program, specific knowledge and resources are necessary for maintaining and managing an occupational health program for home care. State and federal regulations, such as those promulgated by OSHA, mandate certain program components. There are many additional policies and procedures that should also be included in a program. Specific needs and program designs will depend on the size of the organization, the scope of its services, and the types of patients it serves. For example, there may be more emphasis on exposure to childhood diseases in an organization with a pediatric population than in one whose focus is the care of older patients. In designing or reassessing an occupational health program for home care or hospice, the variables listed in Exhibit 13-1 should be considered. Once these factors

195

Exhibit 13-1 Considerations for the Design of an Occupational Health Program

Type of home care or hospice organization (hospital-based or freestanding)
Scope/type of services
Patient population
Size of organization
Number of employees
Number of locations
Specific risks among the population from which employees are drawn
Epidemiology and risk for specific infectious diseases in the geographic area (e.g., tuberculosis)

have been examined, an appropriate and comprehensive occupational health program can be developed and implemented.

Once a program is developed and implemented, its effectiveness should be continuously monitored. The appraisal can be accomplished through tabulating ongoing indicators (e.g., number of needlesticks on the sharps injury log, frequency of exposures to contagious illnesses, and days lost as a result of occupational injuries). Although these monitors should demonstrate continuous improvement through the reduction of exposures and lost days, they may also identify areas that require increased attention and enhancement. Thus the occupational health program is linked to the infection control program, patient and worker safety programs and performance improvement efforts.

The determination of who will provide occupational health services is very important. Although the designated infection control practitioner (ICP) in the home care or hospice organization can administer, maintain, and improve the program through the development and implementation of policies and procedures, this person should not routinely provide occupational health services to colleagues as a health care provider. Although he or she will be called upon to evaluate specific situations (e.g., exposures) and should be available to provide interpretation of policies and direction on procedures, he or she should not render direct care to employees. A registered nurse or infection control practitioner in the home care or hospice organization may perform pre-employment health assessments, administer purified protein derivative (PPD) skin testing and some vaccines (e.g., HBV vaccine), and screen

staff members after a potential exposure to bloodborne pathogens. The individuals involved in administrative duties such as infection control and quality management, however, may not have the skills and experience to provide a full range of occupational health care. In addition, provision of care may create a conflict of interest and lead to confidentiality issues. For example, if an employee is exposed to blood and follow-up serologic testing is performed, the results of those tests must be kept confidential. Most states have specific laws regarding results of HIV testing, as well. In fact, all information about employees and their health history and status must remain confidential.

Physicians with knowledge and experience in occupational health should be retained to provide occupational health services, such as follow-up for exposures and injuries. The initial health assessment that is performed at the time of employment should be limited and can be accomplished in the home care or hospice organization by the ICP or a designated nurse. The employee should be referred to a physician, however, if further assessment of a specific finding is warranted (e.g., a positive PPD skin test). Many of the additional occupational health needs should be outsourced not only because they may be beyond the competencies of the individuals in the organization but also because they frequently require a physician's additional assessment and/or orders for appropriate diagnostic tests, vaccines, or treatments. A hospital-based home care organization can use the employee health services of the hospital. A small home care organization that serves a limited geographic area may arrange for these services through a local hospital or a physician with a specialty in family practice or internal medicine. Ideally, this should be a physician with training and experience in occupational health. Larger agencies with multiple locations may choose to contract for services from a network provider, such as a health plan or preferred provider network, that also provides medical management services for workers' compensation cases. The utilization of a single network may facilitate communication between the organization and the providers, thereby improving the coordination of care. In addition, the network and its providers become familiar with the home care or hospice organization's specific policies and procedures and can establish a working relationship with the infection control practitioner and others involved in workers' compensation management.

Whatever the arrangements for the provision of occupational health care, agreements and expectations should be set in writing and may include the home care or hospice organization's policies and procedures (e.g., the definition of "exposure"). The occupational health services should be evaluated on an annual basis. Evaluation should cover clinical quality (e.g., outcomes of care), the functional status of employees requiring care for injuries, days lost as a result of illness, and compliance with organization procedures and nationally recognized guidelines (e.g., postexposure evaluation and treatment). Service quality should also be considered. This includes practical issues—such as accessibility for appointments (urgent and scheduled), return of phone calls, and written communication and documentation—and the general willingness to work with the organization to coordinate care and minimize lost time.

RECORDKEEPING

Just as each home care or hospice staff member has a personnel file, each staff member also should have a personal health record. This record should be initiated at the time of employment and should include documents such as the initial health assessment, records of immunizations, declinations, annual reassessments such as the results of annual tuberculosis (TB) skin testing, and reports of occupational exposures or injuries, including information about follow-up and results of any other testing. Individual health records must be kept in a secure manner, separate from personnel files—in a separate locked cabinet with a specific person or persons designated to have access to the files. The standards of confidentiality of patient information also apply to the personal health information of home and hospice care staff members.

In addition to individual health records, to meet the requirements of OSHA the home care or hospice organization must maintain a log of occupational illnesses and injuries. The OSHA 300 log must be maintained with records of all work-related injuries and illnesses, including exposures and infections. This may include back injuries, dog bites, and exposures to bloodborne pathogens, TB, and other infections (OSHA, 2001). However, the Needlestick Safety and Prevention Act, which was signed into law in November 2000 and became effective in April 2001, includes additional requirements for recordkeeping. In an effort to improve tracking and trending of exposures to bloodborne

pathogens, an additional sharps injury log is required. At a minimum, for each injury the log should contain the type and brand of device involved in the incident and the work area or department. It should also contain a description of how the exposure occurred. The injury must also be included in the OSHA 300 log. To maintain the privacy of the individuals involved in such exposures, the employer must insert the phrase "privacy case," rather than the employee's name, on the log to which other staff have access. This then requires that the employer maintain a separate, confidential list of employee names, with related case numbers (OSHA, 2001).

HEALTH ASSESSMENT AND IMMUNIZATIONS

The current recommendations regarding the initial health assessment of new employees suggest that this evaluation should be minimal. A full history and physical examination by a physician or physician extender has not proven to be cost effective or generally necessary (Bolyard, 1998). Instead, a general health assessment and functional status evaluation (e.g., ability to meet the physical requirements of the job) are recommended. For home care or hospice staff members who will be directly involved in patient care, the initial assessment should include an infectious disease history. This evaluation should include history of infectious diseases that can be prevented by vaccines (i.e., childhood diseases and HBV), history of any condition that may increase the employee's risk for acquiring or transmitting infection, and selected laboratory testing (where required by organizational policies and procedures or state licensure regulations). The history of infection with TB and administration of a tuberculin skin test (PPD), if appropriate, is discussed later in this chapter. Additional requirements related to state licensure should also be included. There are no recommendations that routine cultures be performed on new home care or hospice.

VACCINE-PREVENTABLE DISEASES

The U.S. Public Health Service provides recommendations regarding the use of vaccines for children and adults through its Advisory Committee on Immunization Practices (ACIP). When the Food and Drug Administration brings a new vaccine to market through its approval process, ACIP examines the data and scientific information about the specific infectious disease and the vaccine and formulates national recommendations. Subsequently, other agencies and organizations, such as the Centers for Disease Control and Prevention (CDC) and the American Academy of Pediatrics, base their recommendations for practice on those of ACIP.

Most adults born in the United States have either experienced an infection with the common childhood diseases listed in Exhibit 13-2 or received a vaccination to prevent those infections. People born outside the United States, however, may not have been immunized or may not have had a vaccine-preventable disease. In addition, OSHA requires that all health care employers provide the HBV vaccine to at-risk employees. Other vaccines, such as that for influenza, may also be offered. The initial health assessment should determine the employee's immune status for these illnesses. A sample infectious disease history form for the employee health record is provided in Exhibit 13-3.

If the employee is immune by virtue of having had the infection or the vaccine, that history should be recorded in the employee's health record. This information could be important in the event of an exposure. If the employee's history indicates a lack of immunity (i.e., no recall or record of having the infection or the vaccine), the employee should be considered susceptible until a vaccination is obtained. Home care or hospice organization policy determines whether a simple verbal history of having a disease or vaccine is adequate for confirming the employee's status. If it is not, the policy may require serologic testing or written documentation from a physician.

The determination as to whether a home care or hospice organization will provide serologic testing and vaccination is based on several considerations: the likelihood of occupational exposure to vaccine-preventable illnesses based on the patient population served; the potential outcome of those exposures and the burden for investigation and follow-up; the actual risk (proportion of employees already immune versus those who are susceptible) in the current employee population; and the cost of performing tests and providing vaccines versus the benefit to the organization, its employees, and its patients.

The question regarding who should pay for serologic testing and immunization (except for HBV) depends on the home care or hospice organization's policy. In a hospital-based home care or hospice organization, these services are frequently provided free of charge through the hospital's employee health program. This may not be reasonable in a freestanding home care or hospice organization, where occupational health services are purchased, however, because it creates an additional operating expense. A more common approach is to require that new employees obtain proof of immunity from their personal physicians. State employment laws must be considered when this policy is formulated.

Varicella

In the case of varicella, the virus that causes chickenpox and shingles, most experts agree that a verbal history of natural immunity (i.e., a report from the employee that he or she had chickenpox as a child) from an adult born in the United States is reliable (97% to 99% of American adults are seropositive for chickenpox) and no serologic testing is required to confirm immunity (Kelley et al., 1991). If an individual born and raised in the United States is not sure or does not know or recall whether he or she ever had chickenpox, additional questions (e.g., the number and ages of siblings as well as the number and ages of their own children) can help determine his or her status. For example, if the employee is a parent and reports that his or her own children had chickenpox and that he or she lived in the home and provided care for the children while they were ill, it is likely that the individual is immune. Likewise, if an individual recalls siblings living in the same home having chickenpox but cannot remember being ill himself or herself, it is likely that he or she was either immune at the time or had a mild, subclinical case that was not recognized. Data indicate that, even when an individual born in the United States cannot recall or does not believe that he or she

Exhibit 13-2 Vaccine-Preventable Childhood Diseases

- Measles
- Mumps
- Rubella
- Polio
- Tetanus
- Diphtheria
- Pertussis
- Varicella

Exhibit 13-3 Preemployment Health Survey/Immunization Status

Name _____ Work Area _____

Do you have contact with residents? ☐ Yes ☐ No   ☐ Face-to-face   ☐ Hands-on

HISTORY OF INFECTIOUS DISEASES/IMMUNIZATION (Check all boxes that apply):

Measles (Please provide physician certification of immunization or immunity.)
I was born before 1957.   ☐ Yes ☐ No
I was born in or after 1957.
  I have had measles and offer physician certification.   ☐ Yes ☐ No
  I have had immunization.   ☐ Yes ☐ No Dates _____
    (Give evidence of two live vaccinations.)   After first birthday? _____
  I have a positive antibody titre and offer written proof.   ☐ Yes ☐ No

Mumps
I was born before 1957.   ☐ Yes ☐ No
I have had mumps.   ☐ Yes ☐ No

Rubella (Please provide physician certification of immunization or immunity.)
I have received live virus immunization after 1969.   ☐ Yes ☐ No Dates _____
I have laboratory evidence of immunity.   ☐ Yes ☐ No
  After first birthday? _____

Chickenpox
I have had chickenpox.   ☐ Yes ☐ No
To my knowledge, I have not had chickenpox.   ☐ Yes ☐ No
I do not know if I have had chickenpox.   ☐ Yes ☐ No
If negative or equivocal chickenpox history:
  Did you have sibling(s) with history of chickenpox
  while you were living together?   ☐ Yes ☐ No
  Did you care for your own child with chickenpox?   ☐ Yes ☐ No
I have had laboratory testing to determine immunity status.   ☐ Yes ☐ No

Miscellaneous   Yes   No   Last Booster Date
I have had the polio vaccine series.   ☐   ☐   _____
I have had the tetanus/diphtheria vaccine series.   ☐   ☐   _____
I have had the hepatitis B vaccine series.   ☐   ☐   _____
I have had the measles-mumps-rubella (MMR) vaccine.   ☐   ☐   _____
I am immune to the hepatitis B virus (per laboratory   ☐   ☐   _____
documentation).

_____   _____
Date   Signature—Employee

Source: Reprinted with permission from Nancy L. Thayer, *Infection Control Program: Policy and Procedure Manual,* Baltimore, Maryland.

---

had chickenpox, a large proportion (71% to 93%) test positive (Bolyard et al., 1998). Finally, a new employee can call his or her parents (if possible) to ask about his or her childhood experience with chickenpox and other diseases.

An individual who was born and raised in a tropical area, such as the Caribbean, is less likely to have had chickenpox as a child. Serologic testing has demon-strated that immunity to varicella is far lower in adults raised in tropical and subtropical climates compared with adults raised in temperate climates, such as the United States and Europe, where the rate of immunity is more than 90% (Longfield et al., 1990; Nassar & Touma, 1986). Consequently, an employee who has immigrated from a tropical area is more likely to be susceptible to primary varicella infection (chickenpox).

The varicella vaccine became available in the United States in 1995 and can be used in the immunization of children and adults. ACIP has recommended the immunization of health care staff members with the varicella vaccine if they are not already immune based on their history (CDC, 1997a). Although blood tests for antibodies for varicella are available, testing of employees before administration of the vaccine is not recommended because it is probably not cost effective. If a home care or hospice organization has a large number of employees who are susceptible to varicella and/or are caring for high-risk children (e.g., pediatric patients with cancer or other immunosuppressive diseases), it may wish to consider providing the vaccine. Other risk-reduction strategies can focus on avoiding the assignment of susceptible employees to high-risk children, which reduces the risk of exposure to both.

Measles

Adults born before 1957 are likely to have natural immunity to measles because the vast majority of children caught measles and developed natural immunity to it before the introduction of the vaccine in 1963. Individuals born in or after 1957 may or may not have naturally acquired immunity. Measles vaccines used between 1957 and 1963 did not always confer immunity, which is why outbreaks of measles have occurred in persons born before 1963, the year the current vaccine was made available and appropriate methods for storage and administration were determined. If any individual (including anyone born before 1957) cannot provide written documentation from a physician of having had a positive blood test for measles or of having received one dose of vaccine after the age of 1 year, serologic testing is necessary. Many states require all health care workers to be immune to measles. Once individuals who are susceptible to measles are identified, they should be immunized. Use of the trivalent vaccine for measles, mumps, and rubella (MMR) is recommended; the MMR vaccine is generally more available than a single vaccine for measles (CDC, 1997a).

Rubella

Rubella is less contagious than measles, and there may be more individuals among home care or hospice staff members who have not had rubella and are susceptible. Most women of childbearing age have been tested for

rubella and may have received the rubella vaccine as a requirement for previous employment in health care or from a primary care or obstetric services provider to eliminate the risk of rubella during pregnancy. Even though most individuals born before 1957 are immune to rubella and many have received the vaccine, written documentation of immunity should be required. As with measles, many states require written proof of immunity to rubella for all health care staff members. Such proof can consist of an immunization record or the results of serological testing from a physician. As with measles, individuals identified as susceptible should be immunized with the MMR vaccine. Pregnancy is a contraindication to vaccination (CDC, 1997a).

Diphtheria, Pertussis, and Tetanus

The incidence of diphtheria in the United States is extremely low, so occupational or nonoccupational exposure is unlikely and health care providers are not considered at any greater risk for diphtheria than the general population. Nevertheless, ACIP recommends that adults receive a tetanus and diphtheria booster every 10 years. If a new employee has not received a booster in the past 10 years, he or she should be reminded of this recommendation. The tetanus and diphtheria vaccine is also recommended for prophylactic treatment of a traumatic wound (CDC, 1997a). The pertussis vaccine is not recommended for use in adults (CDC, 1991a). However, there is risk for exposure to pertussis among health care providers, including home care staff. The definition and treatment of exposed personnel are discussed later in this chapter.

Polio

Many adults have received polio vaccination (oral or by injection). Polio is rarely seen in the United States and is not considered a risk for home or hospice care staff. If there are circumstances that would expose home care personnel to a patient with polio (the virus is excreted through the stool), however, immunization should be provided (CDC, 1997a).

HBV TESTING AND VACCINATION

The OSHA rule on bloodborne pathogens (OSHA, 1991) requires that health care employers offer and provide HBV vaccine at no charge to all employees who are at risk for exposure. The policies and procedures related to HBV vaccination should be part of the organization's exposure control plan and incorporated into the occupational health program. In addition, the exposure control plan should outline the use of personal protective equipment, engineering controls, and policies and procedures for postexposure follow-up. Determination of current HBV status should be incorporated into the new employee health assessment (see Exhibit 13-3).

A new employee who reports that he or she has received three doses of HBV vaccine during a previous employment should obtain a record of the vaccination and the results of any antibody testing that was performed. If no antibody testing was performed, the employee can be tested if there will be continued risk of exposure. The year in which the vaccine series was completed and the antibody test results should be recorded in the employee health record, in case new recommendations for a booster dose are announced. If the employee has not had the vaccine, it must be offered within 10 days of employment, in compliance with the OSHA rule. The employee may accept the vaccine or decline it. If the vaccine is declined, a declination statement should be signed by the employee to document that the vaccine was offered and declined. A sample declination statement is provided in Exhibit 13-4. If the

Exhibit 13-4 Declination Form for Hepatitis B Vaccine

In order to comply with the Bloodborne Pathogens Rule of the Occupational Safety and Health Administration, we have offered you, an employee of _____ (name of home care organization), the hepatitis B vaccination in a series of three injections. We have provided information about the benefits of the vaccine and have offered it to you at no charge. At this time, you have chosen not to receive the vaccine. Please sign below to indicate that you have declined the vaccine at this time. In spite of the declination at this time, however, we will provide the vaccine to you at any time in the future at no charge.

I, _____, (print name) understand that I am eligible to receive the hepatitis B vaccine at no charge. I am declining receipt of the vaccine at this time.

_____ _____
Signature   Date

employee decides not to have the vaccine at this time, the home care or hospice organization's policy must allow the employee to accept the vaccine at any subsequent time during employment.

If the employee decides to accept the vaccine, it must be provided in three doses over 6 months, as prescribed. The first dose is given at a designated time. The second dose must be administered 1 month after the first dose, and the third dose must be given 6 months after the first dose (CDC, 1990). It is important that the employee complete the series of three injections to ensure immunity. Although studies have demonstrated immunity after two doses, the best results have been obtained with three doses given at the prescribed intervals. The home care organization or the occupational health provider (or both) must implement a practical procedure to ensure that the employee gets the second and third doses. For example, the second and third doses may be administered by a nurse in the home care or hospice organization's office so that the employee does not have to travel to the occupational health care provider. If the series is not completed as prescribed, it may need to be reinitiated. If the series is interrupted after the first dose, the second dose should be administered as soon as possible. If the third dose is delayed, it should be given when convenient. Administration of the second and third doses should be separated by an interval of at least 2 months (CDC, 2001).

Serologic antibody testing before initiation of the HBV vaccine series is not required. Each organization can determine whether it wants to test routinely for existing immunity before giving the vaccine or whether it wants to provide testing on an optimal basis to the employee. This decision may be based on the likelihood of identifying employees who already are immune to HBV or are chronic carriers. In most situations, testing for HBV markers before vaccine administration is not cost effective and delays the initiation of the vaccine series.

Testing for anti-HBs after the vaccine series has been completed is recommended by the CDC (CDC, 1997a) for those who will have ongoing risk for potential exposure and required by OSHA (OSHA, 2000). This testing helps assure the employee that the vaccine was effective and that he or she has successfully developed immunity. The antibody test should be performed 1 to 2 months after the administration of the third dose of vaccine, and results of serum levels of 10 mU/mL or greater are considered adequate. If the employee has not developed adequate antibody levels after completing the three-dose series at the prescribed intervals, the CDC recommends that the vaccine series be repeated and that the employee be tested again. If the employee still has not developed measurable antibodies, a test for HBsAg should be obtained to determine whether the individual had a previous HBV infection that may have gone unrecognized and led to chronic carriage of the virus (CDC, 1997b).

There is no current recommendation for a booster dose of HBV vaccine even though up to 60 percent of vaccine recipients who initially develop anti-HBs lose the detectable antibody 8 years after vaccination. A booster dose is not recommended based on the knowledge and experience that, even though the antibody is not detectable in a blood test, an individual who initially developed antibody is still protected and will not become infected if exposed to HBV (CDC, 1997b).

ASSESSMENT FOR TUBERCULOSIS

The issue of routine screening for tuberculosis (TB) in home care and hospice has changed considerably in the past two to three years, with the most significant change being OSHA's determination not to cite any home care organization for failure to conduct TB skin testing (OSHA, 2002).

In the late 1980s and early 1990s there was a significant increase in new cases of TB in the United States, including multidrug-resistant TB (MDR-TB). This increase was related to the epidemic of HIV infections. In 1994 the CDC published "Guidelines for Preventing the Transmission of *Mycobacterium tuberculosis* in Health-Care Facilities" (CDC, 1994). Most home care and hospice organizations followed these guidelines either voluntarily or in response to requirements of their state health departments or OSHA. This comprehensive guideline provides clear directions for assessing a health care organization's risk for occupational exposures to patients with TB as well as strategies and plans for preventing such exposures. Since that time, the CDC has observed and reported a significant decrease in newly active cases of TB in the United States over a ten-year period from 1991 to 2001 (CDC, 2003a). Although the overall incidence has declined 62% among U.S.-born persons, TB continues to occur in greater proportion in certain populations and geographic areas. U.S.-born non-Hispanic blacks comprise 47% of all cases, and foreign-born persons also comprise a large proportion of reported TB cases. Geographically, TB occurs more often in seven states (New York, California, Florida, Illinois, Georgia, New Jersey and Texas) than in other states. These states reported 60% of the new TB cases in 2002 (CDC, 2002b). Although the risk of occupationally acquired TB in health care has decreased, some risk remains and is greater in certain states and when caring for certain populations.

In light of the risk for occupationally-acquired TB in the 1990s, in 1997 OSHA was intending to implement a TB rule to enforce the CDC's recommendations, such as it did for bloodborne pathogens in 1991 (OSHA, 1991b). However, because the risk of TB among health care workers has declined so significantly, OSHA announced in late 2003 that it would not promulgate a TB rule, due to the declining incidence of TB and the success of the 1994 CDC guideline (OSHA, 2003). OSHA will continue support efforts to protect health care workers under the general industry respiratory protection standard. When asked specifically about TB testing in home care, OSHA responded that it would not enforce the requirement for TB skin testing in that setting because it does not fall into a high-risk category (which includes health care facilities, corrections institutions, nursing homes, homeless shelters, and drug treatment centers) (OSHA, 2002).

Although TB skin testing in home care is no longer required by OSHA, home care or hospice organizations should not abandon testing until they ascertain state or local health department requirements and formulate overall organization policies. For example, many hospital-based home care providers still perform TB skin testing in the absence of state or local health department requirements because it is required for all hospital employees. If there are no state or local requirements, organizations should still consider the risk for TB exposure and occupationally-acquired infection in their staff members and maintain TB skin testing policies appropriate to the level of risk, considering their geographic locations and patient populations. Based upon the forgoing considerations, the following content on TB is intended to provide guidance on determining an approach for TB skin testing in a home or hospice care organization.

The initial assessment of a new employee should continue to include a baseline evaluation of past skin testing to identify an infection with *Mycobacterium tuberculosis* (CDC, 1998). This may not be very burdensome since most health care organizations, including home or hospice care, continue to perform skin testing and new employees therefore will likely have been tested in the recent past. The home care or hospice organization then needs to determine its own policy regarding skin testing at the time of employment of persons with previously negative skin tests. The current recommendation for other health care settings is to repeat skin testing annually (CDC, 1994).

Mycobacterium tuberculosis can cause active TB in the lungs (i.e., pulmonary TB) or in other sites (e.g., extrapulmonary TB). Exposure to the TB organism from an actively infected individual, however, does not always cause active infection. In most cases exposure causes the exposed individual's immune system to react even though he or she does not have active disease. This is referred to as a "latent TB infection (LTBI)" and is demonstrated by a positive TB skin test (defined below). A person with a positive skin test should be evaluated for treatment of LTBI in accordance with the most recent recommendations of the American Thoracic Society and the CDC in order to prevent the infection from becoming active in the future (American Thoracic Society, 2000; CDC, 2000b). Even after treatment for LTBI is complete, however, the individual's TB skin test will remain positive. A person who has had an active TB infection will also maintain a positive skin test after treatment. That is because the skin test reflects the immune system's response: unlike a culture, it is not a direct test for infection.

The assessment for TB should be included in the pre-employment infectious disease history to document the history of PPD skin test results and/or the individual's history of an active TB infection. If an individual has had an active TB infection in the past, it can be assumed that he or she will have a positive PPD skin test. Further questions about treatment of the infection should be asked to make sure that adequate treatment was completed and that there are no current signs or symptoms of active infection. If the employee reports a history of a positive skin test but never had an active infection, the history should be recorded in the health record, and the employee should be asked about follow-up and treatment of LTBI. A TB skin test should not be administered if the employee reports a history of treatment for active infection or of a previously positive PPD. The current recommendation for health care workers is that they have a chest radiograph to determine current disease status and provide a baseline for future assessment (CDC, 1994). Annual chest x-rays are not recommended, however. PPD positive

staff should be educated and monitored for any signs and symptoms of active infection.

PPD Skin Testing

For individuals who have a history of negative PPD skin tests or who do not know their skin test status, a test should be administered using the Mantoux technique (0.1 mL PPD via intracutaneous administration on the dorsal surface of the forearm). Pregnant employees and those who have received the Callette-Guerin vaccination (BCG) in the past should not be excluded from skin testing (CDC, 1994). An organization may elect to do PPD testing in house rather than to have the occupational health care provider perform the testing. This is usually more convenient and practical, but it is necessary that the test be administered by trained personnel who have the skill to perform the intradermal injection. An incorrectly administered test can affect the accuracy of the results. There are a number of sources, including instructional videos from the CDC and state health departments, that provide information on administration and interpretation of skin tests. Once the PPD is placed, the employee must return to have it read by the nurse. It is no longer acceptable to allow an employee (even a nurse or physician) to read his or her own skin test and report the results via postcard or other means. A qualified individual must read the test 48 to 72 hours after administration. From a practical standpoint, testing must be scheduled for a day that will allow the employee to return for interpretation 2 or 3 days later. Therefore, Mondays and Tuesdays are the best days to administer PPD skin tests.

A positive PPD test is based on the presence of induration (a palpable raised hardened area) at the injection site. If induration is present, it should be measured transverse to the long axis of the forearm, and the measurement should be recorded in millimeters. Induration must not be estimated; it must be measured with a small ruler calibrated in millimeters. Interpretation of the skin test is currently stratified at three cutoff points, depending upon the individual's risk. These cutoff points are: ≥5 mm, ≥10 mm, and ≥15 mm of induration (American Thoracic Society, 2000) and are applied according to risk. For persons at highest risk for developing a TB infection, the cutoff for a positive interpretation is ≥5 mm of induration. In addition to persons who are HIV positive or are solid organ transplant recipients, this group includes those with a recent exposure to an active TB patient such as a family member or health care worker. This is because a recent exposure increases risk for active infection (American Thoracic Society, 2000). A positive reaction of ≥10 mm induration is interpreted as positive in recent immigrants (within the past 5 years) from countries with a high prevalence of TB; injection drug users; and residents and employees in high-risk settings such as jails and prisons, nursing homes, homeless shelters, and residential care facilities for HIV-positive individuals. If the new employee in home or hospice care has previously worked in one of these high-risk settings, the PPD skin test should be interpreted based upon this exposure. An induration of ≥15 mm is interpreted as positive for all others, who are considered at low risk (CDC, 2000). A health professional performing PPD tests in a home care or hospice organization must be aware of the individual's risk group and interpret the PPD skin test accordingly. All individuals with newly positive reactions, also referred to as "PPD converters," should be directed to an occupational health care provider, their primary care physicians, or the county health department for further interpretation and follow-up.

All positive reactions must have further evaluation by a physician, who will evaluate the employee for signs and symptoms of active TB and obtain a chest radiograph to determine whether there is active pulmonary infection. Physical assessment and additional testing may be needed to detect extrapulmonary TB.

If active infection is detected, treatment will be initiated, and work restrictions should be considered for those with pulmonary or laryngeal TB. If there is no active infection, the individual may be placed on treatment for LTBI (CDC, 2000). In most cities and counties, the local health department provides the medication and monitors the individual for side effects or adverse reactions as well as compliance. Employees with newly positive PPD skin tests do not have to be restricted from patient contact once active disease has been ruled out.

Two-Step Testing

The routine use of a two-step method for PPD skin testing has been recommended for health care workers (CDC, 1994). The two-step method refers to the application of a second PPD skin test 2 to 3 weeks after the initial test, if the initial test is negative. New employees who have documentation of a negative PPD within the previous 12 months can use this PPD as the first step. This approach has been found to increase the identification of true positives through a booster effect to the immune system. The first time the PPD is placed, the immune system may not respond, but the second test "boosts" the reaction. When this occurs, the first test is interpreted as a false negative and the second test as a true positive. Some experts argue that the two-step method is necessary to identify all true positive cases so that they can be provided treatment for LTBI, to reduce their risk of active infection in the future.

Routine use of the two-step method may not always be cost effective, since it requires more administrative time and the application of two PPD tests. To determine the value of two-step skin testing for its staff, a home care or hospice organization should first investigate whether there is a state requirement for such testing. If there is, it must be continued. If there isn't, the home care or hospice organization can determine the probable benefit of the two-step method for its specific employee group by reviewing its own experience. If the two-step testing has detected a significant number of true positives based on the second PPD, then it is worthwhile to continue its use. For example, if 20% or 25% of those testing negative on the first skin test come up positive on the second, the two-step method has detected a significant number of true positives. If few or no positives are detected with the two-step method, consideration should be given to abandoning routine two-step testing unless circumstances change. Relevant changes would include a substantial increase in new staff, a change in the population from which employees are hired, or a significant change in the patient population served.

Annual TB Skin Testing

Once each employee has been assessed for TB status at the time of employment, annual (or more frequent) testing may be performed. In most situations, repeating the PPD tests for all patient care employees every 12 months is adequate. In geographic areas where TB is highly prevalent or in situations where the organization is providing care for patients with active TB, more frequent PPD testing (e.g., every 6 months) may be appropriate. If the organization has identified a number of employees with newly positive PPD tests (three within the past year from either occupational or nonoccupational exposures), semiannual testing should be considered (CDC, 1994).

Annual chest radiographs for employees known to be PPD positive are no longer recommended, because few cases of active pulmonary TB have ever been detected as a result of this expensive examination. Employees with a history of a positive PPD, however, should be evaluated annually for any clinical signs and symptoms of active TB infection. This assessment can be accomplished in several ways. A face-to-face assessment through an interview with the employee by the ICP or the occupational health care provider can be scheduled. A simpler way is to use a questionnaire to remind PPD-positive employees of the signs and symptoms of active TB infection and to request that they report these symptoms if they occur. Follow-up with a physician should be recommended if symptoms are present. To document that an annual assessment of PPD-positive employees has occurred, the organization may require that these employees answer the postcard or questionnaire and return it to the organization for placement the personnel health records.

INFLUENZA VACCINE

Occurrences and types of influenza are tracked around the world by the World Health Organization because the viruses that cause influenza A and B frequently change their antigenic makeup. New vaccines must be formulated for each flu season. To determine the vaccine formulation, the CDC tries to predict the incidence of flu in the United States for the coming season, including which viruses will be predominant. Because the viruses change to some degree each year, annual immunization is recommended.

The influenza season in the United States runs from October through May. Immunization campaigns should begin in October with completion in mid-December. Home care or hospice organizations provide the influenza vaccine to their employees on an annual basis to reduce the incidence of influenza among home care or hospice staff members, reduce lost days due to illness, and avoid exposing patients who may be at risk. Frequently, the vaccine is provided at little or no charge by the state or local health department. Although influenza immunization must be voluntary, home care organizations should encourage all staff providing care for high-risk patients to become immunized (CDC, 1997a; CDC 2003b). This includes patients over

65 years old, those with chronic pulmonary disease, and those with other chronic illnesses, such as acquired immune deficiency syndrome (AIDS), that put them at greater risk. Some agencies provide influenza vaccine to patients at high risk as well. Patients with chronic illnesses may not develop antibodies in response to the immunization, however, leaving them at risk for infection.

If an organization has not planned an influenza vaccination program for employees but influenza occurs in greater than predicted numbers, it can decide at that point to provide vaccination even though the season has begun. It takes about 10 days from the time the vaccine is administered for the recipient to develop immunity.

DEFINING AND MANAGING EXPOSURES

Home care and hospice staff members may be exposed to communicable diseases to which they are susceptible either occupationally (from patients and their families) or nonoccupationally (from their own families and friends or while in the community). In either case, some of these exposures should be reported to the home care or hospice organization and evaluated for necessary follow-up to reduce the risk of transmission to high-risk patients and other employees. Exposures to common community-acquired infections, such as upper respiratory viral infections including colds and flu, should not require reporting to or follow-up by the home care or hospice organization. The course of common upper respiratory infections is usually limited, and there are no recommendations for postexposure follow-up. In addition, it would be impossible to determine whether these infections were the result of occupational or nonoccupational exposure. Employees who are feeling ill (with fatigue and general malaise), and especially those with a fever and severe upper respiratory symptoms of coughing, sneezing, and increased respiratory secretions, should not work. Once the initial signs and symptoms of upper respiratory infection begin to subside and the employee's temperature returns to normal, he or she may return to providing patient care. Over-the-counter medications to reduce coughing and production of respiratory secretions can decrease the risk of transmission to patients and other staff members.

There are certain infectious disease exposures to home care staff or hospice staff members that should be

Exhibit 13-5 Infectious Diseases Requiring Follow-Up for Exposures

• AIDS/HIV	• Meningococcal meningitis
• Hepatitis A	• Rubella
• Hepatitis B	• Pertussis
• Hepatitis C	• Tuberculosis
• Measles	• Varicella

reported to the home care or hospice organization so that investigation and follow-up can be performed to reduce the risk of transmission to other staff and patients. A list of these infections is presented in Exhibit 13-3. These illnesses may require specific interventions, including antimicrobial prophylaxis and/or work restrictions. Specific defininitions of exposure to each of these diseases should be included in the home care or hospice organization's policies and procedures. The written definition of an exposure is necessary not only to provide a reference when a potential exposure occurs but also to ensure that there is consistency in identifying and managing exposures.

Varicella

The varicella zoster virus causes chickenpox as a primary infection and most frequently causes illness in young children. Recurrence of varicella results in shingles and is seen more frequently in older people. Chickenpox is contagious and can be transmitted by via the airborne route. Therefore, anyone who is in direct contact with an individual incubating chickenpox (contagion begins 48 to 72 hours before the development of the vesicular skin rash), has already developed the rash (contagion continues for about 5 days after the appearance of the rash), or has shared the air of a contagious person may have been exposed. An exposure to varicella is defined as face-to-face contact indoors for at least 10 minutes or being in the same room for longer than 10 minutes without the protection of a mask. For a home care or hospice employee who is susceptible to chickenpox, it really does not matter whether the exposure occurs while providing care (oc-

cupational exposure) or during nonworking hours (nonoccupational exposure). If the individual is susceptible, he or she may develop active infection and expose patients or other employees. Therefore, if an employee reports a chickenpox exposure, it must be determined whether he or she is susceptible. This should have been accomplished as part of the preemployment health screen and infectious disease history (CDC, 1997a).

The decision as to whether to restrict the exposed employee's work activities depends on the patients for whom the employee provides care. If the patients are adults who are probably immune to varicella, no restrictions may be necessary. In this case, the employee may be carefully monitored for early signs and symptoms of chickenpox and counseled to stay off work if a fever or prodromal symptoms, such as headache, fever, and malaise, develop. If the employee is caring for children, especially those at risk for varicella, work restriction or reassignment should be seriously considered from day 7 after the first exposure through day 21 after the last exposure. This is the period during which active infection is most likely to occur. If the exposed employee is given varicella zoster immune globulin (VZIG), the incubation period is extended to 28 days after the last exposure. The specific date(s) of exposure must be obtained; in many cases the individual may have been exposed on several different days, including during the incubation period, when the infection was not yet recognized but was contagious. Work restrictions may allow for the staff member to work in the office (providing no patient care) if the other staff members are immune to chickenpox. Otherwise, complete work restriction may be indicated.

Susceptible employees should be encouraged to report exposure to varicella and the other infections listed in Exhibit 13-3. Financial disincentives (lack of sick time or paid time off) should be addressed and avoided to encourage reporting. If the employee develops chickenpox, he or she should remain off duty until all the lesions have crusted. Even though varicella is not contagious after the lesions have crusted, the organization may elect to restrict the employee from patient care if the rash remains to avoid questions or concerns from patients and their families. The individual may safely spend this time working in the office.

Although there are a few reports of health care providers developing chickenpox after direct contact with patients with shingles, most infection control experts would consider risk only in exposures involving patients with disseminated zoster. By definition, disseminated herpes zoster is shingles that involves more than one dermatome. In disseminated zoster, the varicella zoster virus has been isolated from respiratory secretions. This may make the infection transmissible via the respiratory and/or airborne route as well as through direct contact with lesions by a susceptible host. If a susceptible home care staff member is caring for a patient with disseminated zoster and has not used a mask, the same work restrictions as for a chickenpox exposure should be considered.

Measles, Rubella, Pertussis, Meningitis, and Hepatitis A

Measles is considered the most contagious infectious disease. It occurs through airborne transmission; therefore, exposure is similar to that of chickenpox: face-to-face contact with an infected person for at least 10 minutes or presence in the same room for longer than 10 minutes without a mask. Measles is infrequently seen in the United States, but it may occur in unimmunized or improperly immunized children. Home care and hospice staff members should be immune to measles by either natural immunity or vaccination. If for some reason a staff member is not immune, however, and because the virus can be shed from the respiratory tract from 5 days after the initial exposure until 21 days after the last exposure, the staff member should be restricted from working during that period. If a rash occurs, work restriction should continue for 7 days after the development of the rash (Bolyard et al., 1998).

Staff members should also be immune to rubella. An exposure to rubella, which is transmitted by respiratory droplets, may be defined as face-to-face contact without a mask for at least 10 minutes. If an exposure occurs, the infection may be contagious from day 7 after the first exposure to day 21 after the last exposure, and the employee should be restricted from work. If a rash develops, the employee should remain off duty for 5 days after the development of the rash (Bolyard et al., 1998).

Whooping cough or pertussis is transmitted via respiratory droplets. Face-to-face contact with a contagious individual for more than 10 minutes may define exposure. A health care staff member who is exposed to pertussis should receive antimicrobial prophylaxis with erythromycin. If prophylaxis is provided, work re-

strictions may not be necessary. If the exposed individual does not receive antimicrobial prophylaxis, however, and/or develops signs and symptoms of pertussis, including a paroxysmal cough, he or she should be restricted from work until 5 days after the initiation of appropriate therapy (Bolyard et al., 1998).

Exposure to meningococcal meningitis occurs most frequently in emergency care providers, such as ambulance personnel. Nevertheless, an occupational exposure could occur in a home or hospice care staff member. Exposure to meningococcal meningitis requires interaction with the patient beyond face-to-face contact. Exposure should be defined as direct, intimate contact with respiratory secretions, such as would occur in kissing or administration of mouth-to-mouth resuscitation (thus the risk to emergency responders). If an exposure occurs, the exposed individual should be provided with prophylactic antibiotic treatment, usually rifampin. No work restriction is necessary (Bolyard et al., 1998).

Hepatitis A virus (HAV) infection is spread by the oral–fecal route. Home care or hospice staff members may have some risk for exposure if they are caring for a patient with an unrecognized HAV infection or are working in a home where a family member has HAV. Although home and hospice care staff members should be adhering to Standard Precautions and wearing gloves when handling stool, unprotected exposures can occur while they are caring for a patient who is incontinent of stool or if they fail to perform adequate hand hygiene. Eating or drinking in the home of an HAV-infected person may also be considered an exposure. If there is sufficient evidence that exposure to HAV has occurred, the home care staff member should be given an intramuscular injection of immune globulin within 2 weeks of exposure. No work restrictions are necessary unless the staff member develops HAV infection. If infection occurs, the person should be restricted from patient care for 1 week after the onset of illness. HAV vaccine is not routinely recommended for health care providers (CDC, 1997a).

Tuberculosis

Exposure to TB increased among all health care workers in the 1990s with the increase of TB in the general population. However, the incidence of TB began to decline in 1996 and has continued to decline each subsequent year, as mentioned earlier in this chapter (CDC, 2002a). Nonetheless, exposure to TB continues to be a potential risk for home care and hospice staff members, especially in specific states and when dealing with high-risk populations (CDC, 2003a). Exposure to TB is defined as face-to-face contact for more than 10 minutes or remaining in the same room with an individual who has active and contagious pulmonary or laryngeal TB infection for more than 30 minutes without the use of a mask or respirator. In home care or hospice, exposures to TB may occur if the organization has not been informed that the patient or a member of the family or household has active TB.

Although the exposed employee may or may not have had a baseline PPD test, another test should be administered as soon as possible after the exposure if the employee is PPD negative by history. This test serves as a new baseline for the current exposure. Home care and hospice staff members who are known to have positive PPD skin tests should not be retested. A second PPD should be administered 12 weeks after the exposure to determine whether infection has occurred. As stated earlier, a cutoff point of ≥10 mm of induration should be used to define a positive reaction in an individual recently exposed to an active case of TB. If the PPD is negative at 12 weeks, no further testing is necessary. If the PPD is positive, further examination by a physician to assess the presence of active infection or to provide treatment for LTBI is indicated (CDC, 2003a). If the employee is asymptomatic (i.e., if he or she has no fevers, cough, or weight loss), work restriction is not necessary. If active disease is evident, the individual should be restricted from work until appropriate therapy has been initiated and there are three negative sputum smears for acid-fast bacilli obtained on different days (CDC, 1994).

Agents of Bioterrorism

Prior to the events of 2001, public health officials throughout the world declared in 1991 that smallpox had been eradicated. Only a few vials of the virus remained in research labs in the United States and Russia. However, with the threat of bioterrorism now facing the U.S. public health system, as evidenced by the anthrax cases in 2001 and 2002, the CDC has focused significant resources on preparing for potential exposures to and infections from agents of bioterrorism. CDC scientists had actually identified the most likely agents—biological, chemical, and radioactive—in an issue of *Morbidity and Mortality Weekly Report* in 2000 (CDC, 2000a). The following are the most likely infectious agents anticipated for use by terrorists:

- *Variola major* (smallpox)
- *Bacillus anthracis* (anthrax)
- *Yersinia pestis* (plague)
- *Clostridium botulinum* toxin (botulism)
- *Francisella tularensis* (tularemia)
- Filoviruses
  — Ebola hemorrhagic fever
  — Marburg hemorrhagic fever
- Arenaviruses
  — Lassa (Lassa fever)
  — Junin (Argentine hemorrhagic fever) and related viruses

Subsequently, the CDC has dedicated a special section of its website to information about agents of bioterrorism and its preparation for management of exposures and illnesses (see *www.bt.cdc.gov*). This website is continuously updated and serves as an ongoing, accurate, and complete source of information regarding all the agents, vaccines, and public health information on preparedness and response.

Smallpox

Although health care professionals should inform themselves about all agents that could potentially be used in bioterrorism against the United States, the agent that may be of most significance to home care providers is smallpox. In addition to the viruses that cause hemorrhagic fevers and the agent for pneumonic plague, smallpox can be transmitted from person to person. The others require exposure to the agent (e.g., anthrax, botulism) or to vectors that carry the disease (e.g., bubonic plague). The CDC has developed a plan for responding to an outbreak of smallpox (see *www.bt.cdc.gov/agent/smallpox/index.asp*) (CDC, 2003c). Within the plan for identification and containment of smallpox, there are three types of facilities forseen for care of patients and isolation of exposures. Those with active smallpox infection would be cared for in a Type C facility (the "C" standing for contagious), which would probably be a community hospital with appropriate ventilation systems to maintain airborne isolation precautions. All smallpox cases within a geographic area would be cared for in this dedicated type of facility. Exposures with fever could also be placed under observation in a Type C facility, or they could be housed in facilities designated as Type X. It is intended that Type X facilities supplement the capacity of Type C facilities and house exposed individuals who were vaccinated but are febrile without a rash. Basic medical care and monitoring of vital signs would be provided. If an individual develops a rash while in a Type X facility, he or she would be transferred to a Type C facility. A third type of facility is also described in the plan, a Type R facility (the "R" standing for residential). Exposed persons who do not develop fever or rash would be quarantined in their homes or with others in a designated residence. Nonimmune family members would have to live elsewhere until the incubation period ended or for 14 days following the administration of the smallpox vaccine to the exposed person. Others have also recommended that patients with smallpox infection be discharged home for care in that setting as soon as they are well enough to leave the hospital (Henderson et al., 1999).

These potential situations and public health planning may impact home care providers. Should the threat actually occur, home care professionals may be requested to assist in the observation of exposed individuals to monitor their temperature for the identification of fever and rash. They may also be asked to care for smallpox patients discharged from a hospital. Home care staff members should consider this possibility and determine if they will avail themselves of the smallpox vaccine, which was made available to other health care workers in 2003 (CDC, 2003). It must be noted, however, that recent experience with the currently available vaccine, which is a live-virus vaccine, has been problematic. Among the issues were cardiac problems exacerbated by the vaccine in a number of cases; avoidance of the vaccine by those with immunosuppression; and the potential for transmission of the virus from vaccine recipients via virus shedding from the vaccination site.

Home care providers who wish to become immunized against smallpox should review the information on the vaccine found on the CDC website (*http://www.bt.cdc.gov/agent/smallpox/vaccination/va ccine.asp*). A new vaccine, not a live-virus vaccine but rather a vaccine made from a cloned virus, is under development. When this vaccine is available, many of the potential problems related to the current vaccine should be alleviated.

Bloodborne Pathogens

Definitions and follow-up procedures for employees exposed to bloodborne pathogens, including HBV, hepatitis C virus (HCV), and HIV, should be incorporated in the exposure control plan and the policies and procedures for occupational health. Exposure to bloodborne pathogens may occur through the percutaneous route (e.g., from a contaminated needlestick or a sharps injury) or through exposure of the mucus membranes of the mouth, nose, or eyes to infected blood or body fluids. From data on occupationally acquired infections accumulated over a number of years and through various studies, the CDC can now provide estimates of risk (CDC, 2001). Transmission of HBV is related not only to the type and nature of the exposure, but more importantly, also to the presence of HBe (hepatitis E antigen) in the source patient. In needlestick exposures in which the source is both HBsAg and HBeAg positive, the risk of infection is 22% to 31%, whereas the risk of developing serologic evidence of exposure (that is, becoming anti-HBs positive) is estimated at 37% to 62%. If the source is HBe-Ag negative but HBs-Ag positive, the risk for infection is only 1% to 6%, whereas the risk of developing serologic evidence of exposure is 23% to 37%. HCV does not seem to be effectively transmitted in occupational exposures; thus, risk for infection from a needlestick exposure from a HCV-positive source is 1.8% (range 0% to 7%). Finally, occupational risk for HIV transmission via needlestick is estimated at 0.3%, with greater risk associated with exposures involving large bore needles, visible blood contamination, and deep injury (Cardo et al., 1997). Mucus membrane exposure is a lower risk, at 0.09%.

For approximately 10 months in 1996 and 1997, the CDC sponsored a study to gain knowledge about bloodborne exposures among home care staff members. Eleven home care agencies participated; their activities during the period of the study included over 33,000 home care visits and almost 15,000 procedures. In the group of 548 home care staff participating in the study, there were 53 reported blood contacts during home care visits, including 5 percutaneous injuries. This incidence was extrapolated to a rate of 2.8 blood contacts and 0.6 percutaneous injuries per 1000 procedures (Beltrami et al., 2000). Comparing this experience to the study of health care workers in other settings, the authors concluded that the observed incidence of exposure was probably valid and that the risk for exposure to bloodborne pathogens in home care is of real concern.

All exposures must be reported, and appropriate assessment and follow-up must be provided. Although initial assessment to determine whether a significant exposure has occurred can be done in the organization's office, a physician should perform further assessment and follow-up. A significant exposure to bloodborne pathogens occurs when a health care provider experiences a needlestick or percutaneous injury (laceration or puncture wound) with a sharp instrument or object that has been used in the care of a patient and has been contaminated with the patient's blood or other potentially infected body fluids. An exposure also occurs when the mucus membranes of the health care provider's mouth, nose, or eyes are contaminated with blood or other body fluids from a patient through a splash or spill. The body fluids of concern in addition to blood include cerebrospinal fluid, synovial fluid, pleural fluid, peritoneal fluid, pericardial fluid, amniotic fluid, semen, vaginal secretions, and any other body fluid containing visible blood. These are the fluids that have been recognized in the transmission of HBV, HCV, and HIV. It should be noted that the list does not include urine, stool, nasal secretions, sputum, sweat, tears, or vomitus unless they are visibly blood contaminated.

When an employee reports an exposure, the designated individual in the organization should determine whether the circumstances meet the criteria for a significant exposure. For example, if an employee reports that he or she experienced an unprotected splash to the eyes and mouth of visibly bloody vomitus, a significant exposure has occurred. If an employee reports a needlestick from a syringe used to obtain a urine sample in which the urine was not visibly bloody, no significant exposure has occurred. Whether or not the exposure is deemed significant, the home care or hospice organization should eventually investigate why the exposure occurred and whether the employee was complying with Standard Precautions. In addition, the report of the exposure should be noted in the employee's health record and recorded in the OSHA 300 log and the sharps injury log.

Once the significance of the exposure has been determined, the status of the source patient (if known) must be sought, to provide the appropriate prophylaxis. The patient's physician should be contacted to provide the status for HBV, HCV, and HIV if it is not already known by the organization as part of the patient record. If the patient is known to be infected with HBV, HCV, or HIV, specific protocols for testing and prophylaxis, as described below, should be followed. A source patient is considered infected with HBV if he or she currently tests positive for hepatitis B surface antigen (HBsAg). A source patient should be considered infectious for HCV if he or she tests positive for antibodies to HCV. The CDC does not recommend testing for the HCV antigen (CDC, 2001). HCV antibody-positive patients are considered potentially infectious for life. Similarly, a source patient who tests positive for antibody to HIV should be considered infectious.

If the exposure occurs from an unknown source (e.g., a needlestick accident due to a contaminated needle in a sharps container for which the source patient is unknown), it should be assumed that the source is potentially infectious unless there are circumstances to indicate low risk based on the patient population. This type of exposure is less likely to occur in home care or hospice than it is in settings where there are many patients cared for at a single facility and where sharps and infectious waste are collected in common containers.

If exposure to HBV occurs and the exposed employee has received HBV vaccine and is a known responder, the employee should be retested for antibody to anti-HBs to confirm immunity. The report of the exposure and the results of testing should be placed in the employee's health record (CDC, 2001).

If exposure to HBV occurs in an employee who has received HBV vaccine and is a known nonresponder, either two doses of hepatitis B immune globulin (HBIG) should be administered (the first at the time of exposure and the second 1 month later) or a single dose of HBIG should be administered and the employee should be revaccinated. If the employee's response to previous HBV vaccination is not known, an antibody test should be obtained. If the level of anti-HBs is adequate (greater than 10 mU/ml), no additional treatment is necessary. If it is inadequate, the exposed employee should receive a dose of HBIG and a vaccine booster. An unvaccinated employee should receive one dose of HBIG, and the vaccine series should be initiated as soon as possible. The vaccine should be administered even if the source patient tests negative for HbsAg, in light of a clear risk for future exposure (CDC, 2001).

HCV is an increasing risk for health care workers in all settings. There is currently no prophylactic treatment for HCV in the event of exposure. If the source patient is known to be infectious, the exposed employee should be tested for antibody to HCV immediately after exposure to provide a baseline result. Retesting should occur 6 months after the exposure to determine whether infection has occurred (CDC, 2001). If results indicate that the employee is antibody positive, the infected employee should be counseled to seek follow-up care from his or her private physician, who should monitor the employee for development or progression of active infection. Should the disease progress, the employee's health record would confirm occupational exposure, and the employee would be eligible for workers' compensation benefits.

Provision of prophylaxis to employees exposed or potentially exposed to HIV must be immediate to achieve the best outcome. Therefore, a mechanism for reporting exposures and for ensuring that the drugs recommended for postexposure prophylaxis (PEP) are available should be established in all home care and hospice organizations. When a significant exposure has occurred, the HIV status of the source patient must be considered. In many cases, the status will be unknown unless the patient is known to have HIV or AIDS. If the patient has AIDS or is otherwise known to be HIV infected, postexposure prophylaxis should be provided to the employee within 1 to 2 hours of exposure. If the patient's HIV status is not known, potential risk based on current knowledge of his or her history and epidemiological factors must be examined. This may or may not be within the capabilities of the individual in the organization who is responsible for infection control or occupational health issues. Even if this person is capable, enlisting the involvement of the patient's own physician and the physician who will be providing postexposure prophylaxis may be prudent, to broaden the input in making a judgment regarding risk and need for postexposure prophylaxis. Frequently, the level of risk falls into three categories: no risk, questionable risk, or high risk. The level of risk should be assessed based on the patient's medical history and lifestyle. Occasionally a concerned employee who has been exposed may wish to initiate a minimal PEP regimen postexposure prophylaxis. The determination of who will pay for the drugs for postexposure prophylaxis will depend on the organization's policy and/or the state's workers' compensation laws.

If there is some concern that risk factors exist and the source patient may be infected with HIV, the source patient's physician should obtain testing within the pa-

rameters permitted by local laws. In most states, the patient must give written informed consent for testing. Some states allow testing without written consent if a health care provider has been exposed. The home care or hospice organization should be familiar with state laws and incorporate compliance into its exposure investigation policies. Postexposure prophylaxis should not be delayed waiting for test results. Blood samples for baseline testing of the exposed employee should be obtained as soon as possible, and postexposure prophylaxis should be initiated immediately. If there is considerable risk of HIV infection in the source patient but the HIV status is not known, the same steps as described above should be followed.

In 1990, the CDC made its initial recommendations for the use of antiviral agents as postexposure prophylaxis for health care workers occupationally exposed to HIV-infected blood or body fluids (CDC, 1990). At that time, the CDC recommended that zidovudine (ZVD) be provided as soon as possible and that it continue for 4 weeks or as long as tolerated. The CDC recommendations have changed, with updates published in 1998 and 2001 (CDC, 1998, 2001). The more recent recommendations, which include the consideration and use of additional antiviral agents, are based on treatment of HIV-infected patients, however, not on use as postexposure prophylaxis. Therefore, these recommendations remain provisional until more experience and data can be accumulated and examined.

The use of ZVD in postexposure prophylaxis for health care workers after percutaneous exposure to HIV has demonstrated a 79% reduction in the risk of infection. The actual risk of a health care worker acquiring HIV infection if he or she experiences a percutaneous exposure is estimated at 0.3%. This risk is based on a number of factors that should also be considered when postexposure prophylaxis is prescribed. A case-control study has demonstrated that a deep needlestick or sharps injury from a device with visible blood contamination increased risk when the device had been placed in the source patient's vein or artery. Additional risk has been demonstrated when the source patient died of AIDS within 60 days of the exposure. This is due to the increased viral dose in the terminally ill AIDS patient (Cardo et al., 1997).

Consequently, if an exposure of a home care or hospice staff member occurs and the source patient is known to be HIV positive or there is evidence of medium to high risk for infection, the circumstances of the exposure should be examined. If the circumstances increase the risk of infection (e.g., deep percutaneous exposure with a visibly contaminated device or similar circumstances), additional antiviral drugs should be added to the postexposure prophylaxis regimen (CDC, 2001). A physician with knowledge of and experience in the use of antiviral drugs should be consulted.

WORK RESTRICTIONS

There are various infections that occur among health care staff members that may pose a risk of transmission from the provider to the patient and others in the environment. A home or hospice care organization should recognize these conditions and formulate a policy for diagnosis, assessment, and work restriction when they occur in patient care personnel. If they are occupationally acquired infections, workers' compensation bene-

fits may be used to pay the employee who is not permitted to work. If the condition is nonoccupational, paid sick-time benefits must be used, if they are provided. Table 13-1 provides a summary of recommendations for work restrictions for home care and hospice staff exposed to selected infectious diseases.

Some skin infections that occur in home care or hospice staff members may warrant a staff member's exclusion from patient care and food preparation activities. If a patient care provider has a skin infection caused by *Staphylococcus aureus,* the potential for transmission of the infective agent to the patient must be assessed. First, the specific type, location, and extent of infection should be considered. If there is a draining wound on the hands or upper extremities, there may be risk for transmission even if the wound is covered. This may depend also on the extent or size of the wound and the degree of drainage. An extensive

Table 13-1 Summary of Suggested Work Restrictions for Health Care Personnel Exposed to or Infected with Infectious Diseases of Importance in Health Care Settings, in the Absence of State and Local Regulations (modified from ACIP recommendations)

Disease/problem	Work restriction	Duration	Category
Conjunctivitis	Restrict from patient contact and contact with the patient's environment	Until discharge ceases	II
Cytomegalovirus infections	No restriction		II
Diarrheal diseases			
Acute stage (diarrhea with other symptoms)	Restrict from patient contact, contact with the patient's environment, and food handling	Until symptoms resolve	IB
Convalescent stage, *Salmonella* spp.	Restrict from care of high-risk patients	Until symptoms resolve; consult with local and state health authorities regarding need for negative stool cultures	IB
Diphtheria	Exclude from duty	Until antimicrobial therapy completed and 2 cultures obtained ≥24 hours apart are negative	IB
Enteroviral infections	Restrict from care of infants, neonates, and immunocompromised patients and their environments	Until symptoms resolve	II
Hepatitis A	Restrict from patient contact, contact with patient's environment, and food handling	Until 7 days after onset of jaundice	IB
Hepatitis B			
Personnel with acute or chronic hepatitis B surface antigemia who do not perform exposure-prone procedures	No restriction*; refer to state regulations; Standard Precautions should always be observed		II

Table 13-1 continued

Disease/problem	Work restriction	Duration	Category
Personnel with acute or chronic hepatitis B e antigenemia who perform exposure-prone procedures	Do not perform exposure-prone invasive procedures until counsel from an expert review panel has been sought; panel should review and recommend procedures the worker can perform, taking into account specific procedures as well as skill and technique of worker; refer to state regulations	Until hepatitis B e antigen is negative	II
Hepatitis C	No recommendation		Unresolved issue
Herpes simplex			
Genital	No restriction		II
Hands (herpetic whitlow)	Restrict from patient contact and contact with the patient's environment	Until lesions heal	IA
Orofacial	Evaluate for need to restrict from care of high-risk patients		II
Human immunodeficiency virus	Do not perform exposure-prone invasive procedures until counsel from an expert review panel has been sought; panel should review and recommend procedures the worker can perform, taking into account specific procedure as well as skill and technique of the worker; Standard Precautions should always be observed; refer to state regulations		II
Measles			
Active	Exclude from duty	Until 7 days after the rash appears	IA
Postexposure (susceptible personnel)	Exclude from duty	From 5th day after 1st exposure through 21st day after last exposure and/or 4 days after rash appears	IB
Meningococcal infections	Exclude from duty	Until 24 hours after start of effective therapy	IA
Mumps			
Active	Exclude from duty	Until 9 days after onset of parotitis	IB
Postexposure (susceptible personnel)	Exclude from duty	From 12th day after 1st exposure through 26th day after last exposure or until 9 days after onset of parotitis	II
Pediculosis	Restrict from patient contact	Until treated and observed to be free of adult and immature lice	IB
Pertussis			
Active	Exclude from duty	From beginning of catarrhal stage through 3rd week after onset of paroxysms or until 5 days after start of effective antimicrobial therapy	IB

continues

Table 13-1 continued

Disease/problem	Work restriction	Duration	Category
Pertussis (continued)			
Postexposure (asymptomatic personnel)	No restriction, prophylaxis recommended		II
Postexposure (symptomatic personnel)	Exclude from duty	Until 5 days after start of effective antimicrobial therapy	IB
Rubella			
Active	Exclude from duty	Until 5 days after rash appears	IA
Postexposure (susceptible personnel)	Exclude from duty	From 7th day after 1st exposure through 21st day after last exposure	IB
Scabies	Restrict from patient contact	Until cleared by medical evaluation	IB
Staphylococcus aureus infection			
Active, draining skin lesions	Restrict from contact with patients and patient's environment or food handling	Until lesions have resolved	IB
Carrier state	No restriction, unless personnel are epidemiologically linked to transmission of the organism		IB
Streptococcal infection, group A	Restrict from patient care, contact with patient's environment, and food handling	Until 24 hours after adequate treatment started	IB
Tuberculosis			IA
Active disease	Exclude from duty	Until proved noninfectious	IA
PPD converter	No restriction		IA
Varicella			
Active	Exclude from duty	Until all lesions dry and crust	IA
Postexposure (susceptible personnel)	Exclude from duty	From 10th day after 1st exposure through 21st day (28th day if VZIG given) after last exposure	IA
Zoster			
Localized, in healthy person	Cover lesions; restrict from care of high-risk patients†	Until all lesions dry and crust	II
Generalized or localized in immunosuppressed person	Restrict from patient contact	Until all lesions dry and crust	IB
Postexposure (susceptible personnel)	Restrict from patient contact	From 8th day after 1st exposure through 21st day (28th day if VZIG given) after last exposure or, if varicella occurs, until all lesions dry and crust	IA
Viral respiratory infections, acute febrille	Consider excluding from the care of high-risk patients‡ or contact with their environment during community outbreak of RSV and influenza	Until acute symptoms resolved	

*Unless epidemiologically linked to transmission of infection.

†Those susceptible to varicella and who are at increased risk of complications of varicella, such as neonates and immunocompromised persons of any age.

‡High-risk patients as defined by the ACIP for complications of influenza.

Source: Reprinted with permission from B. Bolyard, O. Tablan, W. Williams, M. Pearson, C. Shapiro, & S. Deitchman. CDC guideline for infection control in health care personnel, *American Journal of Infection Control,* Vol. 26, No. 3, pp. 299–301, © 1998, Mosby-Year Book, Inc.

wound on the face or neck may pose risk. A draining wound on the trunk or a lower extremity that is covered and for which the drainage is well contained, however, may not pose such a risk. In any case, the home care or hospice staff member must be attentive to conscientious hand hygiene if he or she is permitted to provide care or be involved in food preparation (Bolyard et al., 1998).

The other variable to consider in determining whether a provider with a staphylococcal skin infection should be providing care is the patient's risk. If the patient requires wound care, central line or urinary catheter care, or other skilled care that involves a potential portal of entry for the bacteria, he or she should not be exposed to the provider. Many home care and hospice patients have needs based on medical conditions, such as cerebrovascular accident, hypertension, or other conditions that do not involve a portal of entry, however. If the patient is immunocompetent and has intact skin, the risk may be minimal. A home care or hospice staff member known to be colonized with *S. aureus* (nasal colonization or skin carriage) should not automatically be excluded from patient care. Any exclusion should be in light of epidemiological evidence of transmission of the organism to patients.

Employees with skin and wound infections caused by *Streptococcus* species should be handled in the same manner as those with staphylococcal infections. With both organisms, if the care provider is restricted, he or she may return to work when adequate treatment has been provided and/or when the wound is no longer draining. The organization may require a negative wound culture before the staff member returns to patient care.

Other skin conditions may not involve specific organisms such as *Staphylococcus aureus,* but an employee may be excluded based on appearance. For example, if a home care or hospice staff member has extensive poison ivy, it may be prudent to restrict patient care and allow the person to work in the office to avoid questions and concerns from patients and families. The same approach may be considered for staff members recovering from illnesses with viral exanthams, such as chickenpox. Although they may have passed the time of contagion, there may be concerns on the part of the patient or family if the rash remains evident.

Scabies may be occupationally or nonoccupationally acquired. The definition for occupational exposure should require skin-to-skin contact with an individual who has untreated scabies. This type of exposure may occur during direct care, such as bathing. If a home care or hospice employee discovers that a patient has scabies, Contact Precautions (gowns and gloves for direct contact with the patient and his or her immediate environment) should be initiated (see Chapter 7). However, if the home care worker has been exposed prior to the recognition of infestation in the patient, he or she should be observed for signs and symptoms of infestation. Should signs and symptoms occur, the staff member should seek treatment from his or her primary care physician. Once the staff member is treated, he or she may return to patient care. Home care and hospice staff members should not receive prophylactic treatment for scabies (Bolyard et al., 1998). When infestation is identified in a home or hospice care patient, the patient's physician should be notified, and treatment for the patient should be ordered and provided.

Herpes simplex virus (HSV) is another skin infection that may occur in home care or hospice staff members. HSV is not usually an occupational infection. However, a home care or hospice staff member may acquire an occupational HSV infection of a finger, known as herpetic whitlow. This infection usually occurs when a staff member with nonintact skin around the nailbed (i.e., a hangnail) contacts oral secretions of a patient who is shedding HSV. A home care or hospice staff member with herpetic whitlow must be restricted from patient care until the lesions have healed and there is no risk of viral shedding. A physician's prescription for antiviral agents is usually necessary (Bolyard et al., 1998).

HSV infections occur more often on the mouth and face, and they may recur frequently. The actual risk of health care workers transmitting oral HSV to patients is not known. Most hospitals allow staff members to continue patient care activities unless their assignment includes patients with severe immunosuppression (e.g., those undergoing organ transplantation) or low-birthweight premature infants. Home care and hospice staff members with oral HSV lesions do not have to be restricted from patient care, but they should be reminded of the importance of careful hand hygiene and avoidance of touching the lesions during patient care activities. Use of antiviral agents should be encouraged to decrease viral shedding and hasten healing of the lesions. If the lesions are extensive, the home care or hospice organization may elect to exclude the staff member from patient care to avoid questions and concerns from the patient and family.

Home care and hospice staff members should be instructed to notify the organization if they are experiencing diarrhea so that the situation can be assessed. If an infectious cause (e.g., viral gastroenteritis or *Salmonella* or *Shigella* infection) is suspected, the staff member should be restricted from patient care or food preparation until he or she is evaluated by a physician or the symptoms subside. Any provider who is experiencing diarrhea must pay careful attention to hand hygiene, especially if he or she is involved in food preparation. A home care staff member experiencing vomiting from a potentially infectious cause, such as viral gastroenteritis, should be excluded from patient care until the symptoms subside (Bolyard et al., 1998).

Occasionally a home care or hospice staff member experiences conjunctivitis that prompts concern regarding potential transmission to patients. Evaluation by an ophthalmologist should be sought if there is purulent drainage or if epidemic keratoconjunctivitis (EKC) is suspected. EKC is caused by an adenovirus, and nosocomial transmission has been associated with outbreaks in eye clinics. Therefore, EKC may be a concern if the home care or hospice staff member recently received optical care. As its name implies, EKC is very contagious. A home care or hospice staff member with bacterial conjunctivitis should be excluded from direct patient care until the infection is treated and no longer contagious or the symptoms have subsided. A home care or hospice staff member suspected of having EKC should be seen by an ophthalmologist and excluded from patient care until it is ruled out (Ford, Nelson, & Warren, 1987).

PREGNANT STAFF MEMBERS

Many home and hospice care staff members are women of childbearing age; therefore, concern about exposure to infectious agents while pregnant and providing patient care often arises. Pregnant staff members are at no greater risk for exposure to and infection with infectious diseases than other staff members. There has been documentation of specific infections that pose some risk to a fetus, but these diseases are no more prevalent in home care or hospice patients than in the general population. All home care and hospice staff members, including women who may become pregnant, should be encouraged to obtain available vaccines, as discussed earlier in this chapter. In addition, all staff members should be instructed in the use of personal protective equipment and should employ precautions for bloodborne pathogens and other infectious agents as prescribed (Bolyard et al., 1998). Table 13-2 provides a summary of issues that may be of concern to pregnant home care staff.

In addition to some of the infectious diseases discussed previously, pregnant personnel may perceive increased risk if they are exposed to patients with cytomegalovirus (CMV) or parvovirus. CMV is a common virus and a member of the herpes virus family. Many people experience asymptomatic CMV infections in childhood. The concern among home care or hospice staff members arises when they are caring for patients chronically infected with and shedding CMV. This may include pediatric patients and patients who are immunosuppressed, such as solid organ transplant recipients. Perinatal CMV infection can cause hearing loss or a congenital syndrome leading to various pathologies in the newborn. Although a susceptible pregnant home care staff member is theoretically at risk for occupational infection with CMV, that risk is no greater than it is for nonoccupational infection. In fact, it may be less because the staff member should be complying with Standard Precautions regarding the use of gowns, gloves, and masks. Pregnant providers should not be excluded from the care of patients known to be infected with CMV (Bolyard et al., 1998).

Parvovirus B19 is a rare cause of fetal loss and hydrops fetalis. Chronic infection with viral shedding may occur in patients with chronic anemia or immunosuppression. As in the case of CMV, pregnant home care staff members do not appear to be at greater risk for occupational infection than others are, and transmission is rare. Expanded precautions should be employed for patients known to be shedding parvovirus B19, to protect all staff members. Pregnant staff members should not be excluded from their care (Bolyard et al., 1998).

Table 13-2 Infectious Diseases of Concern to the Pregnant Employee

Disease	Infection source	Transmission	Precautions (in addition to standard precautions and hand hygiene)	Reassignment of pregnant worker
HIV/AIDS	Blood Body fluid containing blood Cerebrospinal fluid Synovial, pleural, peritoneal, pericardial, and amniotic fluid Vaginal secretion Semen	Parenteral (needlesticks) Mucus membrane Nonintact skin	None	No
Cytomegalovirus (CMV)	Urine Blood Respiratory secretions Transplant patients Day care toddlers	Close intimate contact	None (except mask, if CMV pneumonia). If children at home attend day care center, good hand hygiene at home.	No
Hepatitis A	Feces	Fecal-oral	None	No
Hepatitis B	Blood	Parenteral Mucus membrane Nonintact skin	None Immunization with hepatitis B vaccine (safe during pregnancy).	No
Hepatitis C	Blood	As above	None	No
Herpes simplex types I and II	Lesions/vescular fluid	Direct contact with lesions Respiratory secretions Saliva	None Avoid direct contact with lesions.	No
Herpes zoster (shingles) • Localized • Disseminated	Open, weeping lesions Lesions, possibly respiratory secretions	Direct contact Direct contact Droplet contact	None Masks	The nonimmune health care worker, pregnant or not, should not have patient contact.
Rubella (German Measles)	Respiratory secretions	Droplet contact	Masks Respiratory isolation. Immunization available for nonpregnant worker.	The nonimmune health care worker, pregnant or not, should not care for rubella patients.
Rubeola (Measles)	Respiratory secretions	Airborne Droplet contact	Masks Airborne isolation. Immunization available for nonpregnant worker.	The nonimmune health care worker, pregnant or not, should not care for rubeola patients.
Toxoplasmosis	Cat feces Raw meat Unpasteurized milk	Ingestion	None	No
Tuberculosis	Airborne droplet Nuclei	Airborne	N-95 respirator Airborne isolation	No
Varicella (chickenpox)	Respiratory secretions Lesion secretions	Droplet contact Airborne Contact with lesions	Masks Gowns Airborne/contact isolation	The nonimmune health care worker, pregnant or not, should not have patient contact.

* Standard Precautions are to be followed on all patients. Use gloves for contact with all moist body substances, gowns, masks, and eye shields when needed to prevent splashing.

Courtesy of Scottsdale Healthcare, Scottsdale, Arizona.

REFERENCES

American Thoracic Society. (2000). Targeted tuberculin testing and treatment of latent tuberculosis infection. *American Journal of Respiratory and Critical Care Medicine, 161*(4), S221–S247

Beltrami, E., McArthur, M., Mc Geer, A., Armstrong-Evans, M., Lyons, D., Chamberland, M., & Cardo, D. (2000). The nature and frequency of blood contacts among home healthcare workers. *Infection Control and Hospital Epidemiology, 21*(12), 765–770.

Bolyard, B., Tablan, O., Williams, W., Pearson, M., Shapiro, C., & Deitchman, S. (1998). CDC guideline for infection control in health care personnel. *American Journal of Infection Control, 2,* 289–354.

Cardo, D., Culver, D., Ciesielski, C., Srivastava, P., Marcus, R., Abiteboul, D., Heptonstall, J., Ippolito, G., Lot, L., McKibbon, P., & Bell, D. (1997). A case-control study of HIV seroconversion in health care workers after percutaneous exposure. *New England Journal of Medicine, 337,* 1485–1490.

Centers for Disease Control and Prevention. (2003a). Trends in tuberculosis mortality. *Morbidity and Mortality Weekly Report, 52,* 217-222.

Centers for Disease Control and Prevention. (2003b). Settings where high-risk persons and their contacts may be targeted for vaccination. Retrieved 7/5/04 from *http://www.cdc.gov/flu/professionals/infectioncontrol/settings.htm.*

Centers for Disease Control and Prevention. (2003c). Smallpox response plan and guidelines (version 3.0), Guide C—Infection control measures for healthcare and community settings and quarantine guidelines. Retieved 7/6/04 from *http://www.bt.cdc.gov/agent/smallpox/responseplan/index.asp#guidec.*

Centers for Disease Control and Prevention. (2002b). Progressing toward tuberculosis elimination in low-incidence areas of the United States: Recommendations of the Advisory Council for the Elimination of Tuberculosis. *Morbidity and Mortality Weekly Report, 51*(RR05), 1–16.

Centers for Disease Control and Prevention. (2001). Updated US Public Health Service guidelines for the management of occupational exposures to HBV, HCV, and HIV and recommendations for postexposure prophylaxis. *Morbidity and Mortality Weekly Report, 50*(RR11), 1–42.

Centers for Disease Control and Prevention. (2000a). Biological and chemical terrorism: Strategic plan for preparedness and response. *Morbidity and Mortality Weekly Report, (49)* (RR04); 1–14.

Centers for Disease Control and Prevention. (2000b). Targeted tuberculin testing and treatment of latent tuberculosis. *Morbidity and Mortality Weekly Report, 49*(RR06), 1–54.

Centers for Disease Control and Prevention. (1998). Public Health Service guidelines for the management of health-care worker exposures to HIV and recommendations for postexposure prophylaxis. *Morbidity and Mortality Weekly Report, 47*(RR07), 1–6.

Centers for Disease Control and Prevention (1997a). Immunization of healthcare workers: Recommendations of the Advisory Committee on Immunization Practices (ACIP) and the Hospital Infection Control Practices Advisory Committee (HICPAC). *Morbidity and Mortality Weekly Report, 46*(RR18), 1–42.

Centers for Disease Control and Prevention. (1997b). Recommendations for follow-up of health-care workers after occupational exposure to hepatitis C virus. *Morbidity and Mortality Weekly Report, 46,* 603–606.

Centers for Disease Control and Prevention. (1994). Guidelines for preventing the transmission of *Mycobacterium tuberculosis* in health-care facilities. *Morbidity and Mortality Weekly Report, 43*(RR13), 1–32.

Centers for Disease Control and Prevention. (1991a). Diphtheria, tetanus, pertussis: Recommendations for vaccine use and other preventative measures—Recommendations of the Advisory Committee on Immunization Practices (ACIP). *Morbidity and Mortality Weekly Report, 46*(RR10), 1–28.

Centers for Disease Control and Prevention. (1991b). Hepatitis B virus: A comprehensive strategy for eliminating transmission in the United States through universal childhood vaccination—Recommendation of the Advisory Committee on Immunizations Practices (ACIP). *Morbidity and Mortality Weekly Report, 40*(RR13), 1–25.

Centers for Disease Control and Prevention. (1990). Protection against viral hepatitis: Recommendations of the Advisory Committee on Immunization Practices (ACIP). *Morbidity and Mortality Weekly Report, 39*(Suppl.), 1–26.

Do, A., Ciesielski, C., Metler, R., Hammett, T., Li, J., Fleming, P. (2003). Occupationally acquired human immunodeficiency virus (HIV): National case surveillance data during 20 years of the HIV epidemic in the United States. *Infection Control and Hospital Epidemiology 24 (2)*:86–96.

Ford, E., Nelson, K., & Warren, D. (1987). Epidemiology of epidemic keratoconjunctivitis. *Epidemiology Reviews, 9,* 244–261.

Henderson, D., Inglesby, T., Bartlett, J., Ascher, M., Eitzen, E., Jahrling, P., Hauer, J., Layton, M., McDade, J., Osterholm, M., O'Toole, T., Parker, G., Perl, T., Russell, P., & Tonat, K. (1999). Smallpox as a biological weapon. *Journal of the American Medical Association, 281*(22), 2127–2137.

Kelley, P., Petruccelli, B., Stehr-Green, P., Erickson, R., & Mason, C. (1991). The susceptibility of young adult Americans to vaccine-preventable infections. A national serosurvey of U.S. Army recruits. *Journal of the American Medical Association, 226,* 2724–2729.

Longfield, J., Winn, R., Gibson, R., Juchau, S., & Hoffman, P. (1990). Varicella outbreaks in Army recruits from Puerto Rico: Varicella susceptibility in a population from the tropics. *Archives of Internal Medicine, 150,* 970–973.

Nassar, N., & Touma, H. (1986). Brief report: Susceptibility of Filipino nurses to the varicella zoster virus. *Infection Control, 7,* 71–72.

Occupational Health and Safety Administration. (2003). OSHA withdraws proposal on occupational exposure to tuberculosis. Retrieved 7/6/04 from *http://www.osha.gov/pls/oshaweb/owadisp.show_document?p_table= NEWS_RELEASES&p_id510603.*

Occupational Health and Safety Administration. (2002). Tuberculosis testing procedures for the home health care industry. Retrieved 7/6/04 from *http://www.osha.gov/pls/oshaweb/owadisp.show_document?p_table= INTERPRETATIONS&p_id524249.*

Occupational Health and Safety Administration. (2001a). Occupational exposure to bloodborne pathogens: Needlestick and other sharps injuries; Final rule. 29 CFR part 1910. Retrieved 7/6/04 from *www.OSHA.gov.*

Occupational Health and Safety Administration. (2001b). Recording and reporting occupational injuries and illnesses. CFR 29-1904. Retrieved 7/6/04 from *www.osha.gov.*

Occupational Health and Safety Administration. (2000). HBV antibody testing is required after vaccination series; HBV booster not required. *Standard Interpretations,* 03/10/2000. Retrieved 7/6/04 from *www.OSHA.gov.*

Occupational Health and Safety Administration. (1993). Criteria for recording on OSHA form 200. Washington, DC: Author.

Occupational Health and Safety Administration. (1991). Occupational exposure to bloodborne pathogens: Final rule. CFR part 1910.1030. *Federal Register, 56,* 64004–64182.

Panlilio, A.L., Orelien, J.G., Srivastava, P.U., Jagger, J., Cohn, R.D., Cardo, D.M.; NaSH Surveillance Group; EPINET Data Sharing Network (2004) Estimate of the annual number of percutaneous injuries among hospital-based healthcare workers in the United States, 1997–1998. *Infection Control and Hospital Epidemiology, 25*(7):556-62.

CDC Recommendations for HIV Postexposure Prophylaxis

The following algorithm is intended to guide initial decisions about PEP and should be used in conjunction with other guidance provided in this document.

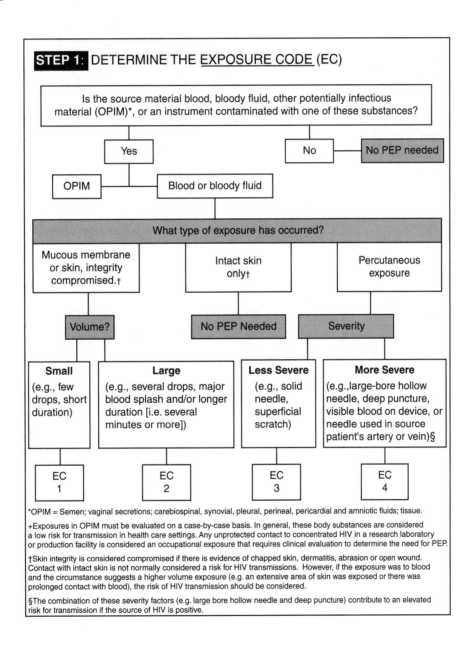

STEP 1: DETERMINE THE <u>EXPOSURE CODE</u> (EC)

Is the source material blood, bloody fluid, other potentially infectious material (OPIM)*, or an instrument contaminated with one of these substances?

Yes → OPIM / Blood or bloody fluid

No → No PEP needed

What type of exposure has occurred?

- Mucous membrane or skin, integrity compromised.†
- Intact skin only† → No PEP Needed
- Percutaneous exposure → Severity

Volume?

Small (e.g., few drops, short duration) → EC 1

Large (e.g., several drops, major blood splash and/or longer duration [i.e. several minutes or more]) → EC 2

Less Severe (e.g., solid needle, superficial scratch) → EC 3

More Severe (e.g.,large-bore hollow needle, deep puncture, visible blood on device, or needle used in source patient's artery or vein)§ → EC 4

*OPIM = Semen; vaginal secretions; carebiospinal, synovial, pleural, perineal, pericardial and amniotic fluids; tissue.

+Exposures in OPIM must be evaluated on a case-by-case basis. In general, these body substances are considered a low risk for transmission in health care settings. Any unprotected contact to concentrated HIV in a research laboratory or production facility is considered an occupational exposure that requires clinical evaluation to determine the need for PEP.

†Skin integrity is considered compromised if there is evidence of chapped skin, dermatitis, abrasion or open wound. Contact with intact skin is not normally considered a risk for HIV transmissions. However, if the exposure was to blood and the circumstance suggests a higher volume exposure (e.g. an extensive area of skin was exposed or there was prolonged contact with blood), the risk of HIV transmission should be considered.

§The combination of these severity factors (e.g. large bore hollow needle and deep puncture) contribute to an elevated risk for transmission if the source of HIV is positive.

Source: Reprinted from *Morbidity and Mortality Weekly Report,* Centers for Disease Control and Prevention, National Institute for Occupational Safety and Health, 1998.

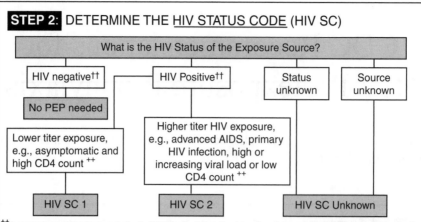

STEP 2: DETERMINE THE <u>HIV STATUS CODE</u> (HIV SC)

What is the HIV Status of the Exposure Source?

| HIV negative†† | HIV Positive†† | Status unknown | Source unknown |

No PEP needed

Lower titer exposure, e.g., asymptomatic and high CD4 count ++

Higher titer HIV exposure, e.g., advanced AIDS, primary HIV infection, high or increasing viral load or low CD4 count ++

HIV SC 1   HIV SC 2   HIV SC Unknown

††A source is considered to be negative for HIV infection if there is a laboratory documentation of a negative HIV antibody, HIV PCR or HIV p24 antigen test result from a specimen collected at or near the time of exposure and there is no clinical evidence of an acute or recent retroviral-like illness. A source is considered to be infected with HIV (HIV Positive) if there has been a positive laboratory result for HIV antibody, HIV PCR or HIV p24 antigen or physician-diagnosed AIDS.

++Examples are used as surrogates to estimate the HIV titer in a exposure source for purposes of considering PEP regimens and do not reflect all clinical situations that may be observed. Although a high HIV titer (status code 2) in a n exposure source has bee associated with an increased risk of transmission, the possibility of transmission from a source with a low HIV titer also must be considered.

STEP 3: DETERMINE THE PEP RECOMMENDATION

EC	HIV SC	PEP recommendation
1	1	PEP may not be warranted. Exposure type does not pose a known risk for HIV transmission. Whether the risk of drug toxicity outweighs the benefit of PEP should be decided between the exposed HCW and treating clinician.
1	2	Consider basic regimen. Exposure type poses a negligible risk for HIV transmission; a high HIV titer in the source may justify consideration of PEP. Whether the risk of drug toxicity outweighs the benefit of PEP should be decided between the HCW and treating clinician.
2	1	Recommend basic regimen. Majority of HIV exposures are in this category; no increased risk of HIV transmission has been observed but use of PEP is appropriate.
2	2	Recommend expanded regimen. Exposure type represents an increased HIV transmission risk.
3	1 or 2	
	Unknown	If the source or, in the case of an unknown source, the setting where the exposure occurred suggests a possible risk for HIV exposure and the EC = 2 or 3, consider PEP basic regimen.

RECOMMENDED PEP REGIMENS

Basic regimen = 4 weeks of ZDV 600 mg/day in two or three divided doses, and 31C, 150 mg, BID

Expanded regimen = Basic regimen plus <u>either</u> indinavir 800 mg qh8 <u>or</u> nelfinavir 750 mg. TID

CHAPTER 14

Developing and Maintaining an Infection Control Program

Several broad influences within the health care industry have increased focus on the importance of infection control programs in home and hospice care. With shortened lengths of in-patient stays, patients are being discharged home in a condition that may require a greater intensity of home care services than has been the case in the past, and more patients and families are taking advantage of the benefits of hospice care. In addition, the majority of surgical procedures are now performed in ambulatory surgery settings, increasing the need for postoperative observation and care in the home. This increase in acuity in the home care population necessitates continuous management efforts and support to assure adequate assessment skills and the ability to provide home care clinical services. Nurses and other home care and hospice staff members must be able to assess patients and identify those clinical problems and issues that require a physician's attention and intervention. This includes the identification of infection risks, signs and symptoms, and risks related to systems of care, such as provision of home infusion therapy.

Additional scrutiny of the entire health care system occurred with the 1999 report from the Institute of Medicine (IOM), "To Err Is Human" (IOM, 1999). Although neither home care nor hospice is specifically mentioned, this publication has had a significant impact on health care delivery, with a major focus on patient safety and the avoidance of medical errors and adverse outcomes. Since the IOM report, there has been additional activity focused on patient safety in home care. The Agency for Healthcare Research and Quality (AHRQ), which is part of the Department of Health and Human Services (HHS), and the National Patient Safety Foundation (NPSF) have both funded grants related to home care safety (Rosati, 2003; NPSF, 2002).

In addition, the Joint Commission on Accreditation of Healthcare Organizations (JCAHO, 2004) has promulgated national patient safety goals (NPSG) for home care (see Exhibit 14-1), which include a goal for the reduction of health care–acquired infections. Goal #7 specifically focuses upon prevention of health care–acquired infections through compliance with the CDC guidelines for hand hygiene and the management of adverse outcomes and unanticipated deaths related to health care–acquired infections.

A home care or hospice organization can develop and manage its infection control program through a variety of approaches depending on the scope of services, patient population, and infection risks. In light of the patient safety focus on health care delivery in the United States, home care and hospice leaders should consider the infection control program in this context, along with the other programs promoting patient and staff safety, such as quality improvement, employee/occupational health, and safety and risk management. These functions should be linked in some fashion—through a management structure, a committee structure, or both—in order to facilitate communication, coordination, and synergy. Many health care organizations are planning to get the most effective benefit from these functions by placing them within a patient safety framework, although there is no "standard" organization plan or template in home care or other types of health care delivery.

Exhibit 14-1 2005 JCAHO Home Care National Patient Safety Goals

1. Improve the accuracy of patient identification.
2. Improve the effectiveness of communication among caregivers.
3. Improve the safety of using medications. (Not applicable in home care.)
4. Improve the safety of using infusion pumps. (Not applicable in home care.)
5. Reduce the risk of health care–acquired infection.
   a) Comply with current CDC hand hygiene guidelines.
   b) Manage as sentinel events all identified cases of unanticipated death or major permanent loss of function associated with a health care–acquired infection.
6. Accurately and completely reconcile medications across the continuum of care.
7. Reduce the risk of patient harm resulting from falls.

Source: Joint Commission on the Accreditation of Healthcare Organizations. (2004). *CAMHC Update 2004.* NPSG-2–NPSG-4. Oakbrook Terrace, IL: Author.

DEFINING THE INFECTION CONTROL PROGRAM

Several organizations have published recommendations for infection control program structure in home care (Friedman, C. et al., 1999; Health Canada, 2004). In addition, the JCAHO has standards that address this issue (Friedman, M., 2004; JCAHO, 2004b). A collaborative position paper developed by the Association for Professionals in Infection Control and Epidemiology (APIC) and the Society for Healthcare Epidemiologists of America (SHEA) (Friedman, C. et al., 1999) outlines the elements these organizations believe are essential for an infection control program in nonhospital settings (see Exhibit 14-2). These include integration of infection control principles and strategies in the policies and procedures for provision of patient care in order to reduce the related risk of infection. This is especially important as more invasive and advanced therapies are provided in the home, including various types of home infusion therapy, and as more acutely ill, vulnerable patients are cared for at home. There is a paucity of published information and data for use in developing and implementing evidence-based infection control practices in home care, however. Rather than directly adopting policies and procedures developed for hospital settings, home and hospice care infection control staff must adapt these procedures, based upon

Exhibit 14-2 Principle Functions of an Infection Control Program

1. To develop and recommend policies and procedures.
2. To obtain and manage data and information for surveillance of health care–acquired infections.
3. To intervene to prevent infections.
4. To educate staff, patients, and families regarding infection control practices and principles.

Source: Adapted from Friedman, C., *et al.,* Requirements for infrastructure and essential activities of infection control and epidemiology in out-of-hospital settings: A consensus panel report. *American Journal of Infection Control, 20,* 695–705.

infection control principles and science. This will help assure the feasibility as well as the effectiveness and efficiency of the clinical approach within the home care or hospice practice setting. Exhibit 14-3 provides a list of the essential infection control subjects that should be addressed by clinical policies and procedures.

To develop more evidence for the effectiveness of home care or hospice infection prevention and control practices, surveillance systems to identify home care–acquired infections and capture the associated risk factors are also a recommended component of an infection control program (Friedman, C. et al., 1999). As discussed in Chapter 11, implementation of surveillance in home care has been challenging (Managan et al., 2002). As home care and hospice leaders determine the best use of their limited resources for an infection-surveillance program, priority should be given to the infection risks posing the greatest threat of adverse outcomes in home care and hospice patients.

Exhibit 14-3 Patient Care Practices, Policies, and Procedures

- Hand hygiene
- Standard Precautions and use of personal protective equipment
- Transmission-based precautions
- Provision of intravenous therapy
- Infection control practices related to wound care, respiratory tract care, and urinary tract care
- Application of clean and sterile techniques
- Food preparation and provision of enteral therapy
- Cleaning and disinfection of medical equipment and supplies
- Handling and transport of medical waste and laboratory specimens

The approach to surveillance should be simple and practical, with the goal not only of identifying the incidence of home care–acquired infections but also of examining the potential risks related to the care provided. If a home care organization provides home infusion therapy services, the surveillance program should include identification of IV catheter–related bloodstream infections and insertion-site infections as a priority. If the organization does not provide home infusion therapy, priorities for surveillance should be determined through identification of other risks for home care–acquired infections related to the use of devices such as urinary tract catheters or the specific population risks. In hospice, focus on pressure ulcers may be a priority.

The surveillance program and its priorities should be examined at least annually. The surveillance plan and approach should be adjusted and revised to reflect changes in population risk, new therapies and procedures, recent information in the published literature, and any newly published definitions for home care–acquired infection that might provide comparison of data and experience (Embry & Chinnes, 2000; Shanz, 2002).

Infection control considerations are also a part of the home and hospice care organization's occupational health and employee safety program. As outlined in Chapter 13, many of these issues are subject to regulation by federal OSHA rules and various state requirements. The infection control program should include and address all issues related to occupational risks for exposure to infectious diseases, disease prevention prior to exposure through provision of vaccines, prevention related to work practices and use of personal protective equipment, and protocols for postexposure management and prophylaxis. Exhibit 14-4 provides a

list of essential components for occupational health as it relates to infection control. External sources, such as hospital-based occupational health departments, free-standing occupational health clinics, or physician offices, may be identified for the provision of these services. If such sources are identified, home care or hospice management should be involved in all contractual agreements and should receive assurance that contractors possess appropriate credentials and licenses as well as professional liability insurance coverage.

Staff education, a key component of the infection control program, must be undertaken on a continuous basis once initial orientation is completed. New staff members must be informed about the organization's infection control program, policies and procedures for provision of clinical care and hand hygiene, procedures related to Standard Precautions and prevention of exposure to bloodborne pathogens, and any additional isolation procedures that are in place to protect staff from occupational exposure to infectious diseases. Exhibit 14-5 provides an outline for infection control orientation in home care; Exhibit 14-6 pro-

Exhibit 14-4 Essential Components of Occupational Health/Infection Control Policies

- Initial assessment and health history
- Confirmation of immunity and/or provision of vaccines
- Initial and annual TB skin testing, as required
- Identification of occupational exposures and follow-up of nonbloodborne pathogen exposures
- Postexposure prophylaxis for exposures to bloodborne pathogens
- Exclusions from patient care activities
- Surveillance of occupational health risks

Exhibit 14-5 Content for Infection Control Orientation Program for Home Care

Role of infection control in home care
- Patient safety
- Patient care
- Occupational health
Patient care practices
- Hand hygiene
- Standard Precautions and selection and application of transmission-based precautions
- Provision of intravenous therapy
- Infection control practices related to wound care, respiratory tract care, and urinary tract care
- Application of clean and sterile techniques
- Food preparation and provision of enteral therapy
- Cleaning and disinfection of medical equipment and supplies
- Handling and transport of medical waste and laboratory specimens
Role of surveillance
- Identification of any home care–acquired infections
Occupational health
- Bloodborne pathogen exposure control plan
- Tuberculosis control plan
- Reporting exposures to bloodborne pathogens and other infectious diseases

Exhibit 14-6 Sample Outline: Annual Education Regarding Bloodborne Pathogens

Exposure control plan
 • Brief review and information on how to obtain a copy
Tasks that may lead to exposure
Definition of an exposure
Use of engineering controls and personal protective equipment
 • Types and provision of personal protective equipment
 • Selection of personal protective equipment
 • Use, decontamination, and disposal of personal protective equipment
 • Limitations of personal protective equipment
Hepatitis B vaccine
 • Benefits, efficacy, safety
 • Method of administration
 • Availability and testing
How to handle emergencies with risk of exposure
Exposure incidents
 • Reporting and evaluation
 • Medical follow-up and testing
 • Postexposure prophylaxis
Questions and answers*

 *A knowledgeable individual must be available to answer questions—even when a video is used.

Exhibit 14-7 Responsibilities of the Infection Control Program Manager

 • Develop and maintain policies and procedures for infection control
 • Review patient care policies and procedures for infection control content
 • Develop and maintain policies and procedures for occupational health related to infection control
 • Identify and maintain infection control references and resources (internal and external)
 • Serve as an organizational resource for infection control practice
 • Perform surveillance of home care–acquired infections
 • Aggregate, report, and analyze surveillance data
 • Facilitate infection control education (initial and continuing)
 • Assist in identifying risk reduction projects for infection control

vides a sample outline for annual training related to bloodborne pathogens and the exposure control plan, as required by OSHA.

DESIGNATION OF AN INFECTION CONTROL PROGRAM MANAGER

Infection control is a specific health care discipline with a growing body of scientific knowledge. Designation of a single individual as the infection control practitioner (ICP) in a home care or hospice organization to serve as an infection control resource and to manage routine infection control issues seems sensible and practical. A registered nurse with significant experience and knowledge in clinical care and, ideally, with a special interest in infection control is a model candidate for this role. This individual may eventually demonstrate his or her competence by becoming certified in infection control through the Certification Board of Infection Control and Epidemiology, Inc. The role of infection control practitioner may be assumed as part of a staff nurse's position and as such may provide an opportunity for advancement. More commonly, it is made part of the responsibilities of an

ICP who is also responsible for patient safety or quality management functions and/or occupational health, safety, workers' compensation, and risk management. The incorporation of the infection control function into another job will depend on who is available and interested in the role as well as how other clinical and support functions are organized. The size and complexity of the home care or hospice organization will dictate the amount of resources allocated to this function. In a multi-location organization, a corporate infection control practitioner may support individuals in the field who manage local infection control issues as part of another role. This model may promote efficient use of internal resources in that one individual would maintain knowledge of current infection control issues and share that information and knowledge with others. Specific responsibilities for an ICP in home care are listed in Exhibit 14-7.

JCAHO ACCREDITATION AND INFECTION CONTROL

The IOM report ("To Err Is Human") was the impetus for the JCAHO forming a special infection control expert panel to review and suggest improvements to the JCAHO's infection control standards. These new standards raise the bar of expectations for home care and hospice organizations. The revised standards address two new issues—emerging antimicrobial resistance and the management of epidemics and emerging pathogens—and require a commitment by the home care or hospice organization's leaders not only to make infection prevention and control a priority, but also to provide adequate resources for the appropriate interventions.

The JCAHO's survey process for home care and hospice recently changed. The new process is based on a concept called "tracer methodology." This methodology focuses the surveyor's activities on areas that the JCAHO has predetermined to be paramount in assuring high-quality, safe home care and hospice services. These are called "priority focus areas (PFAs)" and "clinical service groups (CSGs)" and are preselected by the JCAHO central office. When tracing the patient through his or her home care or hospice experience, the surveyor focuses on standards that are applicable to the PFAs selected. One of the PFAs that can be selected is "infection control." This title can be misleading because the infection control PFA is not limited just to standards in the chapter on surveillance, prevention, and control of infections, but it also includes standards from the chapters on provision of care, treatment and services, improving organizational performance, management of the environment of care, management of human resources, and management of information (Friedman, M. M., 2004a).

Regardless of whether infection control is selected as one of the home care or hospice organization's PFAs, infection control will always be addressed during home visits and patient tracer activities, as it has been in past years. What's different in the new survey process is that at some point in the agenda (i.e., either during the data use system tracer or in a standalone infection control system tracer), time will be spent discussing the implementation of the infection control program. Prior to the selection of tracer patients and during the initial surveyor planning session, the surveyor reviews infection control surveillance data collected for the applicable track record time period (either 4 months or 12 months) and considers the data in the selection of tracer patients. If breaches in infection prevention or control measures were identified during home visits, or if during staff interviews or record review infections identified were not properly reported or staff knowledge deficits were noted related to infection prevention and control measures, these shortcomings will be discussed during the infection control system tracer or during the leadership session (Friedman, M. M., 2004a).

System tracer activities focus on processes, systems, and functions that are influential to the patient's care experience; they also consider the outcomes and findings from the individual tracer activities. Currently, one of the three possible system tracers addresses the topic of infection control. If no problems related to infection control are identified by the surveyor(s), then the individuals participating in the infection control system tracer should be ready to discuss infection control processes in their organization as it pertains to the selected PFAs. Topics that may be discussed include how the leaders:

- Implement and monitor the staff's compliance with the CDC hand hygiene guidelines
- Provide ongoing in-service training and education related to infection control
- Communicate the aggregate results of surveillance activities and the follow-up actions to be taken, if any
- Manage a patient's care when the patient is colonized or infected with a multidrug-resistant organism, such as MRSA or VRE (Friedman, M. M., 2004b)

In a complex organization survey (e.g., a survey for a hospital-based home care program), the discussion arising during the systems tracers is directed towards *all* programs undergoing an accreditation survey. As such, the focus on home care and hospice is not as intensive as it would be if home care were the only program being discussed. A home care or hospice representative should attend these sessions and be prepared to discuss issues that came up during the home care surveyor's patient tracer activity, even if the home care surveyor is not conducting that particular session (Friedman, M. M., 2004c).

If a home care organization has regularly given thoughtful consideration to the infection control strategies, policies, and procedures that need to be in place to provide patient care and to address surveillance activities and occupational health issues, its preparation for an accreditation survey should be minimal. Staff members (employees and contracted individuals and providers) who provide direct patient care should be aware of the organization's policies and procedures and be able to demonstrate compliance during staff interviews and home visits during the survey. For example, when the procedure for wound care requires that gloves be changed after the removal of the wound dressing, home care staff members must follow the organiza-

Exhibit 14-8 Infection Control Indicators

Performance Indicators from Selected CDC Guidelines	Indicators Adapted for Home and Hospice Care
Hand Hygiene	**Hand Hygiene in Home Care**
Periodically monitor and record adherence as the number of hand-hygiene episodes performed by personnel divided by the number of hand-hygiene opportunities, by ward and by service. Provide feedback to personnel regarding their performance.	Periodically monitor staff during routine home care and selected activities (e.g., provision of wound care, home infusion therapy) for appropriate compliance to hand hygiene indications and procedures. Provide feedback regarding performance.
Monitor the volume of alcohol-based hand rub (or detergent used for handwashing or hand antisepsis) used per 1000 patient days.	Monitor volume of alcohol-based hand rub and antibacterial soap issued to home care and hospice staff by month or quarter to identify use patterns.
Monitor adherence to policies dealing with wearing artificial nails.	Monitor adherence to policies dealing with wearing artificial nails.
When outbreaks of infection occur, assess the adequacy of health care worker hand hygiene.	When outbreaks of infection occur, assess the adequacy of home care and hospice staff compliance with hand hygiene.
Intravascular Catheter–Related Infections	**Home Infusion Therapy**
Implement educational programs that include didactic and interactive components for those who insert and maintain catheters.	Implement educational programs that include didactic and interactive components for those who insert and maintain catheters.
Use maximal sterile barrier precautions during catheter placement.	Use maximal sterile barrier precautions during central line placement.
Use chlorhexidine for skin antisepsis.	Use chlorhexidine for skin antisepsis.
Monitor rates of catheter discontinuation when the catheter is no longer essential for medical management.	Monitor rates of catheter discontinuation when the catheter is no longer essential for medical management.
Isolation for Prevention of Transmission in Health Care Settings	**Isolation and Standard Precautions in Home Care**
Monitor appropriateness of transmission-based precautions initiated at the time of admission, based on clinical diagnosis and appropriateness of discontinuation.	Monitor appropriateness of transmission-based precautions initiated at the time of admission or during the course of home care, based on clinical diagnosis and appropriateness of discontinuation.
Periodically audit use of PPE by health care workers when caring for patients on expanded precautions.	Periodically audit use of PPE by home care and hospice staff for compliance with Standard Precautions.
Assess adequacy of supplies of PPE for adherence to recommended expanded and Standard Precautions.	Assess adequacy of supplies of PPE for adherence to Standard Precautions.
Prevention of Pneumonia	**Prevention of Pneumonia**
Establish a standard operating procedure for influenza vaccination and monitor the percentage of eligible patients in acute care settings, or patients or residents in long-term care settings, who receive the vaccine.	Establish a standard operating procedure for influenza vaccination and monitor the percentage of eligible home care patients who receive the vaccine.
Before and during the influenza season, monitor and record the number of eligible health care personnel who receive influenza vaccine, and determine unit- and facility-specific rates.	Before and during the influenza season, monitor and record the number of eligible home care and hospice staff who receive influenza vaccine.

tion's procedure(s). Hand hygiene based on the CDC's hand hygiene guidelines should also be accomplished according to policy and procedures. Staff should be knowledgeable about their roles and responsibilities in surveillance and reporting of potential infections in patients. They should also know which specific exposures or illnesses that they may experience (occupational and nonoccupational) should be reported to the home or hospice care organization and how they should report them, as the surveyor may ask them about this as well.

MAINTAINING AND ADVANCING THE INFECTION CONTROL PROGRAM

As the application of infection control principles and practices in home care and hospice develops and evolves, each home care and hospice organization should continuously examine its own approaches and strategies, track and trend its own experience, and identify new information and data that should be considered. Review of current policies and procedures and response to external data and recommendations are important in maintaining an infection control program that provides optimal benefit to patients and staff.

The effectiveness of efforts directed at patient and staff safety, including infection prevention and control, should be reviewed and evaluated in a continuous manner. Surveillance to identify the incidence of home care–acquired infection would seem to be an obvious method for assessing prevention methods. Additional methods should be considered and implemented, how-

ever. For example, all home health and hospice organizations should track the incidence of needlestick injuries among staff to determine the effectiveness of programs and equipment to prevent these accidents. In addition to these more obvious measures, home care and hospice administrators and those responsible for patient and staff safety should be aware of the performance indicators now routinely incorporated into all CDC guidelines published by the Healthcare Infection control Policy Advisory Committee (HICPAC) (CDC, 2002a; CDC, 2002b; CDC, 2004). Although many of these measures appear to be focused on hospital-based care, they can be adapted to home care and hospice in appropriate, useful ways. Exhibit 14-8 summarizes the performance indicators from the CDC guidelines addressing hand hygiene, intravascular catheter–related infections, and isolation and provides some suggestions for their adaptation to home care. Other measures for determining compliance and effectiveness of procedures can be developed and applied in any agency, especially if there is a perceived problem with infection-prevention efforts.

In the context of patient safety, quality improvement, performance measurement, and infection control, surveillance should not simply include collecting data and reporting them. The results of surveillance and other performance measures must be examined, analyzed, tracked, and trended, and evidence must be available that there has been some conclusion as to how the risks related to adverse outcomes and complications can be reduced.

REFERENCES

Centers for Disease Control and Prevention. (2002a). Guidelines for the prevention of intravascular catheter–related infections. *Morbidity and Mortality Weekly Report, 52*(RR10), 1–36.

Centers for Disease Control and Prevention. (2002b). Guidelines for hand hygiene in healthcare settings. *Morbidity and Mortality Weekly Report, 52*(RR16), 1–56.

Centers for Disease Control and Prevention. (2004). Draft Guideline for Isolation: Preventing Transmission of Infectious Agents in Healthcare Settings. Retrieved 06/15/04 from *http://www.cdc.gov/ncidod/hip/isoguide.htm.*

Embry, F., & Chinnes, L. (2000). Draft definitions for surveillance of infection in home health care. *American Journal of Infection Control, 28,* 449–453.

Friedman, C., Barnett, M., Buck, A., Ham, R., Harris, J., Hoffman, P., Johnson, D., Farrin M., Nicolle, L., Pearson, M., Perl, T., & Solomon, S. (1999). Requirements for infrastructure and essential activities of infection control and epidemiology in out-of-hospital settings: A consensus panel report. *American Journal of Infection Control, 20,* 695–705.

Friedman, M. M. (2004a). Tracer methodology and the new JCAHO home care & hospice survey process (part I). *Home Healthcare Nurse, 22*(10), 710–714.

Friedman, M. M. (2004b). Tracer methodology and the new JCAHO home care & hospice survey process (part II). *Home Healthcare Nurse, 22*(11), 748–752.

Friedman, M. M. (2004c). The JCAHO complex organization survey process and its impact on hospital-based home care and hospice providers. *Home Healthcare Nurse, 22*(12), 854–857.

Friedman, M. M. (2004). What's new in the 2004 Joint Commission home care and hospice standards, Parts 1 and 2. *Home Healthcare Nurse, 22,* 56–59 and 124–128.

Health Canada. (2004). Development of a resource model for infection prevention and control programs in acute, long term, and home care settings: Conference proceedings of the Infection Prevention and Control Alliance. *American Journal of Infection Control, 32,* 2–6.

Institute of Medicine. (1999). *To Err Is Human.* Washington DC: National Academy Press.

Joint Commission on the Accreditation of Healthcare Organizations. (2004a). *CAMHC Update 2004.* NPSG-2–NPSG-4. Oakbrook Terrace, IL.

Joint Commission on the Accreditation of Healthcare Organizations. (2004b). 2005 home care surveillance, prevention and control of infection. Retrieved 7/18/04 from *www.jcaho.org.*

Manangan, L., Pearson, M., Tokars, J., Miller, E., & Jarvis, W. (2002). Feasibility of national surveillance of health-care-associated infection in home-care settings. *Emerging Infectious Diseases, 8,* 233–236.

National Patient Safety Foundation. (2002). Clinical decision support to reduce adverse drug events in high-risk home care patients. Research grants at *http://www.npsf.org.*

Rosati, R., Huang, L., Navaie-Waliser, M., & Feldman, P. (2003). Risk factors for repeating hospitalizations among home healthcare recipients. *Journal for Healthcare Quality, 25,* 4–10.

Schanz, M. (2002). Infection control in the home. *Caring, 21,* 40–43.

Index

page numbers in *italics* denote figures and exhibits; page numbers followed by t denote tables